This Side of
DOCTORING

This Side of
DOCTORING
Reflections From Women in Medicine

Eliza Lo Chin
Editor

Sage Publications
International Educational and Professional Publisher
Thousand Oaks ▪ London ▪ New Delhi

For information:

Sage Publications, Inc.
2455 Teller Road
Thousand Oaks, California 91320
E-mail: order@sagepub.com

Sage Publications Ltd.
6 Bonhill Street
London EC2A 4PU
United Kingdom

Sage Publications India Pvt. Ltd.
M-32 Market
Greater Kailash I
New Delhi 110 048 India

Printed in the United States of America

Library of Congress Cataloging-in-Publication Data

This side of doctoring : reflections from women in medicine / edited by
    Eliza Lo Chin.
        p. cm.
Includes bibliographical references.
    ISBN 0-7619-2354-3 (cloth)
    1. Women physicians.   2. Women physicians—Anecdotes.
I. Chin, Eliza Lo.
    R692.T45 2002
    610'.82—dc21   2001005795

01   02   03   04   05   10   9   8   7   6   5   4   3   2   1

Acquiring Editor: Rolf Janke
Developmental/Production Editor: Claudia A. Hoffman
Copy Editor: Linda Gray
Typesetter/Interior Designer: Janelle LeMaster
Cover Designer: Michelle Lee
Cover photograph copyright © C. A. Hoffman

For the sake of confidentiality, the names of patients have been changed.

For the women and men
whose stories made this book possible
and for my family, who made my story possible.

Human kind might be divided into three groups—
men, women, and women physicians.
— *Sir William Osler**

**L. Welsh, 1925, p. 44.* Reminiscences of thirty years in Baltimore. *Baltimore: Norman, Remington.*

CONTENTS

FOREWORD

I've never been so glad to be proven wrong. When the idea of this anthology was first proposed, I was skeptical and hoped that Eliza wouldn't be too disappointed when so few women responded to her call. That so many physicians put their emotional and creative and feminine sides on hold during training, and never recover them, also seemed likely to doom this project. But behold the assembled voices of more than 140 women physicians, each authentic and strong. While this compendium cannot span equally well the universe of women physicians and underrepresents some, most women will discover in this book connections to a welcome network of like experiences.

Male readers will find this compendium valuable in quite another way. A brief anecdote illustrates why. I'm among the thousands who are grateful for the mentoring of Dr. Carola Eisenberg. Carola was the first woman in a decanal position at MIT prior to becoming the first woman dean of student affairs at Harvard Medical School. During the 1970s, women residents as well as students discovered in Carola a much needed beacon of sanity and support as, despite dramatic increases in the numbers of women trainees, the "gender climate" remained decidedly chilly. She began opening her home on occasional evenings to the residents so they could share with each other their stresses and coping mechanisms. Her fine husband, Dr. Leon Eisenberg (then chair of Harvard's Department of Social Medicine) told me that he did not understand why these very bright and obviously highly competent women needed extra help. But one evening while making himself a cup of tea in the kitchen, he overheard the voices coming from the living room. He remained transfixed for the next hour or so while lightbulbs flashed on. He had flattered himself to be a champion of equal rights for women but had simply failed to see what went on right in front of his eyes in the mostly male faculty groups he was part of every day. Thus, the ancient power of stories to draw in, to educate.

In *Writing a Woman's Life*, Carolyn Heilbrun (1988) urges women to write their stories because "power consists to a large extent in deciding what stories will be told." Women professionals looking for their foremothers' stories find comparatively few published ones. And as Heilbrun notes, the women's stories that have been published "are painful, the price [has been] high, the anxiety is intense, because there is no script to follow . . . let alone any alternative stories." Actually, women seeking to combine family, love, and work still lack anything resembling a script; no journey myth works either (Odysseus?). Each woman is still devising her own path on a far from level playing field, dodging unexpected paradoxes—for example, treating other people's children in the hospital while hers are sick at home or professional isolation whereas the experience for men is highly social and socializing.

Most of this book's entries pose questions that converge around three main themes interweaving across the chapters: Who am I in relation to my family? Who am I in relation to my patients? What about my own plans and ambitions? With regard to the latter, as More (2000) noted in her study of women physicians, the effects of "choice" and "necessity" remain more tangled in women's than in men's careers. As McClelland (1967) observes, "A woman's success is less easily visible [than a man's who is following a single course] . . . because it consists of the sum of all these [part-time] activities." But as Williams (2000) shows in *Unbending Gender*, "women do not prefer marginalization. . . . What is needed is not a mommy track, but work restructured to reflect the legitimate claims of family life."

To focus first on who a woman physician is vis-à-vis her family, tensions around women's multiple roles begin even before medical school. During their medical school interviews, many contributors were asked questions such as, "Why don't you want to be wife and mother?" At the same time, Linda Clever ironically notes, "Being a physician is one of the few socially acceptable reasons to abandon a family." Catherine Chang speaks for many when she says, "I have so much to say, it is difficult to find the words. . . . the struggle to balance my career and family . . . constantly tears at me." Cynthia Kapphahn confesses, "The sheer determination that helped get me through medical school and residency has proven quite useless in my family life. . . . instead, intuition, patience and a form of 'non-effort' are required." Marcia McCrae advises women to give up idea of balance: "Don't be frozen in the middle. . . . learn to prance, slide, skip, skid, and skitter from one end of the see-saw to the other." Laughter is also recommended; Patricia Temple found herself "at the park when the children had runny noses and wet diapers and all I had in my purse was a stethoscope." Linda Clever offers strategies on keeping family glued together and enjoying each other: "negotiate, accommodate, and recreate." Finally finding statement is the emptiness that can occur when women wait too long "to fit the mystical process of reproduction into the unerringly practical cycle of our professional production" (Sayantani DasGupta).

In Barbara Sommer's words, medicine still demonstrates a "pervasive lack of seriousness toward women who want an academic career while providing a loving environment for their family." Thus, most women physicians are still patching together individual solutions and shoehorning their professional and second-shift responsibilities into structures created by men with full-time support at home. The continuing tyranny of dualistic thinking—for example, *either* you're fully available during your 20s to 40s to work *or* you'll never reap academic rewards, *either* you're tenured *or* nontenured—remains beyond the scope of this book (McElvaine, 2001). But such systems issues beg to be addressed, given that (a) youth is associated with neither scientific achievement nor clinical acumen, (b) women physicians (at least in primary care) tend to be most productive between age 50 and 60, and (c) we cannot afford to waste medical careers, involving substantial public investment (Etzkowitz, Kemelgor, & Uzzi, 2000).

As McMurray and Jordan (2000) have written, "Medicine is particularly appealing to women because it offers the opportunity to have significant intellectual stimulation embedded in a relational context." For physicians, family and professional roles can enrich each other in unexpected ways. Daphne Miller remarks, "The moments of talking with patients about my conflicts and challenges [regarding family responsibilities] have helped me become a wiser doctor and mother, and they have bolstered the confidence of my patients in their ability to care for themselves and others." But witness the contrasts between the days when physicians had opportunity to talk with patients along such personal lines and today. As Lucy Candib declares, "I have chosen to remain in one setting for the past 15 years. . . . A doctor used to be a person who came and stayed . . . in the community." Not only is this community orientation much less common now, but the increasing corporatization of medicine can put physicians at war with patients, as Julia McMurray here notes, "New patients are enraged at the more than three months' wait for a physical. They feel betrayed by the slick advertisements . . . there just doesn't seem to be enough time for them to begin to trust me . . . I am simply heartsick."

Negative influences on the patient-physician relationship are indeed disturbing. But one of the strengths of the book is that contributors wear their hearts on their sleeves. The poetry here comes from the heart too: "Babies . . . slippery as chance" (Alison Moll); "Your love cut through the layers of my . . . shield" (Kathleen Franco); "the hospice within, buried in fertile soil, germinates and flowers tubular fruit" (Stephanie Nagy-Agren); and "Rare/restive respite, only briefly restful/the press of things undone still live and warm" (Mary Clark). Nassim Assefi discusses how writing complements her medical work: "We trace anatomical landscapes with our hands and battle pathology with the latest technology . . . the professional culture . . . fosters disagreement with the emotional realm . . . [But] with fiction, I get under the skin and am able to express processes at work in human life that cannot be explained in a medical textbook." Even women who don't consider themselves writers are advised, "Keep a journal of your stories. They are the vitamins that will help you grow as a person and in a profession . . . a roadmap of where you have been and where you are going" (Beth Alexander).

This collection is a vibrant and accurate roadmap of the past and present of women physicians. I also read it as Acts 1 and 2 of a drama with tragic, comic, and poetic elements. Act 3 is about to begin.

— Janet Bickel

Associate Vice President, Institutional Planning and Development
Director of Women's Programs, Association of American Medical Colleges
Author of Women in Medicine: Getting in, Growing, and Advancing *(2000)*

References

Etzkowitz, H., Kemelgor, C., & Uzzi, B. (2000). *Athena unbound: The advancement of women in science and technology*, Cambridge, UK: Cambridge University Press.

Heilbrun, C. (1988). *Writing a woman's life*. New York: Norton.

McClelland, D.C. (1967). Wanted: A new self-image for women. In R. J. Lifton (Ed.), *The woman in America* (pp. 187–188). Boston: Beacon.

McElvaine, R. (2001). *Eve's seed: Biology, the sexes and the course of history.* New York: McGraw-Hill.

McMurray, J. E., & Jordan, J. (2000). *Work in progress: Relational dilemmas of women physicians.* Wellesley College, MA: Stone Center.

More, S. E. (2000). *Restoring the balance: Women physicians and the profession of medicine, 1850–1995.* Cambridge, MA: Harvard University Press.

Williams, J. (2000). *Unbending gender: Why family and work conflict and what to do about it.* New York: Oxford University Press.

ACKNOWLEDGMENTS

I am deeply grateful to the many individuals who helped make this book possible. Rita Charon's initial guidance gave me the courage to transform a mere dream into a distinct reality. Rolf Janke at Sage Publications recognized the potential in my idea, even in its incipient stages, and provided enthusiastic support every step of the way. I cannot thank him enough for his commitment, sincerity, and flexibility during the past two years. Janet Bickel's early encouragement reaffirmed the importance of such a book within the medical literature. Her leadership at the Association of American Medical Colleges and particularly her focus on women in medicine add an important and fitting perspective to the anthology.

My editorial reviewers Annie Armstrong-Coben, Nassim Assefi, Douglas Chin, Sayantani DasGupta, Gayatri Devi, Kathleen Dong, Melissa Fisher, Rebecca Kurth, Joan Lo, Aaron Manson, Julia McMurray, Stephanie Nagy-Agren, Danielle Ofri, Melissa Parisi, and Audrey Shafer graciously read portions of the manuscript, despite their own busy schedules, and offered critical, insightful comments that helped mold the final manuscript. A special thanks to Renda Soylemez, whose fine editorial skills helped turn raw material into a cohesive narrative; to Stephanie Nagy-Agren, who shared with me several wonderful pieces that I would never have found otherwise; and to Danielle Ofri and Kathleen Dong, who provided detailed editorial suggestions, line by line. My acknowledgments also to Michael LaCombe, associate editor of

Annals of Internal Medicine, from whose sections, "On Being a Doctor" and "Ad Libitum," several of these pieces were selected.

The chapter on pioneer women doctors was inspired by Marjorie Sirridge, who first introduced me to the autobiographies of early women physicians—eventually motivating me to begin my own collection. Regina Morantz-Sanchez generously reviewed the historical chapter, lending her expertise on the complex development of 19th- and early 20th-century women physicians. Her groundbreaking publications have greatly enlightened our historical interpretation of women in medicine.

I wish to acknowledge Nora Nercessian (Harvard Medical School) and Peter Wortsman (Columbia University College of Physicians & Surgeons) for their help in contacting an earlier generation of women physicians. Numerous individuals and organizations, including Robert Coombs, Dan Hsiung, Sanjyot Dunung, Beverly Ballaro, Robert Vietrogoski, Kilbourg Reedy, Tara McGloughlin, Sethina Edwards, the Marion Hilliard House, the Bentley Historical Library, the Douglas County Museum, the Owens-Adair Apartments, the Rochester Hills Museum, and the American Medical Women's Association, also provided resourceful information along the way. So many friends and relatives helped spread word of this project to other women physicians, as did medical school deans, chiefs of staff, department chairs, and professional organizational leaders across the country. The encouragement of countless colleagues, staff members, patients, and friends sustained me during the long and busy months. To my long-time assistants, Dorothy, Devina, and Maureen, and to my circle of "mommy friends" in New York and California, a heartfelt thank-you.

This book would never have been finished without the wonderful and sensitive guidance of my editor Claudia Hoffman, whose insightful revisions added clarity and focus to each chapter. I am deeply grateful for her incredible support during this past year. Thanks also to other members of the outstanding Sage team—Anna Howland, who helped locate publishers and secure the missing reprint permissions; Leticia Gutierrez, who coordinated the numerous author contracts; and Linda Gray, copy editor extraordinaire, who painstakingly fixed all the little details and added the final, polishing touches.

I can never express enough gratitude to my family. My mother, Grace Lo, taught me through love and example that career and family are not mutually exclusive entities. She and my father, Wenso Lo, have provided tremendous support and encouragement for this undertaking, as they have in all aspects of my life. My twin sister, Joan Lo, with her husband, Alan Go, were a continual source of practical assistance and sounding boards for the many questions that arose. I also thank my husband's parents, Howard and Olga Chin, and his brothers, Don and David Chin, for their generous help as I scrambled to meet deadlines, and my sister-in-law, Mika Chin, for her fresh editorial perspective during the final stretch.

I am grateful to our nanny Sharma for her dedication and love toward our family, which allowed me the freedom to pursue my work during our years in New York City. I am a better mother for having known her infinite patience with children. My children, Emily, Sarah, and Nathan continue to bless my life with endless joy. Their very existence became the impetus for my desire to write about the double challenge and privilege of being both mother and physician. With much love, I thank my husband Doug for his unwavering support and encouragement in this project—despite the additional chaos it brought into our lives. I am especially grateful for his thoughtful input and for meticulously editing portions of this manuscript.

Most of all, I am deeply indebted to the more than 150 women and men whose stories, poems, and essays have made this book complete. I am privileged and honored to have shared with you in this collaboration.

INTRODUCTION

The idea for this book was borne out of a personal need for mentoring. I embarked on this journey over two years ago, just months after the birth of my second daughter. Being a young mother, physician, and wife, I found myself perpetually struggling to achieve some semblance of balance in my life. As a clinician-educator at Columbia University, I frequently encountered medical students and residents contemplating these very same issues. Yet how had other women physicians managed to structure their lives so admirably? Surely my situation was hardly unique, despite the realities of having two young children and a surgical resident husband. Thus, the notion of collecting written experiences began to take shape.

Perhaps many of my personal conflicts stemmed from the intrinsic dilemmas faced by most working mothers, dilemmas arising from the social liberation that women have achieved in the past century. No longer bound by traditional domestic expectations, women have eagerly and successfully embraced professional careers. Yet reconciling the desire to pursue an all-consuming profession such as medicine with the equally demanding needs of family can be a formidable experience, one inevitably accompanied by some degree of guilt or uncertainty. Reassurance usually comes later, only with the perspective of time.

The idea of compiling an anthology, however, remained dormant for nearly a year following its conception, buried under the frenetic routine of everyday responsibilities. It was Julia McMurray's story "Doctor's

Daughter," published in the *Annals of Internal Medicine* in September 1999, that rekindled my vision and ultimately inspired me to action. A few background phone calls led to a meeting with established writer-colleague, Rita Charon, through whom I contacted Janet Bickel at the American Association of Medical Colleges (AAMC) and eventually Rolf Janke, then-Editorial Director at Sage Publications. Nationwide correspondence to medical schools, hospital centers, professional organizations, and individual physicians soon followed the next month.

The response was overwhelming. Letters of support with stories, poems, and essays streamed through my mailbox over the next six months, laying the foundation for a new network of women colleagues and friends. Reading these letters, I was amazed by the diverse yet somehow common experiences of women across different specialties, ages, and geographic divides. People whom I had never met shared with me their most intimate stories. With relief, I discovered that my daily juggling act was far from unique. Others were also engaged in that same endeavor, living busy but deeply fulfilled lives. The unfolding of their stories echoed my own experience.

This Side of Doctoring brings together a collection of stories, poems, and essays that capture the essence of being a woman physician— reflections on doctoring from a woman's perspective, sketches of personal life from a doctor's perspective. These are poignant narratives of joy, frustration, regret, and fulfillment, a testament to the struggles and triumphs of women in medicine for the past century and a half, from the very early pioneer doctors to the medical students of the 21st century. Among these pages, younger physicians will, hopefully, find guidance as they develop in their personal and professional lives.

Much like an American quilt, this anthology is richly textured by each woman's extraordinary life and career. The assemblage of so many different voices exemplifies the varied paths that women have created within the medical profession. Together they stand as an enduring tribute to the dedication of all women physicians to both their patients and their families.

— *Eliza Lo Chin*

1

HISTORICAL PERSPECTIVE

Eliza Lo Chin

To acknowledge our ancestors means
we are aware that we did not make
ourselves, that the line stretches
all the way back.

— Alice Walker*

Women have practiced the art of medicine and healing for centuries. Barred from the formal education available to men, the early women doctors in America learned primarily through apprenticeships and self-education. These "doctresses" labored on the periphery of mainstream medicine, but over time, a few managed to build thriving practices, catering mostly to women and children. Perhaps the most renowned of these individuals was Harriet Hunt, an ardent feminist and dedicated physician of the 19th century. Never formally trained, she was later awarded an honorary M.D. degree in 1853 by the Women's Medical College of Pennsylvania (Elliot, 1869).

Women's entrance into the medical academy was pioneered by
Elizabeth Blackwell, a bright, young, English immigrant whose decision
to pursue medicine was prompted by a friend who later died from a
serious illness. This friend's confession, "If I could have been treated by
a lady doctor, my worst sufferings would have been spared me" was to
make a lasting impression on the young Elizabeth (Blackwell, 1895).
Undaunted by the obstacles before her, she embarked resolutely on her
mission. After multiple rejections, she was finally accepted quite "by
accident" at the Geneva College of Medicine in New York (Abram, 1985).
The school's administration had actually intended to decline her
admission but, desiring the student body's support, had put the issue to
a vote. Imagine their shock when the class, in a boisterous, joking mood,
voted unanimously to accept her (Smith, 1911). One classmate spoke
years later about Blackwell's first day:

> A lady, on his invitation, entered, whom he formally introduced as
> Miss Elizabeth Blackwell. She was plainly but neatly dressed in
> Quaker style, and carried the usual note-book of the medical
> student.
>
> A hush fell upon the class as if each member had been stricken
> with paralysis. A death-like stillness prevailed during the lecture,
> and only the newly arrived student took notes. She retired with the
> Professor, and thereafter came in with him and sat on the platform
> during the lecture. (pp. 8–9)

Two years later, in 1849, Blackwell graduated first in her class.
Her triumph unleashed a flurry of protests within the medical
establishment. One Boston physician lamented,

> It is much to be regretted that she has been induced to depart from
> the appropriate sphere of her own sex, and led to aspire to honors
> and duties which by the order of nature and the common consent
> of the world devolve alone upon men. . . . As this is the first case
> of the kind that has been perpetrated either in Europe or America,

I hope, for the honor of humanity, that it will be the last. (D. K., 1849)

But a wedge had been driven into the once solid barrier of exclusion. Other pioneer women soon followed suit, notably among them Elizabeth's younger sister, Emily Blackwell, as well as Maria Zakrzewska, Mary Putnam Jacobi, and Ann Preston. The Women's Medical College of Pennsylvania opened in 1850, the first of several institutions devoted primarily to the medical education of women. In 1857, the Blackwell sisters, along with Zakrzewska, founded the New York Infirmary for Women and Children.

By the end of the 19th century, 19 women's medical colleges and 9 women's hospitals had been established through the efforts of this pioneer generation and the leadership of several liberal-minded male colleagues. The struggle for coeducation, however, progressed with much more difficulty, initially successful only in a minority of institutions. A deep-rooted prejudice still pervaded much of the medical establishment, fueled by the theories of Harvard professor Edward H. Clarke (1874) who proclaimed that women who sought advanced education would develop "monstrous brains and puny bodies; abnormally active cerebration and abnormally weak digestion; flowing thought and constipated bowels." As one sympathetic physician commented, "It was almost a disgrace to be seen walking on the street with a woman doctor to say nothing of the enormity of showing her a kindness" (Helga, 1946).

The path to medicine was rough and unpaved for this pioneer generation. Many pursued their goals against the wishes of their families, enduring the hard years of study with little support and often flagrant discrimination (Luchetti, 1998; Morantz-Sanchez, 1985). Mary Putnam Jacobi (1891) wrote fervently of these "obscure heroisms":

Girls have been hissed and stampeded out of hospital wards and amphitheaters where the suffering patient was a woman, and properly claiming the presence of members of her own sex; or where, still more inconsistently, non-medical female nurses were tolerated and welcomed. Women students have been cheated of their time and money, by those paid to instruct them: they have been led into fields of promise, to find only a vanishing mirage. At what sacrifices have they struggled to obtain the elusive prize! They have starved on half rations, shivered in cold rooms, or been poisoned in badly ventilated ones; they have often borne a triple load of ignorance, poverty, and ill health; when they were not permitted to walk, they have crept—where they could not take, they have begged; they have gleaned like Ruth among the harvesters for the scantiest crumbs of knowledge, and been thankful. (pp. 198–199)

Within such a climate of hostility, the early women medical students labored even more diligently to prove their academic merit, often sensing that the future of the entire female gender lay upon their shoulders. Many eventually graduated at or near the top of their class (Morantz-Sanchez, 1985). The success of these efforts was reflected most obviously in the impressive standing achieved by women physicians by the end of the 19th century. They constituted 5% of American physicians and numbered over 7,000 (Morantz-Sanchez, 1985).

Even from the early days, women brought their feminine influences to the practice of medical healing. They stressed the importance of the physician-patient relationship, the need to treat "the spirit as well as the body," and the benefits of preventive medicine (Morantz-Sanchez, 1985). Particularly concerned about the welfare of their own sex, they established numerous dispensaries for women and children that provided not only medical care but also social services and health education. In addition, these clinics created opportunities for practice and training that otherwise were not readily open to women (Moldow, 1987). In 1893, a group of women physicians founded the *Woman's Medical Journal*, an endeavor ultimately leading to the 1915 organization of the Medical Women's National Association (later the American Medical Women's Association). That same year, women finally gained membership into the American Medical Association (AMA).

The advent of the World War II brought an unexpected boon to women's campaign for equal education. In some instances, the number of male applicants had decreased to such an extent that many medical schools began to look more favorably on female medical students. Yet in 1949, just 100 years after Elizabeth Blackwell received her degree, still only 5.5% of entering students were women (Bickel, Clark, & Lawson, 2000). This number remained below 10% until the 1970s, when the first significant increase became apparent.

Why weren't more women entering the medical field? Historians have identified a number of complex historical, cultural, and scientific factors contributing to the weakening of the women's medical movement during the first half of the 20th century. Although discriminatory practices still generally prevailed and several institutions established quotas to limit the number of female students, stronger underlying forces were responsible for the declining numbers of women within the field. Of particular significance was the changing face of medicine itself. With the rise of modern hospitals and advances in scientific theory, a stronger focus was placed on the objective and technical aspects of medicine, perhaps diminishing the appeal to many women drawn to its humanistic potential. Several female physicians spoke publicly of their concerns as the "science" of medicine gained prominence over the "sympathy" of healing (Morantz-Sanchez, 1985). Meanwhile, other, more nurturing fields, such as nursing, public health, and social work, became increasingly attractive. Medical educational reform, empowered by the release of the Flexner report, was another important factor. In his detailed study of medical education, Abraham Flexner identified significant weaknesses within the current system that mandated change, prompting medical schools to upgrade admission requirements and standardize the curriculum to make it more lengthy and rigorous (Morantz-Sanchez, 1985). As historian Regina Morantz-Sanchez (1995) concludes, "Medical professionalization itself . . . was essentially a profoundly 'gendered' phenomenon . . . structured entirely in response to the male life cycle," creating more hardships for women with domestic aspirations or responsibilities. Yet another factor was simply the failure of the women's medical colleges. By 1920, all but one had closed or merged with other institutions because of inadequate financial resources or declining enrollment.

Furthermore, because society in the 1950s viewed women's primary role as that of caring for the family, the social climate discouraged women from working extensively outside the home (More, 1999). Sylvia Hewlett (1986) identifies this period as the "postwar cult of motherhood." "To be a good mother in the fifties was a role that knew no bounds, as mothers became personally responsible for the psychological and cognitive development of their children." This prevailing culture created a painful dilemma for professional women, particularly those with children. As historian Ellen More (1999) aptly states, "The most intractable obstacle for women physicians in these decades was their own deeply rooted ambivalence about their 'right' to a career at all."

The revival of feminism in the 1960s signaled a renewed interest in women's professional careers, a trend reflected by the substantial increase in female medical school applicants by the mid-1970s (Bickel et al., 2000). Furthermore, Title IX of the Higher Education Act, passed in 1972, prevented federally funded educational institutions from discriminating against applicants on the basis of gender. Not surprisingly, 22.4% of new medical school entrants in 1974 were women, up from 9.1% in 1969 (Bickel et al., 2000). Gaining strength in numbers, women physicians became more vocal in their efforts to change the medical establishment. Several national conferences sponsored by the U.S. Government, the American Medical Women's Association (AMWA), and the Josiah Macy Jr. Foundation specifically promoted the advancement of women within the field.

By the latter 20th century, overt discrimination had become less apparent, yet subtle inequities still persisted at all levels within the profession. Dr. Mary Howell's highly controversial book, *Why Would a Girl Go Into Medicine?*, published in 1973 under the pseudonym Margaret Campbell to protect her identity as Associate Dean at Harvard Medical School, criticized the discriminatory practices that still pervaded medical education (Campbell, 1973). AMA data from the 1980s furthermore revealed the disturbing fact that women continued to earn significantly less than their male counterparts (AMA, 1995). And despite their advancement in academic medicine, a "glass ceiling" seemed to prevent further "upward mobility" of women faculty (Lorber, 1993). Not surprisingly, the number of full, tenured, female professors has remained quite low; few women have become department chairs, deans, or medical directors. Even as late as 1991, the highly publicized resignation (later rescinded) of Frances Conley, professor of neurosurgery at Stanford, brought to light charges of sexual harassment at one of the nation's preeminent medical institutions (Conley, 1998).

Recent data suggest, however, that women are increasing their foothold within American medicine. According to the AMA (2000), women now compose 22.8% of U.S. physicians. Within academic institutions, 28% of full-time faculty are women, although their ranks are skewed toward the instructor or assistant professor levels. Only 12% of full professors and 23% of associate professors are women (Bickel et al., 2000). But the future does look promising. Women now make up 45.6% of new entrants to U.S. medical schools and are an entering majority in 36 schools (Bickel et al., 2000).

Despite these numerical gains, what can be said about the women themselves? The literature in this area is just beginning to evolve. Although a recent survey reported general satisfaction among female physicians, a surprising 31% of respondents indicated that they might not choose to follow the same career path again. Predictors influencing this decision included high work stress, history of harassment, increased family responsibilities, younger age, and lack of job autonomy (Frank, McMurray, Linzer, & Elon, 1999). Hopefully, the identification of these factors will provide the impetus for improving the workplace environment to the benefit of all physicians.

Studies of women in academic medicine (Carr et al., 1998; Levinson, Tolle, & Lewis, 1989) have underscored the conflicts that women faculty encounter when choosing to combine career and family. Particularly unique to this setting is the time frame in which promotion and tenure deadlines must be achieved. Some women delay having children in favor of first establishing a career. Most, however, choose to embrace motherhood, even at the expense of increased hardship and slower career development (Levinson et al., 1989). Clearly, the dilemmas have not yet been fully resolved.

Looking back over the past 150 years, women have made tremendous advances within the medical profession, overcoming traditional barriers to establish their rightful place within the profession. No longer considered strange or peripheral, they have become a strong, vital force, achieving a level of prominence that was unimaginable in the mid-19th century. And as the rising numbers suggest, there is every reason to believe that they will continue to succeed. The question that remains is whether this success will translate into happiness and fulfillment for a generation of women balancing the demands of a strenuous but rewarding profession with the equally taxing demands of family life, against a changing backdrop of societal expectations for both women and men.

> No woman studying medicine today will ever
> know how much it has cost the individuals
> personally concerned in bringing about these
> changes; how eagerly they have watched new
> developments and mourned each defeat and rejoiced
> with each success. For with them it meant much
> more than success or failure for the individual,
> it meant the failure or success of a grand cause.
> — Mergler (1896, p. 92)

References

Abram, R. J. (1985). Will there be a monument? Six pioneer women doctors tell their own stories. In R. J. Abram (Ed.), *"Send us a lady physician": Women doctors in America, 1835–1920* (pp. 71–106). New York: Norton.

American Medical Association. (1995). *Women in medicine in America: In the mainstream*. Chicago: Author.

American Medical Association. (2000). *Physician characteristics and distribution in the U.S.* Chicago: Author.

Bickel, J., Clark, V., & Lawson, R. (2000). *Women in U.S. academic medicine statistics 1999–2000*. Washington, DC: Association of American Medical Colleges.

Blackwell, E. (1895). Pioneer work in opening the medical profession to women—autobiographical sketches. London: Longman.

Campbell, M. A. (1973). "Why would a girl go into medicine?" *Medical education in the United States: A guide for women.* Old Westbury, NY: Feminist Press.

Carr, P. L., Ash, A. S., Friedman, R. H., Scaramucci, A., Barnett, R. C., Szalacha, L., Palepu, A., & Moskowitz, M. A. (1998). Relation of family responsibilities and gender to the productivity and career satisfaction of medical faculty. *Annals of Internal Medicine, 129,* 532–538.

Clarke, E. H. (1874). *Sex in education: A fair chance for girls.* Boston: James R. Osgood.

Conley, F. K. (1998). *Walking out on the boys.* New York: Farrar, Straus & Giroux.

D. K. (1849). The late medical degree to a female. *Boston Medical and Surgical Journal, 40,* 58–59.

Elliot, H. B. (1869). Woman as physician. In J. Parton, H. Greeley, T. W. Higginson, J. S. C. Abbott, J. M. Hoppin, W. Winter, T. Tilton, F. Fern, G. Greenwood, E. C. Stanton, et al. (Eds.), *Eminent women of the age: Being narratives of the lives and deeds of the most prominent women of the present generation* (pp. 513–550). Hartford, CT: S. M. Betts.

Frank, E., McMurray, J. E., Linzer, M., & Elon, L. (1999). Career satisfaction of U.S. women physicians: Results from the women physicians' health study. *Archives of Internal Medicine, 159,* 1417–1426.

Helga, M. R. (1946). The women's medical college of Chicago: Later called the Northwestern University Woman's Medical College, 1870–1902. *Medical Woman's Journal, 53,* 42.

Hewlett, S. A. (1986). *A lesser life: The myth of women's liberation in America.* New York: William Morrow.

Jacobi, M. P. (1891). Women in medicine. In A. N. Meyer (Ed.), *Woman's work in America* (pp. 139–205). New York: Henry Holt.

Levinson, W., Tolle, S. W., & Lewis, C. (1989). Women in academic medicine: Combining career and family. *New England Journal of Medicine, 321,* 1511–1517.

Lorber, J. (1993). Why women physicians will never be true equals in the American medical profession. In E. Riska & K. Wegar (Eds.), *Gender, work, and medicine: Women and the medical division of labour.* London: Sage.

Luchetti, C. (1998). *Medicine women: The story of early-American women doctors.* New York: Crown.

Mergler, M. (1896). *History of competitive examinations. In Woman's Medical School, Northwestern University (Woman's Medical College of Chicago) the institution and its founders; Class histories 1870–1896.* Chicago: Cutler.

Moldow, G. (1987). *Women doctors in gilded age Washington: Race, gender, and professionalization.* Urbana & Chicago: University of Illinois Press.

Morantz-Sanchez, R. (1985). *Sympathy and science*. New York: Oxford University Press.

Morantz-Sanchez, R. (1995, Spring). How women made history in medicine. *Harvard Medical Alumni Bulletin*, pp. 17–24.

More, E. S. (1999). *Restoring the balance: Women physicians and the profession of medicine, 1850–1995*. Cambridge, MA: Harvard University Press.

Smith, S. (1911). *In memory of Dr. Elizabeth Blackwell and Dr. Emily Blackwell*. Academy of Medicine, New York & the Women's Medical Association of New York City. New York: Knickerbocker.

Walker, A. (1973). *Revolutionary petunias*. San Diego, CA: Harcourt Brace.

2

EARLY PIONEERS

It must have been a lonely vigil once,
to be a woman in medicine, even at the top.
— Howard Spiro (1979)[1]

Glances and Glimpses[2]

Our business gradually increased. One cure opened the way for other
cases; and an enforcement of dietetic rules, bathing, and so forth, soon
placed on a permanently healthy platform those who consulted us. Our
diagnosis was not copied from that of any eminent M.D. Indeed it
required a strong and determined effort never to speak disparagingly of
the profession, or of physicians, but to be quiet and candid. Very carefully
did we venture out into the broad ocean—preferring, at the outset, to
keep along shore, till experience could trim the sails, and confidence pilot
a larger craft. Soon, opportunities were offered us to visit country towns;
I accepted them cheerfully; my sister remained at home. From these
journeys I gathered rich knowledge; so many "given up cases" were
presented to my notice!—also chronic diseases of an aggravated
character. These last were opportunities for friendly relations and
examinations; but not cases to be accepted professionally. My field of
observations broadened wonderfully;—if hospitals closed their doors to

woman, except as patient and nurse the public were beginning to perceive the inconsistency—nay, injustice—of the act! We had, before long, patients from the highly cultivated, the delicate, and the sensible portions of the community. . . .

I have already said that we perused medical works with much dissatisfaction. This probably arose in great measure from our being entirely shut out from the medical world, having no minds with which to interchange views, compare thoughts, and examine experiences, and whose sympathy would have cheered and encouraged us. We felt the need of a clear, exploring light: at last we found it. George Combe came to this country, and, in October, 1938, commenced a course of lectures in Boston. What can I say of them! Those persons who heard them remember their power; those who did not cannot conceive it. To me they were revelations—bread for a hungry spirit, and water for a thirsty soul. . . . He opened to us the labyrinth of life; he lighted up its mysterious chambers, and bade us enter and explore; he gave us the golden clue of connection between cause and effect and end. His philosophy was not a fragment—it was a complete and consistent system. At whatever point of the great circle of thought we stood with him, there was ever some radius pointing to the central truth that governed all. My experience confirmed all his teachings: I can never forget them.

— Harriet Hunt
One of the early women physicians, never formally trained
General practitioner, feminist

Letters From Elizabeth Blackwell

From a letter to friend Emma Willard, 1847[3]

Dr. Warrington is discouraged and he joins with his medical brethren in advising me to give up the scheme. But a strong idea, long cherished till it has taken deep root in the soul and become an all-absorbing duty, cannot thus be laid aside. I must accomplish my end. I consider it the noblest and most useful path that I can tread, and if one country rejects me I will go to another.

From a letter to an aunt, Barbara Blackwell, 1860[4]

How good work is—work that has a soul in it! I cannot conceive that anything can supply its want to a woman. In all human relations the woman has to yield, to modify her individuality. The strong personality of even the best husband and children compels some daily sacrifice of self, some loving condescension to the less spiritual and more imperious natures. But true work is a perfect freedom, and full satisfaction.

> — Elizabeth Blackwell
> *Geneva Medical College, 1849*
> *First woman to graduate from a U.S. medical school*
> *Cofounder of the New York Infirmary for Women and Children*
> *and the New York Women's Medical College*

In the Words of Mary Putnam Jacobi

Shall Women Practice Medicine?[5]

These ask not, "Is she capable?" but, "Is this fearfully capable person nice? Will she upset our ideal of womanhood, and maidenhood, and the social relations of the sexes? Can a woman physician be lovable; can she marry; can she have children; will she take care of them? If she cannot, what is she?"

Quoted in *Bowery to Bellevue*[6]

Women must be willing to go up, to be knocked down again and again, before the general hospital will finally be opened.

Woman in Medicine[7]

It is perfectly evident from the records, that the opposition to women physicians has rarely been based upon any sincere conviction that women could not be instructed in medicine, but upon an intense dislike to the idea that they should be so capable.

— *Mary Putnam Jacobi*
Female Medical College of Pennsylvania, 1864
Former Professor of Materia Medica and Therapeutics,
Women's Medical College of the New York Infirmary
Founding President of the Women's Medical Association of New York City

The Fortress[8]

I was in the fortress as it were, but alone and likely to be for a good long time.

— *Elizabeth Garrett Anderson*
Licentiate of the Society of Apothecaries (England), 1865
Founder of the present-day Elizabeth Garrett Anderson Hospital
Former Dean, London Medical School for Women
First woman doctor in Britain

Some of My Life Experiences[9]

I had always had a fondness for nursing and had developed such a special capacity in that direction by assisting my neighbors in illness that I was more and more besieged by the entreaties of my friends and doctors, which were hard to refuse, to come to their aid in sickness, oftentimes to the detriment of business, and now that money came easily, a desire began to grow within me for a medical education. One evening I was sent for by a friend with a very sick child. The old physician in my presence attempted to use an instrument for the relief of the little sufferer, and in his long, bungling, and unsuccessful attempt he severely lacerated the tender flesh of the poor little girl. At last, he laid down the instrument to wipe his glasses. I picked it up, saying, "Let me try, Doctor," and passed it instantly, with perfect ease, bring immediate relief to the tortured child. The mother, who was standing by in agony at the sight of her child's mutilation, threw her arms around my neck and sobbed out her thanks. Not so the doctor! He did not appreciate or approve of my interference, and he showed his displeasure at the time most emphatically. This apparently unimportant incident really decided my future course.

A few days later, I called on my friend, Dr. Hamilton, and confiding to him my plans and ambitions, I asked for the loan of medical books. He gave me Gray's Anatomy. I came out of his private office into the drug-store, where I saw Hon. S. F. Chadwick, who had heard the conversation, and who came promptly forward and shook my hand warmly, saying: "Go ahead. It is in you; let it come out. You will win."

The Hon. Jesse Applegate, my dear and revered friend, who had fondled me as a babe, was the one other person who ever gave me a single word of encouragement to study medicine.

In due time, I announced that in two weeks I would leave for Philadelphia, to enter a medical school. As I have said, I expected disapproval from my friends and relatives, but I was not prepared for the storm of opposition that followed. My family felt that they were disgraced, and even my own child was influenced and encouraged to think that I was doing him an irreparable injury, by my course. People sneered and laughed derisively. Most of my friends seemed to consider it their Christian duty to advise against, and endeavor to prevent me taking the "fatal" step. That crucial fortnight was a period in my life never to be forgotten. I was literally kept on the rack. But as all things must have an end, the day of my departure was at last at hand.

Eleven o'clock p.m. arrived at last, and I found myself seated in the California overland stage, beginning my long journey across the continent. It was a dark and stormy night, and I was the only inside passenger. There was no one to divert my thoughts from myself or prevent the full realization of the dreary and desolate sense that I was starting out into an untried world alone, with only my own unaided resources to carry me through. The full moment of what I had undertaken now rose before me, and all I had left behind tugged at my heart-strings. My crushed and over-wrought soul cried out for sympathy, and forced me to give vent to my pent-up feelings in a flood of tears, while the stage floundered on through mud and slush, and the rain came down in torrents, as if sympathizing Nature were weeping a fitting accompaniment to my lonely, sorrowful mood.

And now I had ample opportunity to reason and reflect. I remembered that every great trouble of my life had proved a blessing in disguise and had brought me renewed strength and courage.

> "For so tenderly our sorrows hold the germs of our future joys,
> That even a disappointment brings us more than it destroys."
> I had taken the decisive step, and I would never turn back.

> — *Bethenia A. Owens-Adair*
> *Eclectic School of Medicine, 1873*
> *The first woman graduate in medicine in Oregon*

From More Than Gold in California[10]

A facial operation of such magnitude is far more repellant than one on any other part of the body. As it proceeded, a student fainted. Soon another; then a third. The three men were stretched out on the floor and no further attention was paid to them. As the gruesome operation proceeded I gritted my teeth, clenched my hands, and held on. Next to me stood a senior woman student. I watched her turn a greenish white and sway a little. Contrary to the ethics of an operating room, where silence is the rule, I hissed in her ear, "Don't you dare faint." She jumped, and flushing with anger, turned on me. In turn I flushed with embarrassment. But the return of blood to our heads by blushing saved the situation." The two women students did not faint and thus disgrace the sex. That three men did faint was merely due to a passing circulatory disturbance of no significance; but had the two women medical students fainted, it would have been incontrovertible evidence of the unfitness of the entire sex for the medical profession.

— Mary Bennett Ritter
Cooper Medical College, 1886
General practitioner

From *Mine Eyes Have Seen*[11]

I am often asked, "How did you happen to study medicine? Then I think of that strange "yellow day" in September of 1881, when the whole of the Eastern States were masked in an uncanny, sulphur-colored light—a mysterious, sinister light for which science has given no explanation.

It was on that day that I followed a rude country wagon moving slowly out from the Adirondack woods, over the long rough road homeward—its burden my brother's body. Somehow there was a weird, almost vaguely sympathetic fitness in the strange yellow light, toning with my grief and despair.

I felt completely adrift, my whole plan of life in sudden and overwhelming chaos. The thought kept recurring; if I had known more of illness and the means of combating it, I might have been able to do more for him. Out of these emotions came the decision which set the course of my life.

I would become a doctor.

— Alfreda Withington
Women's Medical College of the New York Infirmary, 1887
General practitioner

Petticoat Surgeon[12]

In all my pre-college experience I had never heard of a woman physician. My freshman curiosity was therefore whetted when I learned that the two young ladies who were living in a boardinghouse across the street from the sorority house were studying medicine.

They were Vassar products. One of them, Mary McLean, a tall, pale, mettlesome young woman, but a cultured Southern lady withal, was religious to a degree that approached bigotry; the other, Harriet Barringer, was refined and dignified, but more than that, an eye-catcher in a college town. She wore for everyday a long ermine cape and a hat made of peacock feathers. Often, when asked why I selected medicine as a career, I have been tempted to reply, "It was a peacock hat and ermine coat that first attracted me to the medical profession."

The fact that these girls were "hen-medics" did not deter me, as it did my sorority sisters, from making their acquaintance at once. Yet it was only after long and cautious consideration where curiosity was the scale-tipping factor, that the die was cast to call on them. Their enthusiasm for their work fired my imagination.

— *Bertha Van Hoosen*
University of Michigan, 1888
Former Professor and Head of Obstetrics, Loyola University School of Medicine
Founder and First President of the American Medical Women's Association

From A *Child Went Forth*[13]

Subjects, bodies for dissection, were divided into five parts—the head, two uppers and two lowers. By some ironical twist of circumstance, the first dissection assigned to me was a lower. The dissection of the pelvic organs was to be done in company with the young man who was assigned to the other lower. It was a male subject.

The two other women of the class were doing their dissection together. There was no way out. Nothing to do but face the music. I waited as long as possible, putting off the evil day. The young man waited, a bit cynical, wholly amused. It came time for the quiz section in anatomy. The quiz master was a dapper young graduate, much impressed with himself and his authority. He was of the group who hated the incursion of women into what he considered the distinctly masculine territory of medicine.

I had studied my anatomy assiduously, but neither the young man nor myself had touched a scalpel to the subject. We met in the dissecting room. All the other subjects were in position and had had more or less work done on them. The quiz master walked over to our dissecting table.

He turned to the young man. "Why has nothing been done on your subject?" he questioned.

The young man hesitated, glancing at me.

The quiz master turned on me. "Have you the other lower on this subject?" His words were like a steel file.

"Yes," I replied, the blood rushing to my face.

"Do you expect to graduate in medicine, or are you just playing around with the idea?"

"I hope to graduate." I tried to make my voice sound firm, but instead I realized it sounded ridiculously weak and feminine.

The group around me were "all eyes," some friendly, some hostile.

"If you have any feelings of delicacy in this matter, young woman, you had better leave college and take them with you, or fold them away in your work basket and be here, on your stool, tomorrow morning. We don't put up with any hysterical feminine nonsense in men's medical schools."

He turned away. The group followed him to be quizzed on another subject where the dissection was well advanced. I bit my tongue and held back the tears. I was trembling with shame and indignation. I clenched my fists and joined the group. When the quiz master asked me a question I was able to answer it clearly and intelligently. I had lived and dined and slept with *Gray's Anatomy*. . . .

The next morning I entered the dissecting room with every nerve tense. I expected to meet a score of mocking eyes. The place was deserted. Our subject was in position, ready to begin work. Rubber gloves and a dissecting case and Gray's manual were placed conveniently near. There was a note on the table. "You had better go ahead. We can't be here for a day or two. We'll show up for the next quiz."

The quiz master came in after his lecture. He hadn't forgotten. I was perched on my stool, working busily. He asked me what had become of the others. I told him I didn't know. The note was tucked securely in my smock. I put my hand in my pocket and felt it. It was as reassuring as the handclasp of a brother.

Something of the difficulties that I encountered must have crept between the lines of my letters to my father. I had never written anything about them. Perhaps the thought of the dissecting room as we had seen it together stimulated him to allow me to give up medicine for something more pleasant. He may have felt that I could not make a success in a profession that was distasteful to me, thereby causing his pride to suffer a fall. Whatever the motive, a letter came quite unexpectedly, saying that I could go across the bay to Berkeley and enter the University proper if I cared to do so.

I was surprised to find that I had no wish to change. I really liked the study of medicine. I wanted to go on with it more than I wanted anything else in the world. I wanted to win out. I wanted to keep the respect that I felt had prompted those young men to do what they had done that morning. I wanted to demonstrate that a woman could be just as good a sport as a man.

From that time forward when the professors told risqué jokes or made scornful allusions to the encroachment of petticoats, I wrapped the cloak of their respect around me and felt secure in its folds.

> — *Helen MacKnight Doyle*
> *University of California, 1893*
> *General practice and anesthesiology*

Fighting for Life[14]

When I encountered only argument and disapproval, my native stubbornness made me decide to study medicine at all costs and in spite of everyone. That is, after all, hardly a rational way to choose one's life work and yet, in a curious way, it seems to hold the secret of whatever success may come to one in later life. I am thoroughly convinced that obstacles to be overcome and disapproval to be lived down are strong motive forces.

— S. Josephine Baker
Women's Medical College of the New York Infirmary, 1898
Former Commissioner of Health in New York City and Director of the
Bureau of Child Hygiene, New York City

From Bowery to Bellevue[15]

After supper we made evening rounds, the staff telling me from time to time of my various duties as they presented themselves in the course of our trip through the wards. Finally we were standing in a group in the hall when the house surgeon turned to me and said casually, "Dr. Dunning, you are on duty tonight for the routine catheterizations in the male surgical ward." I could not quite believe my ears and looked first at him and then at the other members of the staff. There must be some mistake. Could it be possible that the first night they would assign me to this duty in the male ward? I felt as though a stick of dynamite with a burning sputtering fuse had suddenly been placed in my hands. The situation had all the essence of a complete world revolution in it. Since the beginning of time men, and men alone, had dealt with the afflictions and diseases, instrumentation and surgery of the male sexual organs. The earliest and most urgent service has been the relieving of a full bladder by catheterization. Difficulty of urination or total inability to void is peculiarly an affliction of males. This condition is painful and serious, and requires besides delicate instrumentation a complete confidence on the part of the patient in his physician. It is one of the most intimate of all medical ministrations.

Probably it was actually only a question of a few seconds by the clock—time means nothing in the great crises of life. I scrutinized each face carefully and saw that they really and truly meant it! In those moments certain absolute convictions swept over me. First, that my fellow staff mates had conceived a plan wherein I would meet sure disaster the first night I was on duty. These raw young fellows had undoubtedly figured out that by catapulting a young woman physician into a male surgical ward, they would create an erotic reaction on the part of the patients, and probably a riot against the woman doctor would result. Any such happening as this would be material so inflammable for the newspapers that an experiment, which only a small minority of forward looking citizens approved of anyway, would then and there be dubbed a failure. I would probably be forced to resign. I thought of those who were sponsoring the experiment—the reform Mayor, the new President of the Board of Trustees of Bellevue, the gentleman of our own Medical Board, Major Zalinski. I thought of the agony of disappointment for those women, Miss Brackett, Dr. Jacobi, Aunt Emma, my Mother! No, I could not and would not let them down. The blood pounded through my head, as I asked myself, "but how can I accomplish it, this first night when everything is new and strange and I do not know the patients, or the equipment with which I must work?" Suddenly every nerve in my body began to tingle and a second conviction equally strong came to me. "Of course I can do it, I have been trained, I know how." A great flood of gratitude poured out to my professor of urology, Dr. Sam Alexander. Foreseeing this very problem of treating male patients, he had seen to it that I learned the necessary technique, and under him I had developed more than average skill. . . .

. . . The beds were filled with every kind of man one would expect to find a block from the water front—old men, young men barely out of their teens, sailors, longshoremen, hucksters, tramps, bums, and gangsters. Not all needed attention, but the cases were spread all over the ward so it was necessary to cover the entire place. There was a moment of most terrific tension for them and for me. What would they do? I did not know. What would I do? They did not know but they were all waiting to find out, and the place was still as death. Except for my orders and the necessary noise of the instruments, you could have heard a pin drop. I felt thirty or more pairs of eyes watching me from every direction with curiosity, with penetration. . . .

. . . Agility and skill seemed to flow into my fingers that night. Swiftly one after another, the men were made comfortable, and I passed on to the next patient with only one thought in my mind: Would I get through, could I keep up this tremendous pace? We had started systematically on one side of the ward, working down toward the oval end. At last we reached it, turned the curve and started down on the other side, and soon that dreadful ordeal was over. Martin and I had finished our last case, and the patients had maintained a profound and respectful silence! The lights were turned down and the weary men left to rest. I had learned one great lesson that night, and that is that sex does not count when one is sick and in pain; the one who can bring the greatest help and skill is the one who is wanted the most. The problem of the men patients was solved for me that night.

— *Emily Dunning Barringer*
Cornell University Medical College, 1901
New York's first woman ambulance surgeon
Former President, American Medical Women's Association

A Woven Fabric[16]

Life is woven of circumstances and will
circumstances the threads, will the shuttle
weaving ugly rags or fine and beautiful cloth.

Early days of weaving full of knots and smudges,
willfulness, misdirected energy, carelessness.

A cool wind in my face, an inspiration,
    smooth and even.
Color, romance.

Flying fingers push the shuttle.
Joy to love. Joy to be loved.
Unruffled, gently flowing.
I am to be a mother.

A few short months, a tiny morsel in my arms.
I am a mother.

As suddenly,
threads tangle and break.
I cannot see to push the shuttle.
I am a widow.

Not a creature for the world.
I am to carry, to render service.

Not a time for self pity but for weaving.
Broken threads gathered, controlled.

A wide fabric.
Twinkling stars of early morning.
Cobwebs outline a million sparkling dewdrops.
Honey trembles in a primrose challis.
A meadowlark's joyous song.
A hundred prairie chickens feed at daybreak.
Old Prince, my faithful horse, jogs along,
stops in his dusty tracks,
snorts at a firefly in a potato patch.

It was nothing.

The mocking bird sings at midnight.
A vicious stab of lightning,
awesome rolls of thunder
A dusty wind.
The cold of winter.

Old Prince is supplanted.
Engines take me West:
tall firs in cool and luxuriant fern beds
outline the sky,
blue Cascades in a brilliant morning,
clouds in a misty valley.

Nights of patient vigil.
Behold the miracle of childbirth, again and again
ease the pain of passing from this world.

Golden threads of friendship.
Love in return for their constancy.

— *Mary Canaga Rowland*
Women's Medical College of Kansas City, 1901
A frontier woman doctor

Woman at the Gate[17]

On one occasion, I do not know what he [the Dean] thought, but he was jovial and smiling and he immediately said that he was going to show me why women could not be admitted.

First we went to the anatomy dissecting room. Around the walls were several conveniences for men in open view. Then he explained that there were no restrooms suitable for women and no place where women could hang their hats.

However, he said, if we could raise $50,000 to make some improvements in the physical plant, he might consider accepting women. I asked him if he would give us his word of honor that P&S would be opened to women if we fulfilled this condition and he answered yes.

— *Gulli Lindh Muller*
Columbia University, College of Physicians & Surgeons, 1921
Clinical and anatomic pathology

Epilogue

$50,000 was donated to the Columbia University College of Physicians & Surgeons, and Gulli Lindh Muller was among the first group of women admitted in 1917. She graduated in 1921, first in her class.

— *Editor*

A Woman Doctor Looks at Love and Life[18]

I know a lot about marriage, though I've never experienced it, because I have listened to the problems of literally thousands of married women. I also know, even better, the problems of unmarried women. I learned that the bitterest renunciation of all is not a mate—it is motherhood. Looking back on my life, I can chart those moments that were pivotal. The most crucial was the date I had one evening with a man I loved. He was an engineer and had been away on a project for several months. I was interning and missed him dreadfully. There was a tacit understanding that we were engaged. Together we would plan our future and set a date.

He called for me, looking brown and handsome. He had even borrowed a car. We went to dinner—I adored it—dinner away from the hospital was always a thrill. Replete, cosy in the car, waiting for my moment, while he talked of love I fell asleep. I had been on duty in the delivery room for four successive nights preceding this. He drove me home, wakened me, and said a curt good night. How thankful I've always been for that cat nap. A short time later he married someone else. He then provided me with my Gethsemane: He asked me to be his wife's doctor and deliver their first baby. It was a valuable experience. Nothing else in my lifetime has ever or will ever hurt so much. On Mother's Day, in the early morning, that I might miss no overtone of human longing or resignation, the child was born. If I could accept that and survive, and I could, then I could withstand anything.

I have said often that I have never failed to be stirred by the birth of a baby. Even at the instant that I delivered the child that might have been mine, I was moved through my anguish to feel, "This is worth while. What you are doing now is the most worth-while occupation on earth."

It is. Let me tell you about it and of what I know about women.

— *Marion Hilliard*
University of Toronto Faculty of Medicine, 1930
Former Chief of Obstetrics and Gynecology, Women's College Hospital, Toronto

The Antique Roadshow of a 90-Year-Old

1931. The year of my admission to Columbia University, College of Physicians & Surgeons. The George Washington Bridge opened, and MCATs were instituted. Our class was selected on quotas—100 men and 10 women, but only 6 women entered. Bard Hall, the dormitory, opened that year for men only. Since it was not fully occupied, women were later allowed to occupy the first two floors. There we made lifelong friends.

I remember Dr. Loeb, a charming, but intimidating professor of physical diagnosis who was reportedly opposed to women in medicine. He fell in love, however, with a resident in our year. At that time, women were not permitted to marry during residency, but the Chief of Medicine relented and blessed the marriage.

Occupational hazards were a reality in those days. Two of the women contracted active tuberculosis, and one contracted scarlet fever, which progressed to acute mastoiditis. Those were the days we practiced medicine without antibiotics.

When studying pneumococcus pneumonia, one lecture was spent debating whether or not we should digitalize the patient in preparation for the crisis on the ninth day. Later, Dr. Pappenheimer developed a vaccine that was specific for each strain of pneumococcus. It saved my brother's life.

My rotating internship was a most stressful year. I was the first and only woman intern at St. Elizabeth's Hospital in Elizabeth, New Jersey. The male interns ate together in the private dining room while I was relegated to the nurses' dining room.

The only concession made for me as a woman was to ride the ambulance in the summertime, a physically demanding job since it often required carrying stretchers up and down several flights of stairs. As it turned out, the intern assigned to ambulance duty in January became ill, so I replaced him. January 1936 still holds a record for the most brutal January in decades. The driver and I covered a 15-mile radius of mostly unplowed roads, often carrying stretchers down icy, snow-covered steps.

When assigned to the laboratory, we ran the blood counts and chemistries at night. Transfusion compatibility was tested by mixing two bloods on a slide and checking for clotting. Knowing what I know now, it frightens me to think of it!

After internship, I joined my father in general practice and helped run a small hospital, the Swiney Sanitorium, which was attached to our home and offices. During the first year, a child with severe strep throat coughed into my face. Within 6 hours I had a fever, within 12 hours, otitis media, and within 24 hours, acute mastoiditis. An ENT specialist recommended immediately starting a new drug released that week, sulfadiazine. Within 48 hours, my fever broke and the mastoiditis subsided. A miracle! My introduction to antibiotics.

It was difficult keeping up with the rapid advances in medicine while working from 9 a.m. to 11 p.m. with frequent late night house calls. Fortunately, some wonderful postgraduate courses helped keep me abreast of the exciting new discoveries.

Cardiology was making great strides. EKGs were introduced in private offices, coronary occlusion was being recognized, and Dr. Bailey performed the first mitral valve operation. He later told me he didn't know why it worked, but it did. The surgery certainly put my bedridden patients on their feet.

The introduction of Dilantin worked miracles in many previously hopeless epileptic patients. People whose lives had been crippled by seizures could now live more normally.

Pediatric vaccines and TB drugs closed Williard Parker Contagious Disease Hospital and the TB institutions.

The discovery of cortisone revolutionized the treatment of arthritis and allergies. Once considered the practitioner's greatest boon, it became the panacea for a host of different maladies.

I remember being too excited to sleep after hearing Dr. Shinya describe a new invention, the fiberoptic gastroscope and colonoscope.

When my father died after the second world war, we closed the hospital. Three decades later, I retired after practicing 56 years—just at the emergence of the HMOs.

— *Juliana Swiney*
Columbia University College of Physicians & Surgeons, 1935
General practice, Retired, 1986

Sound Investments[19]

I will always remember my pre-admission interview with Dean Rappleye. He stated that each student pays tuition but the school invests far more money in that education. He questioned whether it was a sound investment to educate women in medicine, since their contribution would be short. After 53 years of marriage, my husband, an educator, is retired, but I am still practicing. Is there any way of telling him that the investment was sound?

— *Gertrude Russack Sobel*
Columbia University College of Physicians & Surgeons, 1940
Former Associate Professor of Medicine
State University of New York at Stony Brook
Now retired

The First Women at H.M.S.[20]

When we started medical school in 1945—the first women to enter H.M.S. [Harvard Medical School]—the upperclassmen were sure they knew the reason for which we were invading their sacred male domain —"to get husbands." After having themselves struggled through anatomy, physiology, and biochemistry, they should have known that there must have been easier ways.

Our first contacts with our medical colleagues left us with mixed emotions. Many of the upperclassmen, and some of the faculty, viewed the presence of women at Harvard as a disturbing upheaval of tradition. The upperclassmen subjected us during our first year to mild, but not always good-natured, hazing. We learned to our dismay that men were as gossipy as women, if not worse, and that cattiness was certainly not a female prerogative.

As we progressed through the basic sciences to physical diagnosis, and thence to clinical medicine, we became more secure in our relationship with our colleagues, and acceptance of us as doctors did evolve. Once we entered upon internships and residencies, being women doctors no longer presented any great problem. Occasionally, however, some small incident would occur to make us realize that we did have our limitations. A good example occurred during my internship, when I was called to the accident room by the chief surgical resident to reduce a dislocated shoulder. The patient, a burly truck driver, lay on a cot. I was instructed to place my foot in his axilla and pull on his arm until I heard a snap—indicating that the dislocated humerus had returned to its socket. I followed instructions, pulling until a loud snap was heard. The resident and other interns present congratulated me. Only the patient and I knew that the shoulder was not reduced, but how could I explain to the assemblage that the loud snap had been the noise of a garter dislocating from its girdle?

Now that I am practicing pediatrics my acceptance by colleagues and patients is quite complete. One of my favorite patients is a four-year-old girl, whose pediatrician I have been since her birth. I referred her to a male ophthalmologist, whom she confounded by saying, when she saw him for the first time, "He can't be a doctor—he's a man."

Despite the usual exasperating and, at times, nerve-wracking aspects of pediatrics, I find the most gratifying relationship is with the mothers of my patients. They feel a sense of identification with me, and I with them. Not only can I tell them what to do in case of illness, prescribe medications, make diagnoses, etc., but I can tell them how I conquered certain problems nursing, feeding, or washing diapers—helpful hints which carry authority because they come from both a doctor and a mother.

Just as my patients benefit somewhat because I am a woman, so do my children benefit because I am a doctor. For instance, when I start to scold my daughters because they don't eat their vegetables, I remember my advice to the harassed mother whose Johnny wouldn't eat, and I desist, shrugging my shoulders and saying to myself, "Don't worry, they'll grow." The only one who insists he doesn't benefit from my practice of medicine is my husband, but then, as my mother and I agree, "don't pay attention to husbands—they like to complain, but they don't mean it."

A Postscript[21]

Fifteen years ago I wrote a lighthearted article about the hectic but happy life I was leading trying to combine medicine, marriage, and motherhood. Now, as I look back upon my endeavors, I think I was not only lighthearted—I must have been light-headed as well. Only a chronic case of *Levitas cerebri,* the result of thirty years of intense brainwashing, could have made a person behave as I did then. In 1961 I was the brainwashed product of my culture's view of woman's place in society. Since I had chosen to enter a profession primarily reserved for men, my thirty previous years of cultural indoctrination caused me to feel that I therefore had to prove my femininity—I had to show that I was a woman. In the 1950-1960s my consciousness had not yet been raised. It never occurred to me that as a woman I deserved some liberation from the age-old mores which decreed that it was primarily my responsibility to maintain the home and raise the children. I went all-out to be the good wife and mother that I believed nature had meant me to be.

In addition, as a full-time practicing pediatrician I had office hours, saw hospital patients, made house-calls, and took phone calls. As I write this, I am amazed that neither my family, my home, nor my patients seemed to suffer. I do not feel that I was a hero mother-doctor-wife; in retrospect, I think I was just plain stupid. I have gradually become aware

of a new concept of the woman as a professional person. A woman who
invests just as much of her time, her money, her mind, and her soul in
becoming a doctor as does her male counterpart should be able to realize
an equal return on her investment; she should be able to experience the
joys and responsibilities of marriage and parenthood equally with her
male colleague—but not more equally.

To both husbands and wives the wife's professional involvement is
often looked upon as more of an avocation. To one particular
fellow-alumnus—the one to whom I am married—may I say, "Don't
worry, I still have a fair amount of *Levitas cerebri et cordis,* for which a
cure has yet to be found."

— Doris Rubin Bennett
Harvard Medical School, 1949
Former Chief of Pediatrics at Harvard Community Health Plan (Kenmore)
Among the first group of 12 women admitted to Harvard Medical School

I Will Not Pass Away[22]

I have become the unfortunate anachronism, the unwise one who did
not follow the approved path to psychiatry, pediatrics, radiology, and
research. The rash one who chose general surgery. And after four difficult
years in surgical training at a large Boston general hospital, I am blandly
told, "Statistics show it does not pay to train a woman."

Were the situation less tragic, it would be downright comical. Did it
matter that this hospital had never had a woman in surgery before me
and had no statistics whatsoever regarding the training of such? Did it
matter that four long years had proved the fallacy of the old cry, "The
training is too hard for girls"? Did it matter that my entire life has been
directed toward one professional goal and that nothing short of serious
illness or incapacitating injury could cause me to give up my profession?
Not one whit.

Few realize how devastating it is to be constantly reminded of the
obstacles to one's progress by someone who is in an absolute position to
remove the one then faced. Many have kindly offered to help me go far,

far away, somewhere. And with genuine concern for my interests. But the lesson that Boston is the Hub of the Surgical Universe has been learned too well. I will not pass away.

— *Mildred Fay Jefferson*
Harvard Medical School, 1951
Former Assistant Clinical Professor of Surgery, Boston University School of Medicine
Chairman, Citizens Select Committee on Public Health Oversight

The Beginnings of Women's Health Advocacy

In September 1947, at a welcome reception for the entering class of a prominent Northeastern medical school, a senior faculty member greeted me with the following disclaimer, "Had I been on the admissions committee, you would have never been accepted." In the midst of general hilarity, it sounded like a bad joke. I chuckled and asked, "Why not?" "Because women get married, have children, and waste their education. Now don't laugh, young lady, I am serious."

This was my introduction to medicine.

During the subsequent four years, I heard similar statements from male classmates and faculty alike. The younger men, in particular, enjoyed harassing the women by smirking, jeering, and inappropriate laughter. The faculty made no effort to restrain their boyish high spirits; at times it seemed they liked to provoke it.

With time, I found that women physicians were not the only ones at the butt of their male colleagues' demeaning jokes. Women patients, typically housewives with multiple complaints, were ridiculed, neglected, or given short-shrift workups. Residents tired of the "positive systems reviews" of these patients and what seemed to them constant anxiety-provoked complaints or questions. Businessmen, on the contrary, were managed promptly, with all available measures at the time. They occupied the privileged area on the floor, closely supervised by nurses.

"I had to see another crock in the emergency room last night," complained a resident within the first month of my internship.

"What is a crock?" As the first-year house officer, I was entitled to ignorance and could ask questions without being branded as inadequate.

"A crock is a patient who complains of everything hurting, is always tired or dizzy; does not give a clear history; is obese and therefore difficult to examine; may have a little diabetes, hypertension, or gallstones; and in 9 out of 10 cases is a middle-aged, neurotic, or hysterical woman. She has a 'positive systems review,' a negative workup, and does not believe me when I say that all her pains are just in her head. She unfortunately raises just enough medical suspicion to rouse the tired resident out of bed and keep him working her up until the wee hours of the morning."

Obviously, he considered her appearance in the emergency room as a personal affront, a cross he had to bear as an assistant resident.

"Why do you call these patients "crocks?"

"Because they all have cracked heads."

I was flabbergasted.

In time, I encountered patients with similar symptoms but found that often these pains were well-founded; many even had physical reasons for their complaints. Some had unusual manifestations of ordinary conditions, such as angina, mitral valve prolapse, gall bladder disease, gastroesophageal reflux, and thyroid disease, while others had unusual conditions such as acute intermittent porphyria and other missed diagnoses. In some, the state of panic was induced by traumatic family events; others were going through menopause. A few had clinical depression.

With time, I began to appreciate the varied manifestations of illness in women and tried to treat each patient not only as a challenging diagnostic puzzle but also as a complex human being who needed information, individual management, counseling, and care.

And so began my interest and work in the area of women's health.

— Lila A. Wallis

Columbia University College of Physicians & Surgeons, 1951
Clinical Professor of Medicine, Cornell University Weill Medical College
Past President of the American Medical Women's Association
Founder and first President of the National Council on Women's Health

From Chivalry and Off-Color Jokes to Acceptance and Respect[23]

Numerically we represented 10% of the class. We were regarded as curiosities, but at the same time were resented because, the males insisted, we were taking up the educational slots of men who would use medicine as an income-producing and family-supporting career, whereas we "girls" (as they referred to us) would get married, have families and *waste* this education.

Those were the days of chivalry when doors were held open for us and we were allowed to exit first from elevators. On the other side of the coin, it was common practice for professors to punctuate scientific lectures with "girlie" pictures, to the great glee of the men in the class. The phrase "sexual harassment" was not commonly used then! In the early years, especially in anatomy lab, practical jokes with sexual overtones were sprung on us, but since we did not wince the jokes soon stopped.

Occasionally, our minority gender status was turned to positive use: Dr. Yale Kneeland would call on one of us to detect a subtle tinctorial change in a patient because, he pointed out, the distaff side has a keener color sense.

By the time we reached the fourth year, the males in the class had learned to accept the seriousness of our commitment to our education and profession. In those four years, we all went through a maturation period. Now, when we see each other at reunions, all of us are totally accepted, regarded as equals, and respected.

Time has shown that we *did* use our education to practice the profession of medicine, notwithstanding the fact that we were also able to combine it with marriage and childrearing.

— Marianne Wolff
Columbia University College of Physicians & Surgeons, 1952
Former Professor of Clinical Surgical Pathology, Columbia University
Currently working part-time at a large commercial laboratory
Co-editor of Progress in Surgical Pathology *and* Digestive Disease Pathology

Medicine and Motherhood[24]

When I entered Radcliffe College in 1947, the Dean told our class that we were there for only one purpose: to become educated mothers of our children. Of course, in those days, a woman's highest goal was motherhood. Four years later when I entered medical school, only 394 women (5.3%) in the entire country did so (Johnson, 1983). Had I known how *rara an avis* I was, I would have been too frightened to fly!

Medicine was definitely a man's world in those days. In those years of prefeminist innocence, I accepted without question attitudes and treatments that today would lead to a lawsuit.

On the first day of our obstetrics rotation, the department chair began the introductory lecture thusly: "With apologies to the women attending this lecture in order to become physicians, the function of young women is to have babies." A conscientious student, I dutifully wrote down his words verbatim. It took 18 years for that remark to somehow resurface into my conscious thoughts and enrage me.

I remember the obstetrical call room for male students, a sizeable room with four beds, a desk, and a bathroom with shower, the last a necessity in those days because medical students were on call for one week at a time. Accommodations for women students? I was assigned a cot in a closet-sized room, airless except for one small window opening onto an airshaft. This same airshaft also ventilated the research animal quarters. Many nights I cursed the scientist who experimented with the roosters; no sooner had I fallen asleep after delivering a night's worth of babies than the roosters noticed the dawn.

Even worse than no sleep was the problem of keeping clean. Women students had to use the bathroom down the hall, which did not have a shower. Desperate conditions called for desperate measures, and midweek I found the chutzpah to shoo all of the men out of their call room and take over the shower.

Although I entered pediatrics, one of the traditional women's specialties, I continued to be a pioneer. I was the first woman at Detroit Receiving Hospital to head a department, the first woman to serve as an associate or vice dean at two medical schools, and on more than one occasion, the first woman to chair a committee of a national organization.

But my husband was the *real* pioneer in our family. When he married me, Donna Reed was the sitcom model of wife and mother. My husband not only allowed me to pursue my own goals but has been a source of unconditional encouragement and support, for which I gratefully thank him.

I also thank my children because my profession definitely set them apart from their peers. I was the only mother on the block who worked outside the home. A neighbor once asked me, "How can you bear to leave your adorable daughter at home all day with the colored help?" thereby crowding both racism and sexism into a 17-word question.

Somehow I managed to balance career and family responsibilities but have long thought about this double burden that professional women carry.

What is the double burden? Simply stated, it is career plus motherhood. Everybody knows that women bear the children. But where is it written that women must also bear the sole burden of raising the children?

The relatively recent evolution of Motherhood with a capital M has had a profound effect, not only on women but on all of society. Historians and sociologists know the story well. It began in the 17th century with the weakening of kinship ties and the first stirrings of the nuclear family.

It continued with an emerging focus on childhood, an interest in education, and the moralization of society. Along came industrialization, which geographically separated the workplace from the home. Fathers began to work away from home, entrusting the upbringing of children to their wives. Thus, women became the prime and usually sole rearers of children. The ideology of domesticity glorified this separation of home and public life, extolling the female qualities of nurturing, moral superiority, and maternity. The world of men became the "public sphere," while the world of women remained "private" (Morantz-Sanchez, 1987).

Paradoxically during the 20th century, the size of the female labor force increased first slowly, then exponentially. The largest increase has been in the number of mothers in the workforce; mothers who work full-time and year-round; mothers who juggle careers and children; mothers who are doctors and lawyers, scientists and entrepreneurs; mothers of achievement who have worked hard to get the degrees and experience they need to be leaders in their field. For all women of achievement, the crucial years of career development and mothering coincide.

Today's employed mother is the hardest working person in our society—maybe in history—because of her two jobs. One of these, motherhood, is 24-hours/day, seven days/week, 52 weeks/year with no paid vacation. Mothers of achievement are at the same time trying to get tenured, promoted, or elected. The message to young women who wish to have children and a career is simple: Be superwoman and you can have it all. This is unfair; men can be fathers without missing a beat of their career music.

Some enlightened thinkers have voiced objections to this inequity. Historian Carl Degler wrote, "If women are to have equal opportunities as men, they must not only have the option to have a job and a family— as every man—but they must not be expected to bear the burden of filling both roles simultaneously" (Degler, 1981). Carola Eisenberg (1989) wrote, "The playing field is hardly level if only superwomen, rather than most women, can satisfy the needs of their families and meet their professional goals."

Indifference to the plight of the employed mother permeates the entire institutional fabric of our society. The problem is simply that we hold two opposing ideologies. One says that women should remain at home with the children; children will suffer if women work outside of the home. The other holds that women should have the same opportunities as men; after all this is America, the land of opportunity.

There is no question that fathers must carry more of this double burden. Despite their own careers, working wives still shoulder a large burden of the household work—the so-called asymmetry of marriage (Eisenberg, 1983). Maybe things are getting better. To my amazement, I read a recent personal ad in *New York Magazine*: "Self-supporting househusband with PhD available for career woman wishing to start family."

The woman of achievement herself needs to modify her thinking. We women expect ourselves to be nurturers and caregivers. We're socialized for these roles; we know how self-sacrificing Jane Eyre and Marmee were; we see the way we're supposed to be on both the big and little screens. We nurture and we do it well, so well that we hardly notice our dances of compromise and accommodation.

I have a vision for the new century, a century in which women will continue to advance as the glass ceiling first cracks and then shatters. And there will be an abatement of the double burden carried by women who choose to have both children and a career, because we will stop pretending that all women are at home.

— *Marilyn Heins*
Columbia University, College of Physicians & Surgeons, 1955
Former Vice Dean and Professor of Pediatrics at the
University of Arizona College of Medicine
Author of ParenTips for Effective, Enjoyable Parenting *(1999)*

References

Eisenberg, C. (1983). Women as physicians. *Journal of Medical Education, 58,* 534-540.

Eisenberg, C. (1989). Medicine is no longer a man's profession: Or, when the men's club goes coed it's time to change the regs. *New England Journal of Medicine, 321*, 1542–1544.

Degler, D. (1981). Can we reconcile the demands of family and women's individuality? *National Forum, 61*(4), 22–23.

Johnson, D. G. (1983). *US Medical Students 1950–2000.* Washington, DC: Association of American Medical Colleges.

Morantz-Sanchez, R. (1987, November). *Not feminized but humanized: Reflections on the future of women in the profession.* Presented at the American Association of Medical Colleges' Women in Medicine Program, Washington, DC.

Medical Internship[25]

In 1988 a pediatric resident asked me to tell him something about what it was like to be a house officer at the University of Kansas Medical Center (KUMC) in the "early days." The early days? "Why, I did my internship only a few years ago," I told him. "The memories of that year are still clear in my mind." So much had happened since then, however, that I had to admit that it was clearly more than just a few years ago. Thirty-one to be exact.

There were two of us from Seattle from the graduating class of 1957 of the University of Washington School of Medicine. We came to KUMC for a rotating/mixed internship, my husband Fred and I.

I was determined that year to avoid the white uniformity of the housestaff uniforms. I added to that unimaginative wardrobe some colorful blouses and shirts to replace the white shirts that were issued to me. I received surprised, but approving glances and comments from hospital personnel. It was a small and timid gesture, but in 1957 it constituted a bit of pioneering on my part for women's independent thinking.

We did not have beepers so the housestaff were paged through the hospital public-address system. We had to listen carefully to lists of names being read. If one failed to respond, immediately, the operator sounded impatient on her second page, and finally sounded quite testy. On a few Sunday mornings when we were free to attend church or on occasional dinners out, invariably, Fred or I would suddenly jump to attention, thoroughly convinced that we had heard our page.

One evening a nice young student sought me out. He announced, "I am on call with you tonight in the emergency room and I have a big question. How do we share the interns' bedroom?" I said, "I plan to use it to catch a few winks if it is at all possible." He became flustered and explained, "I'm not sure what to do. I've packed my pajamas and toothbrush, but since you will be using the room, I don't think I'll get dressed in my pajamas."

Attempting to solve his problem, I said, "Why don't you get ready for the evening's work and just put on a scrub suit? Forget about the pajamas. If you are lucky to get some sleep, you can sleep in your scrub suit." But the poor boy was ever so worried. He was very serious and quite insistent, "Don't you think that Dr. Wescoe (the Dean) will be upset with the bedroom arrangement? It might even affect my graduation from medical school." By that time, a bit impatient with his naïveté, I said, "I really don't care what the Dean thinks. My husband trusts me both in and out of the ER. That will have to be good enough for both you and Dr. Wescoe!"

I could see this was not particularly reassuring to him, but the emergency cases took priority and soon kept him too busy to worry and also too busy to put on his pajamas. In fact, he was too busy even to brush his teeth before he stumbled to his ward assignment the next morning. As far as I know, he graduated.

Though times and personnel change, hospital facilities modernize, medical science, skills and therapies revolutionize, and health care organization becomes very complicated, patients don't really change nor does the physician-patient relationship. Caring about and for patients was impressed upon us at KUMC during our internship "in the early days." Even as we approach the twenty-first century, the same ingredients are basic to housestaff training at KUMC. Maybe that's why it seems such a short time ago.

— Grace Foege Holmes
University of Washington School of Medicine, 1957
Professor Emeritus, Pediatrics and Preventive Medicine, University of Kansas
Author of On Safari: A Collection of Stories *(1998)*

Notes

1. Spiro, H. (1979). Myths and mirths. *New England Journal of Medicine*, *292*(7), 354-356.

2. Excerpted from Hunt, H. (1856). *Glances and glimpses; or fifty years social, including twenty years professional life* (pp. 134-135). Boston: John P. Jewett.

3. Excerpted from Blackwell, E. (1895). *Pioneer work in opening the medical profession to women: Autobiographical sketches*. London: Longmans.

4. As quoted in Wilson, D. C. (1970) *Lone woman: The story of Elizabeth Blackwell, the first woman doctor*. Boston: Little, Brown.

5. Excerpted from Jacobi, M. P. (1882, January). Shall women practice medicine? *North American Review*.

6. Excerpted from Barringer, E. D. (1950). *Bowery to Bellevue* (p. 70). New York: Norton. From *BOWERY TO BELLEVUE* by Emily Dunning Barringer. Copyright 1950 by W. W. Norton & Co. Inc. Used by permission of W. W. Norton & Company, Inc.

7. Excerpted from Jacobi, M. P. (1891). Woman in medicine. In *Woman's Work in America* (p. 196). New York: Henry Holt.

8. From Elizabeth Garrett Anderson's speech to the Royal Free Hospital School of Medicine as quoted in Manton, J. (1965). *Elizabeth Garrett Anderson*. New York: E. P. Dutton.

9. From Owens-Adair, B. A. (ca.1906). *Dr. Owens-Adair: Some of her life experiences* (pp. 79-82). Portland, OR: Mann & Beach, Printers.

10. Excerpted from Ritter, M. B. (1933). *More than gold in California, 1849-1933* (p. 161). Berkeley, CA: Professional Press.

11. Excerpted from Withington, A. (1941). *Mine eyes have seen: A woman doctor's saga* (p. 17). New York: E. P. Dutton. Reprinted by permission of Penguin Putnam, Inc.

12. Excerpted from Van Hoosen, B. (1947). *Petticoat surgeon*. Chicago: People's Book Club.

13. Excerpted from Doyle, H. M. (1934). *A child went forth: The autobiography of Dr. Helen MacKnight Doyle with a foreword by Mary Austin* (pp. 247-249, 253). New York: Gotham House. (Republished as *Doctor Nellie: The Autobiography of Dr. Helen MacKnight Doyle*. Palo Alto, CA: Live Oak Press, 1983, 1999). Reprinted by permission.

14. Excerpted from Baker, S. J. (1980). *Fighting for life*. New York: Robert E. Krieger. (Original work published 1939)

15. Excerpted from Barringer, E. D. (1950). *Bowery to Bellevue* (pp. 115-118). New York: Norton. From *BOWERY TO BELLEVUE* by Emily Dunning Barringer. Copyright 1950 by W. W. Norton & Co. Inc. Reprinted by permission of W. W. Norton & Company, Inc.

16. Rowland, M. C. (1994, 1995). *As long as life: The memoirs of a frontier woman doctor* (F. A. Loomis, Ed.; pp. 199-201). New York: Fawcett Crest. Reprinted by permission of F. A. Loomis and Carolyn Madsen Williams.

17. DeBoer, S. (1967, January). Woman at the gate. *P&S Quarterly*, pp. 19-21.

18. Hilliard, M. (1956, 1957). *A woman doctor looks at love and life* (pp. 15–16). Garden City, NY: Doubleday. Used by permission of Doubleday, a division of Random House, Inc.

19. Sobel, G. R. (1994). Women in medicine: "A sound investment." *P&S Journal, 14*(1), 37. Reprinted, with permission from P&S Journal, *The Journal of the College of Physicians & Surgeons of Columbia University,* Winter 1994 (Vol. 14, No. 1).

20. Bennett, D. R. (1961). From *Harvard Medical Alumni Bulletin, 36*(2), 48–49. Reprinted with minor editorial changes by permission of the publisher.

21. Bennett, D. R. (1975). From *Harvard Medical Alumni Bulletin, 50*(1), 36. Reprinted by permission of the publisher.

22. Jefferson, M. (1955). *Harvard Medical Alumni Bulletin, 30*(1). Used by permission of the author.

23. Wolff, M. (1994). From chivalry and off-color jokes to acceptance and respect. *P&S Journal, 14,* 38. Reprinted with minor editorial changes with permission from P&S Journal, *The Journal of the College of Physicians & Surgeons of Columbia University,* Winter 1994 (Vol. 14, No. 1).

24. A version of this paper was originally presented on May 8, 1997, when Dr. Heins was awarded the Woman of Vision Award by the Arizona Region American Committee for the Weizmann Institute of Science.

25. Holmes, G. F. (1998). *On safari: A collection of stories* (pp. 41–48). Lima, OH: Fairway Press. Reprinted and abridged by permission of the author.

3

THE FORMATIVE YEARS

*Somewhere between the time we first put on our
lab coats for anatomy and the day we finished
our subinternships, something about us changed.
Nothing major, it's just that I think we see the world
a little differently now than when we first came here.
Our vision may not be sharper or more perceptive,
but somehow it is different, and I don't think
we can ever see things as we once did.*

— Joseph Rhatigan[1]

A Youthful Encounter

I don't remember the man's name—it was so long ago—but I do
remember that he was short, thick, and smelled of dirty sweat, with black
hair turning gray. His clothes were filthy, his hands oily black from heavy
factory work. On his right forearm was a large red swelling that made
him wince every time he touched it. I was nearly 15 that summer of
1955, working in my father's office while his regular assistant was away.
My father was a solo general practitioner, one of three in that small New
Jersey industrial town, and he handled the majority of the workmen's

comp cases in town, probably because he had gone to grade school with most of the factory managers.

We no longer lived above the office, having moved to a Tudor style home in a nearby "bedroom" community. My parents always joked that we moved to escape the patients who would wander up to our third-story bedrooms and wake my father on Sunday mornings with one complaint or another, but I think it was really because Dad was successful. Our new house was much nicer than this potbellied, 20-room, circa-1810 structure, where my brothers and I always had to use the side entrance to avoid stares or smiles from the patients in the waiting room. Also, we couldn't eat in the dining room during office hours because it was above the X-ray machine.

At 14, I considered myself to be pre-pre-med. My father was happy that summer to be showing me what it was really like to be a doctor. I learned how to examine throats and eardrums, and I met a lot of people he had known when he was a kid. Salk polio vaccine had just become available, and it felt important to give polio shots as one of my tasks. I also measured hemoglobins, performed urinalyses, developed X-rays in the little darkroom, and ran the big basal metabolism machine—everyone came out slightly hypothyroid. Another task was to weigh dieters every two weeks and give them refills of their "diet pills" (pink, white, and brown placebos).

I also sent out all the bills, kept the running ledger, and took the weekly cash receipts to the bank. The charge for an office visit was $3.00, and we saw 30 to 40 patients a day. We made melted-cheese sandwiches for lunch, with an apple and cookies for dessert.

My main job was to greet patients and prepare them for their visits with the doctor. I carefully recorded weights, blood pressures, and temperatures. I wore a white nylon nurse's uniform, quick drying and somewhat translucent, and a stethoscope. The uniform and my new hairdo made me look older than my age, probably by about two years.

Mr.—let's call him Mr. Short—was not only dirty, he was quite a rough character, literally a "dees, dem, and dose-er." I could tell he considered himself a lady-killer, smiling and winking as I went through the motions of checking his vital signs. "All I need is a penicillin shot, Sweety," he announced, as I indicated where he should sit. Instead of sitting, he suddenly pulled down his pants, bent forward 90 degrees and pointed to his right buttock. "Put it right there, baby," he said to me with a grin. I felt my face flush and the skin under my nylon uniform turn pink, but I did my best to remain professional. "The doctor will be in shortly," I said firmly and brightly as I made a quick exit.

I went back to filing papers while my father went in to see Mr. Short. A few minutes later, Dad came out of the room and said he had something very interesting to show me. I kept a straight face as he escorted me back into the room and proudly and quite formally introduced me as his daughter who was interested in studying medicine. Mr. Short nodded politely while I gave him what I thought was a daughterly smile. My father then proceeded to demonstrate the fluctuant mass on Mr. Short's arm and to perform an incision and drainage. I was amazed at the amount of dark green pus that came out. Mr. Short was very quiet, and we did not look at each other's faces. I was then excused while my father gave him a very big shot of penicillin.

My father was proud that I was interested in medicine, and he was a very good teacher. But when I was 14, and for many years after, he was ambivalent about my desire to become a doctor, worried about his delicate daughter having to work so hard and all that I might be exposed to. We were protective of each other: It was at least 40 years before I told him about my encounter with Mr. Short. Even though I have always considered it to be one of the funnier episodes of my adolescence, I never mentioned it until one afternoon of jolly reminiscence over several glasses of wine, shortly before my father died and I myself was close to retirement. That experience certainly did not dissuade me from going into medicine. After all, you never know who, or what, you might encounter behind those office doors.

— *Ann Klompus Lanzerotti*
Currently retired, occasional locum tenens
Internal medicine, Hematology-oncology

From *Kitchen Table Wisdom*[2]

The day it all began stands out in my memory: my father carrying my belongings to my room at the medical student residence, my mother unpacking my clothes and lining my drawers with special paper as always, working as partners until there was nothing left to do.
I remember the uneasy conversation and at last closing the door behind them. How much they had wanted to stay, to share in this last-night-before-the-first-day of medical school. But at twenty, I had wanted to face this momentous thing by myself.

I looked at the carefully folded clothes, the shelves empty of books, the hard and narrow bed, and the bare surface of the desk. The room felt impersonal, monastic even, very different from the feminine bedroom I had slept in the night before. It would be my home for four years. Tonight it felt cold and somehow unsafe.

I felt a familiar doubt, a fear that I was doing the wrong thing, that I was not cut out for this and would fail at it. As a philosophy major, I had barely been admitted to Cornell's school of medicine. The interviewer had looked at my honors degree in Wittgensteinian philosophy, commented that my major was "irrelevant," and entered into a brisk discussion of genetics, his own life work. I had held my own, but secretly I knew I was no scientist. Secretly, I found science colorless and cold. Full of hard edges. Like this room.

Hugging myself, I turned toward the only window. Earlier, I had glanced out and noticed that it looked onto the city street. I had a brief impression of unrelieved grayness. But it was night now, and there across the street was the main entrance of the hospital, one of the best-known in the world. It was blazing with light.

From where I stood I could see the main building and the two wings enclosing the great semicircular driveway. An endless flow of cars came and went, bringing sick people, people in trouble, and those to whom they mattered. I stepped to the window, deciding to watch for a while, just until the lights went out. A little before midnight a crowd of people, many wearing white, arrived, and a little after midnight a great many other white-clad people left and found their way to their cars in the parking lots. The shift had changed. I got the blanket from the bed, wrapped myself in it, and pulled up a chair. Cars, ambulances, taxis, and police cars continued to come and go. I nodded off several times, awakening each time to find nothing had changed. By four a.m. I realized that these lights never went out. People were there, always, for anyone in crisis, anyone in pain. The lights were being passed from hand to hand. And as of this morning, I was a part of this. I knew nothing yet, but I belonged.

In my grandfather's synagogue there was a light that never went out. All synagogues have such an eternal light. It signifies that the unseen presence of God is always in this place. Comforted, I got up and went to sleep. Over the next four years I can't remember ever having the time to look out that window again.

It is not possible to be in a twenty-four-hour-a-day intensive training program for many years and not be changed by it. We worked seven days a week, thirty-six straight hours on and twelve hours off, for most of it. When we were off, we slept. Denial of the body, its needs for sleep, comfort, and even food, was the very foundation of the schedule. No one complained. It was just the way that we all lived. Many of the rooms I worked and studied in had no windows. Often I did not know what day it was or even the time. I remember watching the nursing shift going past me, day after day. I would look up and see Miss Harrison and know it must be morning again. Often I had not slept since I had last seen her. Once during my internship, my mother, visiting me in the house staff residence, was horrified to open my closet and find that I did not have a winter coat. "Where is your coat?" she gasped. I had not known it was winter. I had not been outside the hospital and its underground tunnel systems in over a year.

On one very rare summer afternoon off, I remember traveling home to visit my parents on the subway, realizing only after a while that I had been unconsciously scanning the veins of the bare-armed people around me, wondering whether my skills with a needle were good enough to allow me to successfully draw blood from them. This sort of training changes the way you see things, the way you think. Gradually things that had been central in my previous life became vague and faded into

the background, and other things more heavily rewarded became
overdeveloped. After a time I just forgot many important things.

Thirty-five years ago, I was one of a few women in my training
program, and my male colleagues generally assumed that, as a woman,
I had a greater comfort and skill in meeting the emotional needs of
patients. Actually, at the time nothing could have been farther from the
truth. In many ways I was emotionally less well developed than some
of the men I worked with daily. Throughout four years of medical school
I had competed successfully with men and had fiercely and single-
mindedly cultivated the very qualities of decisiveness, objectivity,
competence, judgment, and analytical thinking that were most respected
in this culture. These qualities had become even more important to me
than to the men as I struggled to overcome what was widely perceived
by them to be a gender handicap.

Yet sometimes the same teammates who so painstakingly treated me
as if I were a man called on me in situations that made them
uncomfortable. When we were all working the clinic or the emergency
room, each seeing patients in our own examining rooms, there would be
a knock on my door. Opening it, I would find another doctor standing
there ill at ease, who would say something like, "My patient is crying . . .
can you come?" I was no more comfortable than he in such situations,
but I realized early that this was part of my ticket to acceptance, and so
I would go and listen while someone shared with me their concerns and
their experience of actually living with the disease we had diagnosed.

At first, I was surprised that people with the same disease had such
very different stories. Later I became deeply moved by these stories, by
the people and the meaning they found in their problems, by the
unsuspected strengths, the depths of love and devotion, the rich and
human tapestry initiated by the pathology I was studying and treating.
Eventually, these stories would become far more compelling to me than
the disease process. I would come to feel more personally enriched by

them than by making the correct diagnosis. They would make me proud to be a human being.

These stories engaged me at another, more hidden point. I too suffer from an illness, Crohn's disease, a chronic, progressive intestinal disease which I had developed at the age of fifteen. So for me, these conversations eased a certain loneliness. This was a different sort of connection than the easy banter and camaraderie I enjoyed with the other medical residents. This was the conversation of people in bomb shelters, people under siege, people in times of common crisis everywhere. I listened to human beings who were suffering and responding to their suffering in ways as unique as their fingerprints. Their stories were inspiring, moving, important. In time, the truth in them began to heal me.

— *Rachel Naomi Remen*
Clinical Professor, University of California San Francisco
Founding Director, Institute for the Study of Health and Illness
Author of Kitchen Table Wisdom *(1996),* My Grandfather's Blessings *(2000)*

Anatomy Lesson

Near the end of my first month of medical school, I sneaked my boyfriend into the anatomy lab. Our professor had specifically instructed us never to do this, never permit nonmedical students to gawk at our cadavers. Dissecting a human body was a privilege, not a curiosity, and the first rite of passage in becoming a doctor. While I agreed with this wholeheartedly, it was for precisely this same reason that I needed to have my boyfriend at my side—not to gawk but to share with him what was profoundly affecting me. My cadaver was almost symbolic, representing many of my conflicted feelings about what it takes to become a doctor. And Jean-Paul—well, I was considering marrying him; he was, after all, moving to New York for me. I found myself watching him closely in different situations to see how he reacted. And, of course, I was also allowing him to see me, allowing him a closer look at what moves me, letting him in—a bit. In any case, it all felt very important, worth borrowing a classmate's ID and strolling past the security guard, up to the 10th floor.

The lights were out in the lab. I felt the adrenaline surge through my body, the rush of doing something so deliberately against what I had been told. That, combined with going into a dark room filled with 40 partially dissected dead bodies made me jumpy. Table 15. There it was. I pulled back the yellow tarp, then the flannel cover. Usually, my lab mates did this unveiling part while I, always needing a minute of adjustment, watched on the sidelines. I had never noticed how soft the blanket was.

Jean-Paul stared down, still, unblinking, registering no expression of shock. He reached back for the metal lab stool behind him. As he pulled it under him, the legs screeched on the floor. I felt irritated, as if the noise betrayed the solemnity the moment required.

"So," I said.

"So," he echoed. He looked over at me and smiled.

"What do you think?" I asked expectantly, waiting,

"It doesn't really look very human, actually," he said, perfunctorily.

I stared at him for a moment, feeling the disappointment welling up in me. Doesn't he get it? Doesn't he see how important this is? Is he that shallow, to not feel the enormity of it all? I looked back down at the body, and suddenly, surprising myself, saw what he saw.

Her flesh seemed matted to her bones, unpliable. It had a yellowish, cheeselike color to it. She appeared to have no eyes under her stiff, frozen half-open lids—the sockets sunken and empty. Her rib cage was gone, sawed off in lab that afternoon. The smell of preserving chemicals was pervasive and impossible to ignore. That very first lab, the first time I had seen her (can I say met her?), it had all seemed so very different.

We had been sternly lectured that day on the history of anatomy, the oldest medical science, and about the responsibility and professional respect we must show to the people who had donated their bodies. Then all 156 students were led into the laboratory, to 40 shiny steel tables; each with a body on it draped in a yellow plastic sheet. There was no mistaking the fact that there were bodies under these sheets. You could tell they were lying on their backs, toes pointing up, you could even make out a rough profile and get a sense of how big each person was. Each student was showing or denying his or her uneasiness in 156 different ways. One of my four lab partners rubbed his hands together, clapped them once, and dramatically pulled back the yellow sheet.

I didn't even know her name, nor did I know how old she was. What I did know was that she died on July 13, 1992, from cardiopulmonary arrest and that she or her family agreed to donate her body for medical school training. It may have been entirely altruistic; it may have been because they couldn't afford to pay for burial or cremation services. In any case, there lay a person who had died over a year ago whose life I knew nothing about.

That first day, we were instructed to wrap her hands and feet in moist flannel and then plastic to prevent drying. I wrapped one of her hands; it was lying on her breast—large sagging breasts covered with age spots. The hands were perfectly manicured. Red polish to match her toenails. Her hair was dressed in tight, gray, freshly permed curls. The same lab partner who had done the unveiling was loudly chewing gum, popping and cracking it, and was being quite rough with the body. He would say, "OK, lets fit this little puppy into the baggy-o" as he shoved her foot into the plastic bag. Every time he touched the body he sang, "Doo-dee-doo."

Our first assignment was to remove her breasts. I was just as aggressive and forceful as the others. We all wanted to do the cutting, to be the one holding the scalpel, rather than the one passing it. Then the breast was removed, and I was holding it—this piece of flesh from a nameless woman who had died over a year ago and whose body had been preserved all this time for this very purpose. I kept having the urge to say thank you to her or to someone. Privately I vowed to honor this body, to learn all that there was to know and to be fascinated with her every vein and tendon and cell and follicle.

But now, here with Jean-Paul, I suddenly felt overwhelmed and defeated by it all. I started to cry. Jean-Paul had flown in from California that day. The last time he had seen me was three weeks earlier, when he had taken me to the airport the day I left for medical school. Since then, we had spoken every day on the phone, sometimes twice a day, and once, five times. Often, I had been emotional and tearful, yet unable to articulate why. He hadn't known this side of me before and wasn't sure what to make of it or what to say. Establishing a phone relationship had been difficult; we had both decided it was important for him to come out for a visit.

"Rebecca," he paused, "what is it? Did I say the wrong thing?"

"No, no," I smiled, "it's nothing."

He came around to my side of the lab table and, facing me, rested his arms on my shoulders. I didn't move, didn't speak. He pulled me into his chest. At first I didn't breathe, then my body began to shake and heave with enormous sobs. He said nothing. Later, when my crying slowed, he turned me around, and we looked out over the remarkable breathtaking view of New York City's night-lit skyline from the anatomy lab. We stayed like that for a very long time, looking out over the city where three months later we would start our life together.

Before we left, he helped me drape her in the flannel blanket and plastic sheet. I had shared my experience with Jean-Paul, and although his reaction did not mirror mine, it had somehow grounded me. I was on the journey of becoming a doctor, and I was very much alive.

— Rebecca Tennant
Stay-at-home mom and writer

Cold Hands

7/17/98

Dear Mr. Perez,

Two weeks ago I went to talk to you before they wheeled you in. You were full of lines and hot with a fever we couldn't make leave you. Your belly was swollen and blocked with tumor. I spoke to you for a minute.

Then I thought about my hands. My constantly cold hands that my husband pushes away. The hands that patients hate to have examine them. Hands I try to warm with water that just don't warm. And I thought about you and your burning skin. So I laid my cold hands flat against your chest. You moaned a sigh of relief, the only sign of comfort I had seen, and I felt good that these hands of mine had a purpose—a purpose of extreme importance.

They came and wheeled you away. Your wife called after you, "Love you babe." Thirty-four years old. I spoke to you in the operating room, but soon you were down. No more speaking.

From the minute I entered the OR, I was scared. From the CT, the tumor was everywhere. Even the doctors were scared. They wanted to get you unblocked so you could go home in peace. Your tumor burst forth the instant the knife touched your skin. A fountain came out of you. A crate full of tumor we put in a pan. Blood spilled.

Your tumor was too much for us—just as it was too much for you. It tied your intestines in knots. It stuck to everything. The surgeons snipped and tied, snipped and tied. I was amazed by their calm and persistence. I felt afraid. Still, we had to leave most of it behind.

They took you to the unit. Every morning, sometimes night, I saw you. We looked at your wound and all your numbers, charting them diligently. Everyone was trying, Mr. Perez. Teams of doctors were trying. We wanted you to wake up, to be able to talk. Once in a while, your eyes would open. Did you recognize me? I'm the one with the cold hands.

Today they said they were "withdrawing support." You may not make it to the morning. I went to you to say good-bye. I said I'm sorry. I hope you find peace and comfort from your pain. I put my hands on you for the last time. Did you feel them?

I left you with tears and saw your family in the waiting room. Your wife reached out to me. I embraced her and we cried. Your children are beautiful, Mr. Perez, I met them both tonight. Your little girl has quite a handshake. Warm.

Good-bye, Mr. Perez. I'm sorry.

— *Jennifer Hyde*
Pediatric resident, Boston Combined Residency Program

Here Is What I Learned

in medical school: that babies
are slippery as chance; no matter
how much coffee one drinks,
the body demands rest
after thirty hours. I fell
asleep standing in a hall
waiting for the elevator.
Elevators
always climb more slowly
when you're responding to a code.
If you take the stairs,
you arrive and can't speak
till you've spent three minutes
gasping and panting.
I learned
that I'm blessed to have small breasts.
No man, my friend told me,
had ever looked her in the eye.
That hospitals are places
where those who have been hurt
harm and heal each other.
I learned that knowledge and wisdom
are unrelated things.
That everyone is bleeding,
whether it shows or not.

— *Alison Moll*
Preceptor at York Hospital's Family Practice Residency Program
Author of Miracles Like Breathing *(1997)*

Jane

Fatigue from 36 hours on call makes the three-mile bike ride home
dangerous. In the dark I think I see moving shapes in my peripheral

vision. I get home too tired to eat, almost too tired to go to the bathroom. I say hi to my husband but am too tired to tell him about my day (and night and day).

I head to the bedroom and lay on top of the covers, still in my scrubs. Ahhh, it feels so good.

Rachel runs in the room and jumps on the bed. "Mommy!" she squeals. "We went on a walking trip to the store and . . . " She chatters on. I try so hard to listen. I sit up. Shake my head hard. I cuddle her on my lap. She smells so good, feels so alive and full of energy. It is such a stark contrast to the death and illness that seem to hang on my scrubs and sweaty body. I feel like I should wash before I hold her.

But I am too tired. I am just going to lay my head down for a minute. I'm not going to sleep yet. I'll just to listen to Rachel talk and rest my head.

An hour later, I wake up to find myself surrounded by stuffed animals. They are set up in a semicircle. There is a cup from a play tea set in my hand. Rachel is talking for me. She has been moving me around like one of her animals. Pretending she has a mommy who talks and plays and listens to her. Hot tears of shame come to my eyes. I feel like a complete failure.

In the hospital, someone else's daughter is dying. Jane is my age—24. She is a psychology Ph.D. student who probably ate the wrong thing at a restaurant and had a severe asthma attack on the subway. By the time the paramedics could get air into her lungs, her brain had turned into the salt and pepper we saw on the CT scan.

The ICU waiting room is next to my locker. Her family is from another city, across the country. They are camping in the waiting room. Her father talks to me when I go to my locker.

He is intelligent, a professor of English. He wants to learn what we are doing with his daughter. What do the lines on the EEG machine mean? What do they actually measure? How is her potassium? Her sodium? Is she overbreathing the ventilator? What level of intracranial pressure is dangerous? He follows me down to the candy machine. It is two in the morning, and I need a Snickers to keep me awake.

He asks me about medical school. What is it like? How long before I become a doctor? When did I last get to sleep? He acts concerned. Fatherly.

Every morning, I go to Jane's room and look at her body, which looks dead. The top of her head is shaved, and there is a "bolt" in place to monitor the pressure inside. Her face is pale and waxy. A tube in her mouth breathes for her. A tube in her nose sucks out her stomach contents. Her body is thin, covered with patches and catheters and wires. Her toenails are painted pink, grown out a bit. She needs a pedicure. Her mother has come in and washed her hair, braided it. Perhaps she will fix her toenails.

As a medical student, I hear both sides. The family accepts me among them and has discussions about what they think and feel and see. The medical team has discussions about what they think and feel and see. The two perspectives are so different that it seems unreal.

Her uncle asks us blunt questions. Is she going to be a vegetable? What are the chances she will wake up? Should we just stop all of this? The attending physician answers that there is a less than a 1% chance she will wake up, based on how she is doing now. But I have also read the paper from which he quotes, a paper written by authors who list less than 1% in the tables when, in fact, there was zero percentage.

We do everything. Monitor every function we can. We adjust her electrolytes, urine output, and intracranial pressure. She stabilizes. Her brainstem seems relatively intact. She will likely be able to breathe on her own soon. But still she does not wake up. No brainwave activity suggests that she is going to.

After several weeks, her father tells me in the hallway, "We don't have much hope, but if there is a one in one hundred chance she will wake up, we need to keep going. Besides, nothing we are doing hurts anything. We have everything to gain and nothing to lose." I usually just listen. But today I am tired and have been thinking too much. Feeling too much. Perhaps empathizing too much with Jane. I tell him what I see. What the physician team says among themselves but not to the family.

"Look," I say, "Jane is not likely to wake up. But in a week or so, if it is decided to stop the life support, she may live without it. She may live just as she is now but without the breathing machine or monitors. She may live like this for a long time. That is the risk of continuing." My heart pounds as I realize what I have said. I should have kept quiet. There must be a reason the team is not telling the family what we see.

"Nobody told me that," he says quietly. "I was just thinking that we could keep trying until there was no hope, and then she would die quietly, peacefully." This is the first time I have seen tears in his eyes. "I don't think she would want to live like this. I have to go speak to my family."

The next morning, Jane's uncle confronts the attending doctor about what I have said. He does not say where he got the information. The attending tells him it is probably true. Her uncle asks him what should be done. "That is up to you," the attending says. The attending seems angry and cuts the meeting off abruptly when his beeper goes off. The team rounds on Jane, but the family's questions are not discussed. I feel like everyone knows I was the one who told the family. I must have betrayed some sort of awful secret.

Two days later, that attending changes services, as scheduled. The new attending assigns me the job of talking to the family "because they know you better than they know me." No one comes with me. The intern says, "I don't do that family stuff."

Four days later, the family decides to withdraw life support.

I am so racked with guilt and uncertainty that I can barely stand to be myself. I have never felt so responsible, so full of power to do harm, so alone. I obsessively read books on death and dying. I need to know that what I said to Jane's father was the right thing. But I don't think that it was. I feel so ashamed that I cannot talk to anyone about it. And all along, I am taking call every third night, 36 hours with only occasional sleep, and becoming profoundly depressed and fatigued. I have insomnia even when I am allowed to sleep.

Jane's father has been talking to me about Jane. Who she is, what she has done, her likes and dislikes, what she was like as a little girl. He and his wife clear out her apartment, close her checking account, move her things back to their house. More family comes. They are waiting for a last family member, her grandfather, to come from India, and then they want to stop the breathing machine. I can feel their hope that she will wake up before the grandfather is able to travel.

Jane has begun to posture. She coughs when the tube is suctioned and draws her arms into her body in an unnatural way. The residents have been spending less and less time rounding on her. No one talks to the family but me.

It is the last day of my rotation and my last night on call. The grandfather arrives and seems to pull the family together. "It is time to let Jane die. She is ready," he tells me. I get the resident on call, who calls the attending. The attending isn't coming in. We are to have the respiratory therapist "pull the vent." But the family wants all the tubes removed and the bolt out of her head. The neurosurgery resident is busy and doesn't have time to come. He has patients to attend to who may live. We wait for hours until the nurses get angry and start paging him with trivial questions, over and over again. He finally removes the bolt at 11:00 p.m. The respiratory therapist then disconnects the ventilator.

Jane coughs and postures and makes terrible noises. It terrifies me, and I back into the corner. Her mother swoons. Jane's brother takes their mother from the room. The nurse gives morphine, and Jane quiets. I stand there for a long time. Finally, I ask Jane's father if he would like me to stay. He wants me to go. The family will notify a nurse if they need anything.

I get a Snickers and a Pepsi and sit at the nurses' station, watching the door. Two hours later (I must have dozed off), Jane's father comes out and tells me, "She died an hour ago, in case you need to know the time." He walks toward the waiting room with his family. The nurses start making calls. The resident comes and listens with a stethoscope in order to "pronounce death." I think, "You don't need to do that, her father already did." Absurdly, this strikes me as funny. I have to suppress a giggle. I feel I am losing my mind.

The body is cleaned; the last IV removed. I watch and realize that she did not look dead before. Now she looks dead. It is not as disturbing as the way she looked weeks ago. Now I feel that there is no one in that body. It is just an empty shell, a cadaver, like the ones I dissected in anatomy. Something I am comfortable with. I watch them put her into a bag. It is close to 3:00 a.m., and I have a final exam tomorrow. I need to sleep.

I walk past the waiting room, and Jane's uncle, the one who always asked the blunt questions, rushes out at me. "Now what do we do?" he asks. "Are there papers or something to sign? Where is the body? What will they do with her?" I answer his questions, but he keeps asking them over and over, seemingly not hearing the answers. I am beginning to feel frustrated. What does he want from me? I am tired. I just want to sleep. I have given all I have, yet he seems to want more of me.

Eventually, I realize he is asking a deeper question. One I have no way to answer. What do they do now that their young, bright, hopeful Jane is dead? What do they do now?

I don't know what they should do now. But I know I should sleep. I go to the call room and turn off my beeper. I am finished with this rotation, I decide. I am not going to answer any more pages.

I have terrible nightmares that I am dying. That they are pulling the tube from my throat. I am alive but cannot breathe. I am awake but cannot move. I can see everyone in the room. I feel myself dying, and somehow I know it is going to hurt terribly. I wake up sweating and shaking.

I bike to school early, and for the first time in my life, I flunk an exam.

— *Ambur L. Economou*
Family practice and obstetrics

Circumstance

Stepping through the door to the office
The patient seemed a normal size
Yet cowering on the cold metal stirrups
Her knees straining across the chasm of air,
She is swallowed by the snow white sheet.

Or maybe it is the swollen belly of the nurse who
Stands beside her that has reduced her
To a quaking child-size figure.
Two women, both would-be mothers, a bond
That might unite them in talk of
Strollers and baby bonnets and that first precious smile
Were it not for circumstance in this life.
Instead, a nurse clasps the hand of a patient
As her embryo is scraped out of her body
On a freeing gush of blood.

Did a current pass between them with that grasp?
Was it the dazzling radiance of those nine months
So close to her supine head that stung the patient's eyes
To tears? Perhaps it jolted the nurse back to
Other hands clasped, the marching feet in DC, the
Swaying crowds, the sunny days when her
Slender abdomen did not so trouble the women
She was trying to help.

And afterwards, the gynecologist shows me, her student,
The tiny fetal sac — the abortion a success —
Swirling in the sterile pan, my thoughts are themselves
Dragged into the eddy despite my best intentions.
The ad had read, "Wanted: pro-choice women in medicine."
But were your eyes acute enough to catch the
Fine, fine print: "Those wanting a family need not apply."

Yet each daughter today believes it will be different.
I stand at the precipice, peering at that line
Of expectant patients extending to the horizon,
Hoping that the weight of my stethoscope around
My neck will not render me too weary for the
Tug of my future toddler's small hand.
Hoping that I will never be the one to lie on that
Table, abandoning one dream for another.

— Renda Soylemez
Internal medicine resident
New York–Presbyterian Hospital (Columbia University)

From the Deccan Plateau

I place one hand on my patient's shoulder and the other on the bell of my stethoscope as I listen intently to distinguish pathological murmurs or a "whispered pectoriloquy" in his lungs. The story of his illness echoes in my head and I, a third-year medical student, glimpse the scars within when he exhales.

My path to neuropsychiatry is not the conventional one. I was born on the Deccan plateau of southern India, the second of twins. At age four, I wandered out of the chill New England winter and into my first classroom. I spoke no English but listened carefully to the words around me. There began my fascination with cultural difference and the unfamiliar, as I began a life utterly distinct from the one I would have lived in India. I returned often and then wrote stories for my classmates in America of the monsoons and the exhilaration with which we used to run into the rain, letting our feet sink into the wet red mud as the grasses whipped behind. I read with them, on the first page of my biology textbook, the words of Curtis and Barnes: "You and I are flesh and blood, but we are also stardust." I hoped to one day become a physician, one who might heal both mental and physical illness.

I matriculated at Brown University to study medicine but along the way pursued degrees in English and American literature. In retrospect,

I realize that my dialogue with literature gives definition to my own experience. I questioned in Descartes "l'ame raisonable," the flaw of asserting mind and body as separate entities. I found, in the existentialism of Sartre and the surrealism of Breton, an inspiration to transcend beyond scientific parameters to find my own truth. These philosophers became my companions in the study of medicine.

Virginia Woolf wrote in *A Room of One's Own* that, although "there is nothing to prevent a woman from being a doctor, a lawyer, a civil servant—there are many phantoms and obstacles, as I believe, looming in her way." Although I have been born into a century and existence eliminating a great many of the obstacles to which Woolf alludes, I have hoped to achieve what was not given to my mother, grandmother, and the women in my family before me, whose lives were ordained at birth, and who contended with phantoms of tradition condemning any aspiration beyond the domestic.

I am inclined to think that I inherited some of their unlived passions by the way in which I live my own life. Each opportunity is singularly valuable, for I am grateful that I can do what they could not. I examine the possibilities of my education and attempt to become a physician who can treat beyond the abstract definition of illness itself to the depth of the person who suffers behind it. Medical school has left me clutching at least a few more fragments of that stardust existence I am still trying to understand.

— *Teena Shetty*
Neurology resident, New York–Presbyterian Hospital (Cornell University)

Song of the Dying Ova[3]

It's the dilemma of all young, professional women, I suppose. How, where, *when* to fit the mystical process of reproduction into the unerringly practical cycle of our professional production. It's the call of success versus the bleatings of our unfertilized ova as they plummet to their doom. As a woman in her mid-twenties entering the good-old-boys profession of medicine, I've come to realize that the more entrenched I become in my training, the louder those bleatings get. In fact, much to my boyfriend's chagrin, the cries of my dying eggs had become almost deafening during the months I completed my rotation through the field of pediatrics.

Taking care of other people's children is actually a mixed blessing for a mamma-wanna-be like myself. Even though many of the mothers I meet are my age and younger, the fact that I have not had children makes giving parenting advice an awkward and often ridiculous undertaking. "You mean, you do all that with your kids?" asked one young mother incredulously after I barraged her with intricate, and perhaps impossible, parenting tips I had read about only moments before seeing her child. When I told her that, in fact, I did not have any children of my own, her face cleared. "No wonder," she blurted out with relief.

I had always thought I would have children by now. My own mother was 21 when she had me, and carted me around throughout her education, from undergraduate through Ph.D. She was lucky enough to have the flexibility to sit me next to her in classes or leave me to play in the graduate student offices with other doctoral candidates in search of distraction. As I grew older, we grew more like close friends, sisters, than mere mother and daughter. Our proximities in age and our inseparability forged a bond closer than nannies and baby-sitters could ever allow. It's a pattern that's not really replicable in the world of medicine. Getting beeped to have your baby-sitter tell you that your child spoke her first word is not really the same as being there. I remember a female pathology professor of mine grumbling about not being able to understand what her children were saying anymore. This wasn't, as I had first guessed, due to some generation gap, but because her children were more comfortable speaking Spanish, the mother tongue of their nanny, than speaking English with their own mother.

While my fascination with motherhood probably stems from the tick-tock of the same biologic clock that beats out a rhythm in most American professional women, it also originates from my heritage. As a daughter of Indian immigrants, I come from a culture that venerates motherhood above all else. Bengal, the region of India from which my parents originate, is actually one of the few places in the world where goddesses still reign supreme and mothers, earthly equivalents of the great goddesses, play a central cultural role. For example, when Indira Ghandi was prime minister, the most popular street graffiti in Calcutta portrayed "Mother Indira" as "Mother India"—dressed as the warrior goddess Durga, riding a fearsome lion, brandishing a sword against all demonic and parliamentarian foes. The image puts American icons of apple-pie-ness to shame.

So, while these primal forces of procreation are making images of babies dance in my head, ironic fate places me in a pediatric ward. It's the perfect torture for fertility-minded women: make them take care of children all day while constantly reminding them of how much more training they must endure before having any of their own. Indeed, during the mornings, after our predominantly female team of doctors had left their own sleeping children to make rounds through the ward, we would catch families at their most vulnerable. Mothers sleeping in the C-shaped posture of protectiveness while their tubed, monitored, and IV-ed children slumbered in the nest of their arms. When we drew blood from or placed IVs in our pediatric patients, it was often the mothers who cried out in empathetic pain as their children's skin was pierced. It's more than a symbiotic relationship, I realized. These were people who used to inhabit one body.

Medicine, like raising children, is hard work, demanding toil, frustration, and heart. As more women enter the field, it will not be acceptable anymore to penalize a pregnant resident who takes maternity leave, look down upon a physician who is late because her child is ill, or equate a good doctor with one who cares more about her patients than her personal life. Indeed, as more pregnant senior residents waddle around the hospital, making major medical decisions with extra large scrubs tied around their protuberant bellies, younger women like myself are gaining role models to look to and learn from.

There were no women with children in my medical school class. However, in the classes below me, there appear to be more and more women who are both mothers and future physicians. I recently saw a woman I know in the hospital, dressed in the requisite white coat, with a stethoscope around her neck, her pockets bulging with papers, tongue depressors, gauze, and the bevy of other medical goodies. There was one difference, however, because besides all of her medical equipment, she also had a baby strapped to her back. Although her husband was to shortly pick up the child, it was encouraging to see a medical student who was more than just a nervous trainee eager to please. Clearly, the times are changing.

While I look forward to the day I can combine motherhood and medicine, the song of the dying ova continues. It's actually got a pretty good beat. And the beat goes on.

— *Sayantani DasGupta*
Research Fellow, Columbia University Department of Pediatrics
Author of Her Own Medicine: A Woman's Journey from Student to Doctor *(1999)*

How I'll Become a Good Physician

We are wives, friends, sisters, daughters, moms, lovers, employees, and volunteers. We are medical students.

Our day-to-day lives seem caught up in memorizing minute details or striving for "honors" in every rotation. But what is our ultimate goal?

Mine is to become a good physician. One who is smart as well as compassionate. One who listens and cures.

In medical school, they'll teach us about science and how to pass the boards. But we must look outside for balance—and go outside, be outside. We must nurture relationships as diligently as we study our books. We must live, love, and learn with those around us.

My Aunt Mary is 42. She has a husband, a 10-year-old daughter, and metastatic breast cancer that now resides in her lungs and brain. She has fought valiantly, and her doctors have been technically wonderful. That she is alive 18 months past our most optimistic expectations is a miracle not because of medicine, but because her nine siblings, parents, in-laws, neighbors and friends have fought along with her. When she could no longer drive to the supermarket, her mom arranged for others to give her a ride. When Mary's legs lost the strength to stand at her daughter's softball games, the team bought her a padded lawn chair. When her health insurance was canceled, the church held a spaghetti dinner to raise money. When she forgot how to do simple chores such as laundry, her sisters helped her to remember. Now that she cannot bathe herself, her parents have sadly yet lovingly reclaimed that obligation. Mary's sisters fill in the words that she forgets while telling her infamous stories and write the notes that she dictates. Her friends listen to her tears but take her gambling when she is laughing. No one does *for* Mary. Despite the extra time and hassle, people do *with* Mary.

Not in my classes, in the library or in the lab will I learn about this love, this generosity of spirit. I cannot use my hard-earned knowledge to make Mary's last months bearable. But I can watch the experts—her family and friends—and learn from them.

And that is how I will become a good physician.

— *Amy L. Dryer*
Medical student, Columbia University, College of Physicians & Surgeons

A Gift

He must love you very much,
I think as I enter the OR
where a woman is being prepared
to receive a kidney from the man
already in surgery next door.

I feel like a Martian placed
carefully in a blue space suit,
breathing in the uncomfortably hot air
under my surgical mask.
The plastic eye shield steams up
and my nose runs.
I try to sniffle surreptitiously,
my hands obedient within the sterile field.

I am given your history—
58-year-old white female
Polycystic kidney disease
Hypertension
End stage renal failure
Dialysis since September
And the live-donor, your husband
a surgery date set
so you can both be home by Valentine's Day.

The surgical resident
who taught me how to scrub in,
and get all of my hair under the hat
comfortably,
makes an incision.
Red, yellow, pink—
Your belly is open.
The flesh retracted
and the contents of your right lower quadrant
are revealed.

Now I know why someone would give you an organ.
You are breathtaking.
The cadavers we studied
never looked like you.
I am overwhelmed
with the beauty and the pulse
of your external iliac artery
and almost miss
the surgeon's voice
begin a battery of anatomy questions.

— *Michelle Monje*
Medical student, Stanford University School of Medicine

Thirtysomething Meets ER[4]

Most medical students choose a medical school for its prestige or price tag. I chose one where I wouldn't be the only student born before 1970. Two years ago, at 32, I traded in my Hollywood executive's black blazer for the opportunity to wear a doctor's white coat. Thirty-two may seem young, but in the world of medical education, where training can last more than a decade, it's often considered over the hill.

That attitude is changing. In 2000, for the first time, U.S. med-school applicants ages 24 and older outnumbered those who applied at the traditional ages of 21 to 23. And admissions committees at some "nontraditional friendly" medical schools—Stanford, Northwestern, the University of California at San Francisco, and Yale, to name a few—are starting to believe that there's something to be said for doctors who enter the profession with real-world experience. I wasn't sure that my background of doing fancy lunches and schmoozing at star-studded movie premieres qualified as "real world," but because I'd be joining several other second-career students, I high-tailed up to Palo Alto.

Yet even at Stanford, a divide existed between Us—a tax policy adviser, Wall Street trader, film executive, lawyer, actress, ecologist, and single mom peppered among the student body like beneficiaries of some geezer affirmative-action program—and Them—22-year-old biochemistry majors who spent their undergraduate years holed up in research labs, fretting over exam scores, and pouring through the latest issue of *JAMA*. At orientation, a 21-year-old classmate, astounded that I was in my 30s, commented, "Wow, by the time you start practicing, you'll be almost menopausal!"

After that, I made an effort to assimilate. I felt like Cameron Crowe when he went back to high school in his 20s and tried to blend in with a bunch of teenagers. So what if my Big Sister, the sophomore mentor with whom each freshman is paired, was five years younger than I was? I joined in our prelecture ritual of singing "Happy Birthday" to our classmates (you could pick Us from the roster because we listed our birthdays minus the year). I traded dresses with a 23-year-old before the school's formal dance. I wrote our anatomy group's freshman skit. I kept

up with the who's-dating-whom gossip circulating near the lockers.
I even went to a few Saturday night keg parties. As far as They were
concerned, I'd become part of the gang.

In truth though, we "nontrads" didn't quite fit in. We weren't exactly
geezers, but we'd definitely outgrown our college-age antics. Instead of
joining our younger classmates for late-Thursday bar nights—a study
break for those who could effortlessly stay awake until 4:00 a.m.— we
opted for a sedate 10 o'clock viewing of *ER* before bed. We replaced their
mantra, "Highest score rocks," with one of our own: "Lowest pass wins."
We were the poster children for slackers in scrubs. One 34-year-old
friend, an ecologist, even stopped coming to our *ER* gatherings when his
wife complained that she wasn't seeing him enough. "If he stays home,
he traces the tendons in my arm as he's studying, and I'm just happy to
be touched," she explained. While our younger colleagues chain-smoked,
hypercaffeinated, and placed exercising, eating, and sleeping at the
bottom of their priority lists, we worked hard but opted for some balance
in our lives.

Great for Us, but what about our future patients?

As part of our first-quarter final exam in "Patient-Doctor," each
student was videotaped taking a medical history. In evaluating my exam,
my professor commented that I was the only student in her group who
bothered to introduce myself when I walked into the patient's room. I was
also, as it turns out, the only second-career student.

Coincidence? She didn't think so. One younger student, she said, had
dutifully memorized the list of 10 "nonverbal communication skills" from
our handout (vary your gaze, lean toward the patient, nod frequently, use
hand gestures) and performed them all in rote sequence, prompting her
concerned patient to ask, "Are *you* okay, honey?" Another younger
student, in a rush to get through the sexual history portion before his
exam time ran out, asked his patient bluntly, "Do you have sex with
men, women, or both?" This line may work at last call in a bar, but the
grandmother of three, recovering from a heart condition, simply stared
back dumbfounded.

Still, I wondered, what about the fact that this kid guessed the
diagnosis? Are the more open-minded programs making a mistake by

admitting those with nonscience backgrounds? "You haven't learned that pathology yet," my professor reassured me. "By the time you're a doctor, you'll know everything you need to take care of patients. Extra knowledge might make him a star at medical conferences, but it won't necessarily make him a better clinician." As I was walking out the door, she added, "It's much harder to teach social skills than science. Just ask yourself: Which doctor would *you* choose?"

After the exam, I went to the anatomy lab and ran into my ecologist friend. He was peering into a cadaver while a classmate who still used a fake ID tested him on various nerves and vessels. "And what's this?" the younger student asked. Each time, my friend shot back the correct answer. Then the grandstanding young science whiz pointed to something never covered in class and asked, "And this structure is beneath what?" Without missing a beat, the 34-year-old replied, "It's beneath . . . my level of interest." Hmm, I thought. Between those two, I'd pick the older guy, hands down. Maybe those admissions committees are on to something after all.

— Lori Gottlieb
Medical student, Stanford University School of Medicine
Author of Stick Figure: A Diary of My Former Self *(2000)*

Freckles[5]

I noticed the freckles on your shoulders this afternoon,
as a black plastic bag was pulled from your arm.
And I stood in awe of things bigger than myself as I gripped the table
for support,
occasionally remembering to breathe.

In anticipation of this day, we made some decisions.
You, to teach
and I, to be taught.
Here we are, together now, in a marriage of circumstance.
Your body the classroom.

I, your strange new pupil, fumbling with parts of you that few, if any,
of your closest friends ever saw.
Finally face to face,
what do you see when you look at me now?
Am I what you thought I'd be?
Eager? Anxious? Do I look as tired as I suddenly feel?
Can you see the lump that rises in my throat
as I struggle to fix my eyes anywhere but on your face
Where what you once were looms largest?
Can you see the tears that fill my eyes as I grieve the loss of someone
I've never met and
struggle for composure in a room full of people I hardly know?

You did not choose me,
yet you trusted me.
And I will never know you,
Although somewhere, a family mourns the passing of one they love.

I need time, that's all.
Time to think about what this means for both of us.
Brother,
Son,
Father,
Husband,
Neighbor,
Cadaver.

I noticed the freckles on your shoulders this afternoon.
Tonight I noticed the freckles on my own.
We're the same, you and I,
only you've been There,
and I haven't.

— *Jennifer Best*
Internal medicine resident, University of Washington

Summers With My Aunt

When I was growing up, I spent every summer on my aunt's farm in North Carolina. Those were lazy days—swimming in the muddy pond, playing *Life* with my brother in the musty cabin out back, chasing the litter of kittens that seemed to be around every year, finally falling asleep in front of Miss America pageants. Those were the years that witnessed the formation of the close relationship my aunt and I share. We passed the days making milkshakes and cinnamon toast, riding our bikes up the dirt road in search of wild blackberries, and shucking corn, feeding the husks to the cow I had named Sweetie Pie. We stayed up late at night talking over a background of falling rain and croaking frogs. My aunt loved to tell me stories of her life, her memories of being swept away by her first husband, a young soldier; of her more mature courtship with her second husband; and of her struggles as an English teacher to barely literate teenagers. She also loved to speculate whimsically on my future.

"Maybe you'll be a doctor one day," she would muse. "I'll come to you with my cane and my thick, thick glasses and I'll say, 'Doctor RD, I need some more pills. My back hurts, and I'm sure my arthritis is getting worse. Won't you take care of me?"

Only my laughter could drown out her quivering but insistent whine when she transformed herself into a contorted elderly patient. I could scarcely imagine my aunt as an old woman hunched over with osteoporosis, supporting herself with a cane and complaining to her doctor. Not my aunt, who had been so strong through the loss of her first husband in the Korean War, her teenage son to a drunk driver's recklessness, and her second husband to a fatal asthma attack miles away from a hospital. Surely my aunt would always be the one to care for me rather than the other way around. At any rate, I certainly felt her predictions of my becoming a doctor were ridiculous, because I intended to be a journalist.

One thing led to another, though, and at 25 I find myself one year short of achieving my MD. Meanwhile, my aunt remains as strong as ever in character, but, ironically, her body has begun to resemble that of the elderly woman she once caricatured. On my last visit, she proudly pointed out the framed image from her most recent cardiac catheterization adorning her kitchen wall, and I was concerned by the triple vessel disease before me. At breakfast, I noticed her pillbox overflowing with its array of antihypertensives, and for the first time, I realized the extent to which my invincible aunt relies on medications. It amazes and relieves me that medicine today is so advanced that, despite her significant heart disease, the only hindrance to my aunt's life is her morning pill regimen. She fills the rest of her day serving as a volunteer advocate for abused children and the president of her gardening society.

My aunt and I still have the long conversations I have always cherished, but now we have new ground to cover. She asks me about her medications, the symptoms she has had, the procedures her doctor recommends. She talks about her cardiologist, how she respects and trusts this man who has literally kept her heart beating. He has eased her panic over the procedures she has had, and he has become her friend as well as her physician. I would like to become that to my patients one day, and I like to think that, to some, I already have.

I still think back fondly to a patient I met during my internal medicine clerkship more than a year ago. From the moment I saw him, he was bound to survive in my memory, for his jaundice was far more striking than the mild yellow tinge I had remarked in other patients. Weakened by illness and fear, his voice was barely audible. Yet I found myself drawn into his tale, intrigued but concerned. He described desperate and incessant vomiting, with diarrhea until he was sure he was empty inside, fever and chills leaving him alternating between burning and clamoring for blankets, all the while coughing until his head throbbed. The man was terrified by his symptoms. A 30-year-old police officer, he had faced death at gunpoint but had never before been betrayed by his own body. Perhaps because he was so frightened, perhaps because he was trying so hard to smile bravely, perhaps because he really was quite ill, I tried to spend a little extra time with him each morning. Over the days that he was in-house, I heard about the charming town in Guyana where he was from and the home he hoped one day to build there, I heard one or two adventures from police life, and I came to know his dedicated mother and dark-eyed son. When the time came for his discharge, he shook my hand and said, "God bless you."

Medicine is a wonderful marriage of the personal connection and intellectual challenge that each unique patient offers. The opportunity to forge these bonds is the essence of why I wanted to become a doctor. What higher privilege than keeping a woman like my aunt alive or restoring that sick police officer to health and having the chance to get to know these remarkable people in the process.

— Renda Soylemez
Internal medicine resident,
New York–Presbyterian Hospital (Columbia University)

The Discovery Clinic[6]

I was only 16 at the time. A cheerleader and honor roll student who wanted to become a doctor. Then one day, everything changed.

I remember vividly that visit to the local health clinic, just down the street from my high school. The Discovery Clinic, it was called, a dull, brown structure that I passed nearly every day. But this time, I went alone, too scared to tell even my closest friends. *Only a pregnancy test,* I reassured myself, *nothing to worry about.*

The free clinic was stocked with only the bare essentials—a couple of examining rooms and a small laboratory. No carpet. The cream-colored walls were undecorated save for one black and white poster with a young woman and baby. The caption underneath read, "Having a baby is like being grounded for 18 years." I was trying not to look at it when the nurse called my name. I walked nervously to the back room. One glance at her concerned expression and my heart sank. Handing me a slip of paper, she reminded me gently, "Never, ever give up on your dreams."

I could barely contain the anxiety I felt growing in my stomach, rising into my chest, trying to come forth as a sound. How would I ever finish high school, much less go to medical school? What means had I to support a child? My boyfriend, not surprisingly, did not stay around. Five years older than I, he was unwilling to face the responsibility of becoming a father. The rush and excitement of his coming into my life seemed oddly dissonant with the way he faded out of my life.

Even my own mother turned away. A single mom herself, she knew only too well how difficult the road would be. She had "raised all the children she was going to raise" and had no intentions of raising any more. The sense of failure was overwhelming—from my family, friends, and teachers. But in time I was able to share the news with others (*had* to share—by six months, it was obvious). More people, including my mother, became supportive during the later months of my pregnancy.

I gave birth the night of my senior prom, just three weeks before my high school graduation. Another lonely, frightening experience. To the hospital staff I was just another minority teenage mom on Medicaid. The nurses chatted across my bed about the latest soap opera gossip, barely acknowledging my existence. I felt like screaming, but a sense of shame kept me silent. How I longed for some kind person just to hold my hand and comfort me. That feeling of isolation and abandonment became the drive to sustain my medical dream: I wanted to give other women the support I never received.

I am now a third-year medical student at Stanford University. My son Jonathan is six. It has been a long struggle, plagued with undercurrents of doubt and uncertainty. Keeping up with both my studies and my family seemed nearly impossible at times, not to mention the problem of never having enough money. I eventually applied for public assistance, and somehow through a combination of food stamps, welfare, Medicaid, public housing, and work-study, we made it. It was not an easy time, and more than once, I was tempted just to quit.

I found innovative ways to provide for my family. I pay for child care by offering free rent, instead of money. After posting an ad in the student union, I met and hired a wonderful man to care for Jonathan after school. Given the premium on housing in Palo Alto, we both benefit by this arrangement. Most important, he is a positive male role model and a good companion for my son.

Along the way, my life has been touched by the generosity of so many friends, colleagues, and mentors. Many have voluntarily baby-sat, giving me a chance to focus on my studies or take care of my own needs.

Several professors were so inspired by my story that they offered to help me pay for child care. One even took Jonathan to Disneyland with his own family. I also draw much support from my African American community and church. In turn, I try to help other young mothers by speaking at programs or counseling pregnant teens.

While not by choice, single parenting has been a gift to both myself and my son. Jonathan is surprisingly mature for his age, especially in his willingness to help and his understanding of my commitments. Furthermore, he has not grown up with rigid gender stereotypes. As for me, being a single mother has presented a unique set of challenges that will hopefully make me a more caring, competent physician.

I often think back to the nurse at the health clinic, wondering sometimes how different my life might have been had our paths not crossed that day. And I am reminded again of the powerful influence with which we as health care providers are entrusted. Our ability to change people's lives is a wondrous responsibility and gift in itself.

— *Melanie M. Watkins*
Medical student, Stanford University School of Medicine

Notes

1. Excerpted from Rhatigan, J. (1992). What matters most. *Harvard Medical Alumni Bulletin, 66*(3), 21–23. Reprinted by permission of the author.

2. Excerpted from Remen, R. N. (1996). *Kitchen table wisdom: Stories that heal* (pp. xxii–xxvii). New York: Riverhead. "Introduction" from *Kitchen Table Wisdom* by Rachel Naomi Remen, MD, copyright © 1996 by Rachel Naomi Remen, MD. Used by permission of Riverhead Books, a division of Penguin Putnam, Inc.

3. DasGupta, S. (1995, December). Song of the dying ova. *Contemporary Pediatrics* [Resident suppl.], pp. 10–11. Abridged and reprinted by permission of the Medical Economics Company.

4. A version of this piece appeared in *TIME* Magazine, April 9, 2001. Used by permission of the author.

5. Excerpted from Best, J. (1999). Freckles. *Annals of Internal Medicine, 130*(7), 612. Reprinted by permission of the American College of Physicians-American Society of Internal Medicine.

6. A version of this piece was published in *MomMD Newsletter*, Issue 9, December 2000 / January 2001 (www.mommd.com). Edited and reprinted with permission.

4

LIFE IN THE TRENCHES
Internship and Residency

*I packed my bags with my papers, my sutures,
my clogs and goggles. I closed the door that I had
opened I know not how often. I recognized its click
as the tumblers fell into place. My training was over.
My soul was conditioned. I turned and walked the
hallways I had walked so many times in the past and then,
suddenly, emerged in the sunlight never to return again.*
— *Crawford C. Campbell*[1]

Unknown Alpha

Gazing out of the tinted glass windows at the New Orleans skyline, I
could barely discern the outline of the Mississippi's banks in the distance.
The water looked angry and brown, and rain was beginning to pelt the
16th-floor call room windows. Beneath the glowering haze of clouds,
the city appeared innocent and small. Not even the distant lights of the
French Quarter could counteract the grayness enveloping the city. For
once, the thought of being confined to the hospital was more favorable
than the freedom to meander about the enchanting streets of the Quarter.

As I hurriedly finished the scut work left over from the long day on our neurosurgery service, I prayed for an easy, quiet night on call. Outside, the storming weather provided little solace. I had hoped for some midweek shut-eye, as I felt like I had not slept in days. Our inpatient service was full, clinics and operating rooms were overbooked, and as usual, we were short on residents. Each morning, I found myself groaning as I rolled out of bed. Like most junior neurosurgical residents at large, urban trauma centers, I was simply trying to take one day at a time. Already, I felt burned out and sometimes wondered how I ended up here, when all my friends had chosen careers more compatible with seeing the sun. I also worried about not learning enough, simply because our inpatients were too sick to be left alone. Some days, I felt like people expected me to be in at least two places at the same time. I was beginning to doubt my skills and stamina, wondering how I would ever make it through the next six years of training at the rate I was going.

With no emergency room calls by 7:00 p.m., I ambled down to the cafeteria with the medical student, anxious for a coveted chance to relax. Five minutes later, in mid-bite, we were called to the ER to see a young child who had fallen out of a second-story window. He had apparently reached over the sill to touch a butterfly, and although his father was watching him, his three-year-old movements were much too swift. His parents wasted no time in getting him to their local hospital, a small suburban facility without trauma services. After the initial evaluation, he was transferred immediately to our facility for further management.

When we entered the trauma bay, the first thing I saw was a fair-headed little boy laying quietly on a stretcher, his sobbing father embracing him. The ER buzzed like a madhouse around them, with loudspeaker announcements against the background drone of nurses, technicians, residents, medical students, and patients. Two gunshot wounds to the chest had arrived shortly after our patient, and most of those amassed in the small area were busy dealing with them. Unlike his father, Unknown Alpha (the name our patient was expeditiously assigned on arrival) appeared stable, with reactive pupils and appropriate crying upon palpation of his scalp hematoma. He had come with an outside CT, which was essentially negative for hemorrhage or fractures. His father, a well-dressed, middle-aged man, was berating himself for having let such a terrible thing happen. After explaining the CT findings to him and the likelihood that all would be OK with his son, he calmed down slightly. I, too, began to breathe easier and called for a pediatric observation bed in the step-down unit.

It was an ER nurse who first noticed the subtle change in Unknown Alpha's left pupil, from 4 mm to 5 mm in just a few minutes' time. I was on my way out of the ER when I heard the news. I ran back to the bedside and peered at the little boy. His eyes were doing something crazy, something I couldn't quite pinpoint—they appeared to be fluttering and roving from side to side, despite the fact that he was responding appropriately to our questions and crying from all of the excitement. The pupillary change was minute but present. With the initial CT negative, I had already mentally placed him in the category of "non-operative." Was he seizing? Was he just tired, with the events of the day catching up to him? I couldn't tell. Having no children of my own yet, their normal antics often perplexed me. Unsure of what else to do, I called CT and told them to make room for us, that we were on our way with a kid. People tend to be a tad quicker when it comes to having a child's well-being at stake, a secret I'd learned in my few but intensive years of training in an overcrowded facility.

We raced upstairs to the scanner, with little time to do much else than place oxygen on our patient. I sat behind the CT technician, literally breathing down her neck as we both watched sequential images flash onto the screen. It seemed to take forever. My heart skipped a beat when I saw the large semilunar hyperdensity, classic for epidural hematoma, blossom onto the screen. One thought stuck in my mind at that moment: *Waste no time.* I called my attending and chief, mincing no words.

The nurse and I raced to transfer Unknown Alpha onto the stretcher, but the stretcher was old and a wheel became stuck. Rather than lose precious time, we picked up Alpha and the oxygen tank ourselves and raced to the OR, his sobbing father running behind us, begging us to save his baby.

Once in the OR, it was hard not to notice the uniform concern that emanated from each person bustling about. For once, no one complained when I impatiently donned my own gown without waiting for the scrub tech. I called for a drill set. Anesthesia was still intubating Unknown Alpha when I began to scrub the left side of his head. I again called for a drill, which was nowhere to be found. Where was my chief? We couldn't wait much longer. Glancing out the window, I realized that the rain was still coming down hard. That meant the streets would be starting to flood and my back-up backup might be delayed.

I had never opened a craniotomy on my own, but we didn't have time to wait. Alpha's left pupil was fully dilated and nonreactive. I certainly did not want a child, or anyone for that matter, to die because I had not acted soon enough. I also did not want to do the wrong thing. With this in mind, and still no drill with which to get through the skull, I numbly cut a large curved flap over the left temporal region. After hemostasis was achieved, a splintered skull fracture stared back at me. I could see the enemy, a hint of dark red clot peeking out from between the two edges of splintered bone.

I asked again for someone to page my chief, wondering if anyone in the room could tell that I was not quite sure of what to do next. Apparently, the last clean drill was in another wing of the building. Examining the array of instruments from which to choose, I grabbed a medium-sized rongeur and began biting away at the bone edge. Momentarily, I was able to make enough of a raggedy hole to allow removal of the clot. There was more to it than I had thought as I pressed on delicate dura underneath, which was probably still actively bleeding. The important part was out, however, and impending herniation thwarted.

After what seemed like eternity but in reality was only minutes, both my chief and the drill materialized, followed by our attending. I breathed a sigh of relief, thankful that I had not caused harm to our patient, and watched as a quick craniotomy was completed and the oozing middle meningeal artery buzzed with the cautery. The anesthesia team joyfully announced that the left pupil was once again reactive, and everyone relaxed. Within an hour, we were wheeling our patient to recovery.

We had forgotten about our patient's parents waiting in the hallway. His tearful father embraced us both and, turning to his wife, pointed to

me and announced, "This lady saved Andrew's life—she is an angel."
Their profuse thanks allowed the pent-up emotions of the evening to hit
us full force, with even my usually stoic chief displaying tears on his
cheeks. Sometimes all it takes is a simple display of gratitude from a
patient or their family to make us realize the ultimate reason why we
choose to do what we do, day in and day out. That one sentence, uttered
by a thankful father, literally erased the mental fatigue that I had felt for
the past few months.

As the year progressed, I saw Andrew and his family several times in
our clinic. Their gratitude toward us never waned. Proudly pointing to his
healed, albeit slightly asymmetric, scar, they would identify me
unabashedly, much to my embarrassment, as the "angel."

— Lori E. Summers
Resident in neurological surgery at Tulane University

Birthday

It was one of my first months of medical internship. I was far from home,
my relationship was on the rocks, it was the day before my birthday, and
I was on call. That night, we were fortunate to have night float, which
meant that we'd get no overnight admissions and that I might leave at a
reasonable time the next day, Saturday, my 30th birthday. Thirty may
sound old for an intern, but I'd taken the longer route to medicine, by
way of a bachelor's degree in English literature, soul-searching
postgraduate courses, work, and after a special hospice experience, finally
a postbaccalaureate premedical program. The hospice program was what
had sold me on medicine. There I witnessed the depths of the physical
and emotional impact of disease. We approached patients and their
families on their own level, shared stories, held hands, and changed
dressings. Helping people live as they wished until the last moment made
us active participants in this deep human dialogue.

But I was not thinking about any of this when I got paged for my
first admission that day. I was thinking "not already and not in the ICU."
The patient was a young woman in her early 30s, married without

children. She had advanced cirrhosis and ascites and had come to the hospital earlier complaining of increasing abdominal pain. She had refused admission, leaving against medical advice. Hours later, she returned with still worsening pain. A paracentesis yielded bloody fluid. This time she agreed to stay.

I remained at her bedside for nearly 30 straight hours, leaving only to talk with her husband, grab a bite to eat, or use the bathroom. At midnight, after hours of struggling to stabilize her, liters of blood products, and two paracenteses, she became agitated and hypoxic. We knew we would lose her airway. We called anesthesia who intubated her as my team whispered happy birthday.

I left her side once more to speak with her husband, an ex-marine about my age. I told him that we had controlled her bleeding with medications, blood products, and arterial embolization but that the shock required intubation, and her condition remained critical. She was young, I said. That would help her. We would continue to do everything we could, and she might come through.

I sat in a chair a few feet from him. Years ago when I had had no medical responsibility for my patients, I'd found it easy to express emotion, to hold hands, to offer a hug of support. But he was young, and I felt the gap between us widen as I struggled to live up to a professional image. I wanted instinctively to reach out—to offer the physical contact that had been so helpful to my hospice patients and their families. Somehow I could not. Although older than many interns, I had always looked young, worn my long hair loose, and maintained an informal air. Having worked so hard to achieve my new role as physician, I didn't want to compromise his confidence in my professional skills by filling the traditional female role of nurturer.

Over the next few days, we watched helplessly as her condition worsened. I knew from the numbers that her chances of survival were minimal—with liver, lung, heart, and kidney failure, her mortality risk approached 100%. Her body became bloated and swollen, no longer resembling the woman I'd seen on admission. I met with her husband several times a day in the courtyard just outside the ICU. We talked openly about her condition, their marriage, and her wishes. Each time

I reached out to him in some way—a word of support, a hand on his shoulder. We cried together. I held his hand as we discussed withdrawing life support and guided him to his wife's bedside for the last time.

The day after she died, my team met him again in the hospital courtyard. He embraced us with tears, thanking each of us for the care we'd given both his wife and him.

This ex-marine gave me a birthday gift that I would never forget. He taught me an important tenet of doctoring—to trust my instincts. I realized that patients would come to respect me as their physician, despite my youth or gender. And in the end, I would serve them better by simply being myself. I learned that showing compassion would only augment, not undermine, my professional abilities—that by sharing their pain, I was helping them to accept, to grieve, and finally, to heal.

— Melissa Fischer
Ambulatory Care Fellow, Veterans Affairs Palo Alto, Stanford University

How I Survived Residency

In our daily work, we witness intimate stories of pain, courage, and physical malfunction. We're acquainted with miracles and tragedies on a regular basis. Our hands trace anatomical topography while our minds apply science. As doctors, we must be complex caretakers, tending to the body and spirit, even as the medical establishment often fosters disengagement with anything beyond the physical realm.

The senseless endurance test of residency, followed by increasing pressure to see more patients in less time, results in a system whereby it's easier to continue hierarchical, patriarchal doctor-patient relationships than to nurture the kind of healing that honors the unique needs and values of each patient. Through an unspoken code of expectations, we learn to hold back tears, be "strong," stay emotionally detached, and squelch what is often called the feminine sides of ourselves.

Writing fiction has been my tool for nurturing personal reflection, exploring profound experiences, and seeing beyond my own narrow perspective. It is my coping mechanism, my response to traditional models of medical education that frequently neglect the spiritual and emotional dimensions of doctoring. With fiction, I get under the skin and am able to understand processes at work in human life that can't be explained in a medical textbook or a 15-minute patient "encounter."

My preferred genre is the letter, and indeed, my first novel —*The Blood of Pomegranates*—is almost exclusively epistolary. As a child, these small packages of creative nonfiction were sent to friends, foreign pen pals, and when terribly lonely, even myself. Until entering medical school, I was able to be a religious correspondent. Now, I take great pleasure in enclosing the occasional handwritten note to my patients when sending them test results.

Recently, I've realized that I can't just produce my next piece of fiction the way I would order an electrocardiogram. It's been humbling to acknowledge that my writing can't be scheduled, that I don't always have control over what emerges on the computer screen from my fingertips. My best writing currently demands unhurried cycles of gestation and percolation. It requires that I overcome the emotional anesthesia of my recently completed residency and allow myself to fully experience the joy and pain of caring for people. Writing fiction has changed the way I practice medicine; it has freed me from mainstream medical culture and connected me to the woman and physician I want to be.

— *Nassim Assefi*
Acting Instructor of Medicine and OB/GYN,
University of Washington School of Medicine

Necessary Journeys[2]

The first adult decision I made was to get married at the age of twenty-four, after I finished medical school. It was also the first decision I had ever made without my father's approval and, at the time, I honestly believed that my choice marked a turning point in a newfound, more confident independence.

I married for love in more ways than one. I had known the man I married since kindergarten and had gone to grade school, junior high, and high school with him. Our parents had known each other for many years, and he'd grown up in a beautiful two-story brick house right near mine, across the street from the big fir tree. We each went off to different colleges, and then, the summer between our first and second years in graduate school (he was in law school while I was in medical school), we suddenly saw each other with new eyes. He was smart, well-read, and witty, and I loved the challenge of talking to him, being with him. He was sexy and ambitious and fun.

I don't think I spent a moment thinking about what marriage really meant. My parents' marriage was a happy one, and since I was still seeing them through a daughter's eyes, I didn't even begin to fathom what combination of love, patience, and sacrifice they'd managed to summon to make it work. I didn't know anyone who had been divorced, and it never occurred to me that the model of my parents' marriage, or any marriage, for that matter, in the small world we'd both grown up in—traditional marriages with a stay-at-home wife—would be no help to us, the young doctor and lawyer, as we tried to find our way.

The honeymoon over, we settled down to real life in Pittsburgh, on what would prove to be a collision course with one another. I had gotten married, but my real commitment was to medicine, one which intensified when, after two years, I switched my residency from pediatrics to, first, general surgery and then to ear, nose, and throat surgery, thereby lengthening my time of training. My husband spent more and more time alone as I spent more and more time at the hospital. I was on call three days a week, working and staying up twenty-four hours. Ambitious and excited by medicine, I honestly didn't see why I should go home for dinner if I could first assist on a surgery that started at eight p.m. Nothing in my husband's childhood had prepared him for living with a wife who wasn't on call for him.

I wrapped medicine around me like a warm, protective blanket. Working with patients opened up a new world where my common sense, my compassion, and my knowledge combined to really let me shine at something. Within the hospital walls where the sick needed help, I discovered my talents and a self-confidence that eluded me elsewhere. Inside the white coat, I was somebody: Dr. Nancy Snyderman. The white coat off, I was a self-conscious young woman who was failing at her marriage.

My husband felt increasingly left out (he was) and depressed. He wanted more of a wife, not to mention more of a life. Neither of us was capable of giving an inch, and the ways in which we connected to each other became darker, full of shadows. Unable to budge me, he began to badger me in self-defense. And the more frustrated he became, the more I withdrew into my ambition and my work, my attention focused on the one place in my life where I actually felt good, even terrific, about myself. He was angry at what he perceived as my betrayal and, in the end, became accusatory. It was a dark time.

And so, disappointed and hurt, I ended it. It seemed simple on the surface: We separated almost immediately after five years of marriage and divorced, leaving with the belongings we brought into the union. I returned the engagement ring, which had belonged to his grandmother, but kept the beautiful piece of French luggage my parents had given us as a wedding gift. It was civilized, as these things go, but hugely painful.

My sense of personal failure was enormous and a source of great embarrassment: I'd gotten an F in the first truly adult thing I'd tried and everyone—family, friends, even casual acquaintances—knew it. And after I moved from Pittsburgh, I just casually edited it out of my personal history, a five-year stretch no one needed to know about. Once again, I turned away from what I needed to look at—that inner self, eager for validation and hungry for love—which was so markedly different from the exterior I allowed the world to see, the ambitious and successful young doctor.

All that meant was that I didn't learn what I needed to be able to choose a different path the next time. Looking away pretty much ensured that I would end up making another bad choice.

I did. But the next time, I would take a much harder fall.

— *Nancy L. Snyderman*

Associate Clinical Professor, Department of Otolaryngology,
University of California San Francisco
Medical correspondent for ABC News
Author of Necessary Journeys: Letting Ourselves Learn From Life *(2000)*

Post-Call[3]

Night,
I stumble in the house
And lock the door.
My tired scrubs
Cry themselves
Into a puddle on the floor.
My thoughts
Falling soft as silence
Down the deep curve of the night.
Sleep
Won't come,
I lay and wonder,
In progress notes
And ER green.
Then dreaming,
I must be dreaming.
In a spinning well of sleep
These children's shadows
Wash away.
Then dreaming,
I must be dreaming.
Sleep
Has come,
I dream and wonder.
These children's shadows
Fall away
Like rings of spinning water
Falling softly down
The deep curve of the night,
The deep curve of the well.

— *Sheri Ann Hunt*
Psychiatry private practice
Candidate, The Seattle Psychoanalytic Society

We're Not in Kansas Anymore:
Men as Medical Mentors

A young woman travels down a mysterious, winding, obstacle-ridden road toward a longed-for goal. Let's say that goal is medicine, and the path, yellow-bricked or otherwise, winds through the obstacles of pre-med, medical school, and postgraduate training. She has left behind family, friends, and perhaps a blossoming singing career, to learn the mysteries of the human body, mind, and soul. For her gender, she's a pathbreaker. Her motley crew of companions are all male. The "Oz" toward which she heads, physicianhood in all its glory, is a construct created and controlled by the wizard of patriarchy. It's an all-male game that Dr. Dorothy has entered, and what she really needs is a mentor—one more practical than a chick in a pink frock accompanied by a village of munchkins.

Perhaps the metaphor is a bit of a stretch. But if Dorothy's Auntie Em had, in fact, been Emma Goldman—the 19th-century anarchist who is the author of my favorite saying, "If I can't dance, I don't want to be a part of your revolution"—then perhaps Dorothy wouldn't have been so content to ease on down the road. She would have demanded female representation. She would probably have begun her journey toward Oz to further the cause of Kansas women.

As the daughter of a feminist activist, some of my earliest memories are of "Take Back the Night" marches, sitting in on my mother's consciousness-raising groups, and participating as a pint-size member of various pro-women's rallies. I was surrounded by images of women's strength: My bedroom walls were decorated with posters from Elizabeth Cady Stanton to Sojourner Truth; my mother's women's group colleagues became my baby-sitters; and even silken saris couldn't hide the steely backbones of my Indian aunties. A liberal New England education only served to further these progressive ideas. I actually came to medicine out of this political understanding. In my naïveté, I saw medicine as a concrete tool for social change and followed my rainbow to medical school. There, my ideals fell flat.

I often compare medicine to militarism and medical school to boot camp. There is a combative language to medicine: where antibiotics "bomb" infections, where doctors work "on the front lines" and "in the trenches," where "incoming" patients are "hits" to be avoided. Like boot camp, medical school strips away individual identities; herds students from class to class, rotation to rotation; dresses us in the uniform of our white coats; teaches us a new vocabulary and even a new way of approaching the world. Taking too much time with a patient, becoming emotionally involved, or recognizing one's personal needs is "weak" (i.e., feminine?). Being "strong," on the other hand, involves sacrificing family for patient responsibility, not questioning hierarchy, and buying into macho rituals such as "pimping"—that is, the ritual humiliation of students and residents with rapid-fire unanswerable questions from supervisory doctors.

As a medical student, I grew to loath medicine. I saw it corroding not only my energy and interest for other subjects (music, theater, literature, travel) but also my relationships with friends and family. (As my husband is fond of saying, "Medicine makes a jealous mistress.") I grew to believe that the root of my problems was the lack of female mentorship. If only I had an older woman physician I could look up to, I thought, I would be happy in my white coat.

While historically, on the yellow brick road of medical training, we women have had few footsteps to follow, these days, the problem is not merely one of numbers. My 1998 graduating medical school class was almost 50% women, and there were many female physician-teachers around—yet not one single female mentor could I call my own. Indeed, the female physicians I met during medical school seemed to embody the same patriarchal ideals of physicanhood as their male colleagues. Perhaps by necessity, they had molded themselves to the image upheld by mainstream medicine.

In my search for this elusive goal of female mentorship, my own personal Oz, I came to the Residency Program in Social Pediatrics at Montefiore Hospital, a unique program in which cultural competency, community-based care, and progressive politics are treated as rigorous and necessary adjuncts to medical learning. It's not surprising, therefore, that after the desert that was medical school, I have found a few mentors in residency. What is surprising, however, is that among the three mentors that I can call my own, only one is a woman. I have discovered that if the culture of mentoring is a feminist one—valuing humanity, interpersonal relationships, and a conscious analysis of power and culture—then the particular sex of the mentor becomes less relevant. To explain, I'll take the Dorothean metaphor one step further.

My first mentor, let's call her "Dr. Tin," is a female physician with no presumptions at adhering to some patriarchal norm. This middle-aged, gentle-voiced woman makes her politics very clear, yet mentors with a motherly touch. The month she was my floor attending, she brought treats for us—cakes, brownies, cookies, fruit—each and every morning for attending rounds. "It's important to let residents know that you care about them as whole people, not just as workers," she would say. By recognizing our humanity, our need to eat, sleep, and bathe, Dr. Tin was enabling us, in turn, to be more humane practitioners.

If I found the heart of mentorship through Dr. Tin, it's "Dr. Lion" who has taught me about courage. Like many medical institutions, Montefiore cares for an urban, impoverished inner-city population. Issues such as gang and family violence, substance use, sex work, and other risk-taking behaviors pepper day-to-day pediatric practice even in the strictly inpatient setting. Yet, Dr. Lion, a soft-spoken white man, steps beyond the boundary of hospital or clinic to make home visits to patients throughout the Bronx and takes residents along with him. And so, in run-down neighborhoods, through graffiti-darkened hallways, into cramped, chaotic, and overpopulated apartments, I have visited patients. I have witnessed the enormous respect with which this physician mentor treats the primarily African American mothers and children we visit; his ease of manner, his clear-eyed lack of censure, his firm but never condescending advice, and most important, his sharp, yet critical eye for detail. Through example, Dr. Lion has taught me the courage to both care and critique.

Ultimately, at the root of this metaphor is my primary mentor, a man I'll call "Dr. Oz." An extremely intellectual sort (in fact, he's the kind of statistics-quoting, latest-study-knowing, pressed-white-coat-wearing doc I would have found intimidating in medical school), this is no man of straw. My gentle-smiled mentor can actually be quite ferocious when he feels an injustice is being done to one of his residents or patients. As a teacher, he is a wealth of information. As a mentor, he mothers with the best of them, even checking up on me when I'm sick. Most important, Dr. Oz has allowed the tables of hierarchy to be turned upside down. That is, he allows me, in my own way, to mentor him, sharing with him ideas about our program's policies and their political implications, about any gendered overtones, about the feelings of the housestaff toward the faculty. He has created an atmosphere of mentorship that allows me to do something I never could in medical school: argue, disagree, and, in turn, readily accept critique of my actions. The most important thing that Dr. Oz has done for me as a mentor is to treat me as though I'm a colleague.

At the end of her journey, when Dorothy gets to Oz, she learns a valuable lesson: not to trust things at face value. As the frightening wizard turns out to be a little man behind a great mask, so, too, might women medical trainees' quest for female mentorship be a search for an elusive goal. We should be cautious not to essentialize gender—that is, to say that a female physician is the best mentor for a younger woman by mere virtue of her biology. In many situations, the best female mentor may be, as in my case, the male one. Ideally, both men and women should work together to create a new, nontraditional culture of mentorship and subsequently of medicine that nurtures rather than punishes, respects rather than ridicules, learns from trainees rather than merely lecturing to them. It's an idea that brings all of us Dr. Dorothies back from over the rainbow, and much, much closer to home.

— *Sayantani DasGupta*
Research Fellow, Columbia University Department of Pediatrics
Author of Her Own Medicine: A Woman's Journey from Student to Doctor *(1999)*

Whine List[4]

I'm not much fun to have around the house this year. No intern is much fun, male or female. I'm gone for long periods of time, and then I reappear and I fall asleep on the couch while my son builds Lego towers on my back. I'm totally unreliable, always arriving after the dinner guests are already there or without the milk I promised to pick up. The smallest request—could you please pick Benjamin up at day care today?—is a major big deal. The night I promised to pick him up, I was all done and signed out of the hospital in good time, but then, sure enough, as I was going down the hall I ran into a group of doctors who wanted to talk about one of my patients (it was only 5 p.m. on a Friday, the perfect time for a long conference), and then when I got away from them, I ran into the mother of one of my other patients who had a few questions she'd forgotten to ask me earlier in the day.

I was polite and friendly to all these people, despite the furious impassioned speech boiling up within me about how I had been in the hospital for thirty-five hours straight, and for just once this year I wanted to pick up my kid and pick him up on time and he was waiting for me and he was only three and he wouldn't know what it meant if I didn't show up.

I know what I sound like, and I know it isn't pretty. Still, I can't get away from the feeling that I am feeling sorry for everyone else in the world, and no one is feeling sorry for me—so I have to do that too. I worry for my patients, I worry for my own kid, and I feel sad when things go wrong for anyone else—and so I manage to feel permanently mournful. That is what sleep deprivation does, too; it makes you into a not particularly appetizing person. I run around with a perpetual refrain of my own grievances pounding in my brain, and I think one reason for that is the pervasive sense in my life that I am meeting other people's needs, all the time, day and night, without relief, and it's just too much. I get a sense sometimes of being nibbled at from all directions.

On the other hand, I'm doing exactly what I wanted to do. Mine is the whine of ambition fulfilled, of privilege and choice. There are certainly things wrong with the way young doctors are trained, with the demands and the schedules we have to put up with. Still, I wanted to do this. And I wanted to have a child. I want more children, and I want to be a pediatrician.

That means, among other things, that I am going to do a lot of nurturing. There will always be parents depending on me, and there will be children to whom I am professionally tied, and there will also be my own children. So the different kinds of succor I provide will mirror each other in interesting ways, as I try to offer help to parents and also to function as a parent myself, as I reassure other people about their children and worry about my own. This seems like a worthwhile kind of life; it is certainly not grounds for self-pity, and I have to recognize most of my current grousing as born of the stress of the moment, the sense that I do not have quite enough time or quite enough vigor to do the things I have to do and do them properly. That doesn't mean they're the wrong things to be doing.

My son asks me what I do at the hospital. I tell him that I take care of children. He asks, working it out in his head according to three-year-old rules, "Do you put Band-Aids on them?" Yes, I tell him. "And does it make them all better?" Well, sometimes, I tell him. When I come home from the hospital, I tell my son, "I missed you." "I missed you too," he assures me, though his tone is the kindly tone of a child obediently parroting into the phone, "I love you, Grandma." "Do you know what I said to everyone all day at the hospital?" I ask him. With enthusiasm, he answers, "You said, 'I miss my little boy, Benjamin.'" "Right," I tell him.

So this is one of the lessons I am choosing to teach my son, by choosing the kind of life we are leading. I would like him to learn that you can do an important job, a job in which you help people in need. And I would like him to learn that just because you are helping people who need you, you don't stop missing the people you love best of all, and you don't have to be ashamed to admit it, either. And best of all I would like him to learn how to do all this without a lot of whining, how to carry it off with style, but he will have to learn that on his own. I only hope that while he is studying wit, grace, and style, no one will wake me up; I'll be the one asleep on the couch with the Lego brick tower on her back.

— *Perri Klass*
Assistant Professor of Pediatrics, Boston University School of Medicine
Medical Director, Reach Out and Read National Center
Author of Love and Modern Medicine *(2001)*

The Only Night I Cried

It was my second month of internship. A dramatic change from the bustling service of chest pain and transplants found me on the service of chemotherapy protocols and antiemetics. As it was, I hated cancer—what seemed at times a slow, insidious decline punctuated occasionally by palliative measures that seemed to do more harm than good. I was often the first to tell patients that their lung, pancreatic, or colon cancer was now metastatic. Sometimes I was not the first, but denial and hope can cause selective deafness.

I recall vividly the young woman with pancreatic cancer—we had no biopsy tissue, but the CT scans and her clinical picture made us certain. I, being so bad with names, cannot recall hers. But I do remember her husband and her three beautiful daughters, each with curly blonde hair. And I remember how her church group visited daily, filling her final days with prayers and song.

As an intern, I had little time to spend with the families. The routine tasks of checking labs, ordering transfusions, tracking down CT scans, and writing endless progress notes more than filled my 14-hour days. Secretly, I was thankful for the distance—it shielded me from the heavy emotional burden that I witnessed on a daily basis.

But this family had engaged me, and it was impossible not to become involved, not to become a little vulnerable. So through casual snippets of conversation with her daughters, I began to know the woman who once was—her likes, her dislikes, her way of living life.

Over the weeks that followed, she slipped into unconsciousness. The decline was rapid, almost relentless. As fate would have it, I was on call for the dreaded 3 a.m. page.

I had faced death before but never in a patient with whom I had been close. *Why me, and why tonight?* Only five weeks ago, this patient had been singing in her church choir. I was overwhelmed by the unfairness of it all.

The room was filled with family members and close friends, an unusual gathering for that early hour. The flickering of three solitary candles offered warmth and tranquility in spite of the cold, dark air. I walked slowly toward the bed. Fumbling for my stethoscope and pen light, I began the exam. Her pupils were fixed; her heart and lung sounds absent.

"I'm . . . so sorry," I faltered, my eyes barely able to make contact.

Her husband was the first to speak. "Thank you for being here. We feel as if you are a member of our family."

Tears streamed down my face. In the background, I could hear them whisper, "She's a good doctor. She really cares." Words that only added to my feelings of futility for what I couldn't change.

My call schedule did not permit me to attend the funeral. Yet in some way, I was relieved. At that stage in my career I could not handle the emotions surrounding this event—my own sense of helplessness and one family's generosity during a time of great sorrow. And how, in the hands of healing, death can still prevail.

— *Sondra Vazirani*
Assistant Clinical Professor of Medicine
University of California, Los Angeles

A Long Road

I graduated from Geneva Medical School in Switzerland, and before starting residency, I took some electives in the United States to broaden my clinical experience and improve my English. During a hand surgery conference in New York, shortly before I was to return to Switzerland, a very attractive fellow approached me and asked me out on a date. Initially I declined, but he persisted until I finally agreed to venture out with him. We immediately fell in love. At the time, he was finishing his orthopedic training at New York University (NYU). Although I had strong feelings for him, I was eager to return home to familiar surroundings and my prearranged residency in plastic surgery.

Through countless letters and phone calls, our overseas love only grew stronger. Months later, he arranged to attend an orthopedic course in Davos, Switzerland, and during the same trip, met my family in Geneva. We traveled to Paris together, where we decided to get married. Because his transfer to Switzerland would have been impossible for administrative reasons, I had to be the one to move. As soon as I completed my general surgery internship in Switzerland, I packed up and moved over.

I enrolled in the general surgery program at NYU. The majority of our rotations were at Bellevue, the largest and busiest city hospital in New York City. Most rotations entailed being on call every other night, although, on some services, I worked until midnight on my "off" nights as well. Realizing that I could not maintain this pace for another five years, I began considering other options. Ophthalmology and oculoplastic surgery were appealing fields, but quite honestly, after six months at Bellevue, anything else seemed attractive. We were also thinking of starting a family in the near future, and a more achievable career goal for me seemed like a good idea at the time.

After obtaining a research grant in ophthalmology, I completed a residency at New York Eye and Ear and enthusiastically embarked on an oculoplastic fellowship at Children's Hospital in Pennsylvania. During the fellowship, however, I realized the shortcomings of the field: I could offer my patients only limited surgical options or refer them out. I sadly remembered my original career goal and became angry with myself for having surrendered my dream so easily. Amid all the changes in my life—moving to a new country, getting married, trying to navigate a foreign medical system, I had somehow lost myself, lost a little of the momentum. So many of my women doctor friends described similar experiences. When they married and moved to other countries, most ended up becoming housewives. I just couldn't let the same thing happen to me.

Eventually, through several contacts, I obtained a position with the Pittsburgh plastic surgery department. Simply needing to take a chance,

I left Philadelphia in the middle of my oculoplastic fellowship. My husband was extremely understanding, having seen me desperately trying to find my way.

The Pittsburgh plastic surgery program offered a wide variety of surgical cases, and I found myself learning quickly while taking on major reconstructive procedures. Although this was a time of professional fulfillment, I was lonely living in a strange city without my husband. An unexpected pregnancy came along to complicate matters. I now had to face both a grueling schedule and morning sickness alone. I also realized that, according to the requirements of the American Board of Plastic Surgery, I still needed to complete the three years of general surgery at NYU as originally planned. When I called NYU, the residency program director tried to dissuade me saying, "You know things haven't changed much around here." After repeated assurances that I would not leave prematurely this time, we signed a mutual contract for two years.

I returned to New York for the birth of our child, leaving Pittsburgh just two weeks before the due date. Our first daughter brought us enormous joy, but my maternity leave soon came to an end, and I was back at Bellevue, essentially taking call as a surgical intern. Those first three months were extremely trying, with a newborn at home and a physically demanding job, in addition to the psychological stress of being ordered around by younger residents. But I never had any second thoughts and continued to pursue my goal. After all, the mountain climber achieves the summit only after risking his life many times during the ascent. Furthermore, my young daughter's smiles and loving eyes put it all in perspective.

Three months after our first daughter's birth, I found myself pregnant again despite planned parenthood. This time I was a bit frightened—as if the challenge of having a newborn at home wasn't enough, I would now have to endure general surgery at NYU while pregnant. Fortunately, this second pregnancy was much easier. I even completed a rotation in cardiac surgery while six months pregnant. During the last trimester, however, I developed signs of oligohydramnios, and my obstetrician advised that I stay off my feet as much as possible. Unfortunately, everyone within the surgery department was already overworked and stretched to the limit, so there was little support. For the remainder of my pregnancy, I trudged through the hospital with pitting edema in both legs despite compressive stockings.

Finally, our second daughter was born, and to our relief, she was perfectly healthy. With two babies at home, this maternity leave was much busier. I could never have managed without a great support team: my husband, who would immediately assume parental responsibilities even after a full day in the operating room; my wonderful, indispensable nanny; and my mother, who flew in from Switzerland. Even so, the transition back to work was much harder this second time. I will never forget that first night on call, my breasts filling with milk, my heart aching for my little baby. As with everything else in life, it became easier with time.

I am presently completing my first year of plastic surgery residency at New York Hospital, a delightful program with knowledgeable and caring people. I am enjoying every bit of it because I know how hard it was to get here. Most important, I have regained a feeling of self-worth that somehow I lost when I first came to this country. The girls are now two and three years old and seem perfectly happy and well-adjusted. My husband has now been in practice for 11 years, and he reminds me to enjoy the climb, no matter how long it may be. I think I can finally see the mountain's summit just up ahead.

— *Elsa Raskin*
Clinical instructor, Cornell University
Plastic surgery private practice

A Time for Change: Innovative Pathways for Residency Training[5]

I began my pediatric internship at Children's Hospital in Boston along with 27 other somewhat nervous but enthusiastic interns. After five days of orientation lectures, demonstrations, and even a canoe trip, my fellow interns began their work on the wards. I went home and did not start my internship until one month later. This arrangement was by design, for a friend and I shared our internship. In an innovative arrangement, we alternated months on clinical rotations, leaving time available for our families and other commitments.

I investigated part-time and shared-residency opportunities because flexibility was important for my own situation. Medicine is my second career. I came to this field after an eight-year career in social work, as a director, researcher, clinician, and faculty member. During medical school, my husband and I had two children. Our daughter was 18 months and our son 5 years old when I began internship.

In my determination to find a residency partner, I created a national clearinghouse called Pediatric Residency Partners[6] to match individuals interested in sharing a residency and to serve as a resource to help people arrange flexible training schedules. Interest existed nationwide; I heard from medical students from as far away as Hawaii, Texas, Wisconsin, Arkansas, and California. Many, but not all, were parents seeking residency arrangements in which they could spend more time with their families. Others wanted time for research or other pursuits.

My residency partner and I initially shared one position, alternating four weeks of work with four weeks off, fitting into the rotation schedule that all interns at Children's Hospital follow. When not formally scheduled, I saw patients in my continuity clinic one half-day each week and attended teaching conferences almost every day. In contrast to the months during which I worked full-time, I had time to read, write papers, and attend meetings. Most importantly, I could reconnect with my family—spending extra time with my son as he began school and with my daughter as she made the transition into the toddler class at her day care center.

On other rotations, I left home each morning before my children awoke and returned at night after they had gone to bed, not seeing them for several days at a time. It helped knowing this schedule was time-limited and that I could again parent my children on a more consistent basis when the rotation ended.

Are there disadvantages? When I rotated onto a new service, there were times when I was at a different level of experience than my fellow residents. It becomes important for attending physicians and supervising residents to be sensitive to these differences and, perhaps, to individualize their teaching to a greater degree. My residency took me five years instead of three, and my paycheck was half that of my colleagues—not quite enough to cover my daughter's day care expenses.

Was it worth it? Yes. Although temporarily I was on a different track than most of my colleagues, the flexible residency allowed richness in my life while preserving energy and enthusiasm for my patients and family. I could be the kind of parent I desired to be while learning to become a good doctor.

Part-time and shared residencies are not just for parents or married residents. Residents with satisfying personal lives are better able to give of themselves. Ultimately, patients will benefit as training programs become increasingly sensitive to the needs of their residents.

— Elizabeth A. Rider
Codirector, Academies of Medical Educators Collaborative
Harvard Medical School, Pediatric private practice

Lamentation of the Female Academician

When I was 22 years old and fresh out of college, I thought that my career was the most important thing in the world. I had been raised in the feminist decades of the 60s and 70s, and my parents taught me that I could be anything I wanted to be. I believed them. As a child, I dabbled in astronomy but realized I was too nearsighted and awkward to be an astronaut. I went through an artistic period, but the realities of mediocre talent and the need to eat regularly blotted out that career dalliance. I contemplated mathematics in college, but my head wasn't round and bald and male enough to fit in; besides, I needed a little more people contact than that provided by calculus and trigonometry. I guess I wasn't deferential enough for the differential equations.

The biological sciences seemed a reasonable career path. I liked bacteria; my dad had shown me proper culture techniques, and besides, this molecular biology stuff was pretty cool. Maybe I could screen a library, clone a gene, and express a protein. Dutifully noting my father's frustration with his lack of clinical credentials and indecisive to an extreme, I thought I would check out these new combined M.D.-Ph.D. programs. I liked science, had always figured I would get a Ph.D., and the practice of medicine seemed interesting—but hopefully not too people oriented. I did the requisite volunteer work at the VA hospital, but instead of serving as a nurse's aid or escort, I worked in the pathology lab, sorting blood and urine specimens, appreciating the meaning of the word, "STAT." I had seen the fliers about the Medical Scientist Training Program posted around the medical center at the University of Missouri as a sophomore, and I told myself I would apply. This was when I still had the confidence to do anything I set my mind to. So I did, and wound up at Stanford University School of Medicine, a naïve kid from the Midwest hell bent on becoming a physician-scientist, whatever that meant.

My first year as a medical student was traumatic. Really, it was my first time away from home. At least I knew one of my roommates, but the other was an "older" woman who didn't eat meat, didn't like science, and preferred the company of women to men. Clueless would be a better descriptor for my first real exposure to lesbianism, but the irony is that we ended up good friends. Within a few weeks, my anatomy dissecting partner came out to me as well, and I guess I figured if surrounded by lesbians, get to know them. My eyes were opened a little wider by the credentials of my colleagues. Fellow medical students from Ivy League schools, with Oxford memoirs, South American cultural exchanges, and readily flowing sunny California idealism abounded. I had the ubiquitous sense of "oh my god, they made a mistake in admitting me. I don't belong here. I'm outclassed, outsmarted, and undone." But somehow I survived the first year, and the second, and found a lab to pursue research.

I could probably wax poetic about the glorious experience of graduate studies, but it really wasn't that wonderful. There were positive aspects, like dictating my own schedule, wearing jeans and T-shirts every day to work, riding my bike to school, and playing volleyball every Friday and Sunday in the Oval. We were hard-core about our science and our volleyball. But there were plenty of times that the senior graduate student in the lab made me cry with his cruelty, impatience, and miserable misanthropism. My adviser didn't want to be bothered. If you could talk football with him, you were a golden boy. Funny, there weren't any golden girls. And more ironic, there hadn't been any successful female grad students in his lab. Ever. I don't know why I never noticed, since I scrutinized all the potential labs before choosing his, and searched in vain for a female mentor who wasn't worse than all the good ol' boys she had tried so hard to emulate. The one female faculty member I seriously considered scared me away, and she was not happy that I chose not to join her lab. A close call.

My dad died while I was in graduate school. I went home before he died to try and calm him through his final battle with cancer. It was the first time in my life that I understood with crystal-clear clarity what the most important thing in the world is: the people in your life. I left my research project at a low point, when I doubted I would ever make it scientifically. And I went home to a mother who could barely cope and a father who was in denial for the both of them. I stayed for 40 days, celebrated Easter mass by myself, and went back to California for a week until my dad crumpled and finally gave up.

I found the gene I was looking for within a month after my dad died. Bittersweet victory. It's hard to streak bacteria when you're crying. But my research career was on the upswing from there on. I would get the Ph.D. The question became, What about the M.D.? That was a terror—going onto the wards. I was older and wiser in some ways but ignorant with regard to clinical medicine. During my OB rotation, I was convinced that every woman who delivered a baby was going to bleed to death. I fell asleep holding retractors during surgery. I was terrified of the crazy VA patients on my psychiatry rotation. I was fascinated by neurology, but found neurologists rather odd. I watched a woman die of necrotizing fasciitis—the horrible "flesh-eating bacteria"—during my medicine subinternship, and when I had to present her at morbidity and mortality rounds, I decided I couldn't take care of big people. I liked kids and their innocence and thought pediatricians were more benign than the average physician, so I took the plunge into pediatrics.

Pediatric residency taught me two things: how to eat poorly and how to not sleep enough. I fell asleep once in mid-sentence while asking an attending a question during a teaching conference in spite of diet Coke. I was so wired that by the end of my third year, I couldn't sit still. A heightened state of awareness may be helpful for dealing with the barrage of ER patients during a shift, but it's not conducive to living a life. The one bright spot was meeting my future husband during internship. He somehow survived my residency as well and kept me sane. I have some fond memories of it, but a lot is blocked out. I can't watch *ER* without getting worked up about the way a patient was handled. My blood pressure probably rises 20 points during that show. I think it's called posttraumatic stress disorder.

Trying to chart a course for the postresidency period was hard. I thought I still wanted to do scientific research but where and in what? I fell in love with genetics and the sheer intellectual fascination of seeing what one gene gone awry can do. I looked for mentors and found a few. One had four kids perfectly spaced throughout residency and fellowship and was back at work the next day after delivery. Another is an accomplished poet and mother of two in her spare time. So I figured I could do it if I set my mind to it. I decided to pursue a genetics fellowship—prolong the training for just another round—and become an academician. Besides, I couldn't look in squirming, screaming children's ears for the rest of my life.

So now, in my third year of fellowship, what have I accomplished? I have been out of the lab for six years, and everything I used to do by hand can now be done faster and more efficiently by a kit. Science has become big business, and if you don't broker power with the movers and shakers in the university setting or the biotech biggies, forget it. My department chair insists on calling me "young lady" and wielding arbitrary, heavy-handed dictums disguised as advice. I write grants and struggle for survival. I am competing with scientists who devote 100% of their professional time and thoughts to the pursuit of fundamental scientific discoveries, not helping a little girl with neurofibromatosis. I work in a clinic a theoretical 10% of my time, which expands to fill a 30% chunk of reality, doing the only thing I feel minimally competent to do these days: diagnose and treat genetics patients. I help teach a course in human genetics for medical students. I go to seminars and meetings because it is expected of me. And for all this, with two advanced degrees, 12 years of advanced education beyond college, I am an "acting instructor" with no benefits, no retirement plan, and a parking space in outer Mongolia—*if* I get there by 8:30 am.

I am now 35 years old. I have a wonderful husband, two adoring dogs, and a mother who is slowly degenerating in a horrible way. I think I want to have a career in academic medicine, but at times I'm not so sure. What I really want is a family, because deep down inside, I know that is the only thing that matters. My biological clock is ticking louder, and my tenure clock hasn't even been started up. Which one will I pay attention to?

— *Melissa A. Parisi*
Acting Instructor and Attending Physician
University of Washington School of Medicine

But I Do Care

I fought so hard to become a physician, sacrificing time, money, and even dignity to go through medical school—the years of delayed gratification set aside for something so much more worthwhile. Then as a resident, I endured the long hours on call, the sleep deprivation, the humiliation of being "pimped" by superiors, and the stress of managing up to 40 patients at a time while being paged at all hours of the night.

When did I first sense that something had gone terribly wrong? Perhaps it was the time I was called by a family member that their father, an elderly man who had recently left the nursing home, had just died. I expressed my sympathy but couldn't help feeling just a little relieved— one less complicated patient to see. Not only did this man have an endless list of health problems, but he was extremely uncooperative during clinic visits. Our practice allowed only 15 minutes per patient, yet he required almost an hour, half of which was spent just coaxing him to let us take his blood pressure.

When did I stop being the compassionate person I once was? My practice of Nichiren Daishonin's Buddhism didn't teach me this feeling of indifference. What happened? Where did I go wrong? Looking for answers, I sought guidance like a cactus seeking water and found refuge in the wise Buddhist teachings. Now I chant to preserve my humanity within a callous, unforgiving health care system. I chant so I may become the compassionate person I once was, the one who wept for others as if their suffering were my own. I chant so people will understand that physicians like myself do care but may be too overwhelmed or tired to show it. I chant with all my heart that the business of healing becomes the business of caring.

And that starts with me.

— Joan Stroud
Family practitioner, Community Healthcare Network
Brooklyn, New York

Notes

1. Campbell, C. C. (1993). The last day. *Harvard Medical Alumni Bulletin, 67*(2), 66–67. Reprinted by permission of the author.

2. Excerpted from Snyderman, N. L. (2000). *Necessary journeys: Letting ourselves learn from life.* New York: Hyperion. Reprinted and abridged with permission.

3. Hunt, S. H. (2001). Post-call. *Wisconsin Medical Journal, 100*(1), 4. Reprinted by permission of the Wisconsin Medical Journal.

4. Excerpted from Klass, P. (1992). *Baby doctor: A pediatrician's training* (pp. 112–114). New York: Random House. Used with permission.

5. Earlier versions of this piece were published in the *Harvard Medical Alumni Bulletin* and *The Resident in Pediatrics.* Used with permission of the author.

6. Pediatric Residency Partners is no longer in operation. The AMA's FREIDA Online (Fellowship and Residency Electronic Database) at http://www.ama-assn.org/cgi-bin/freida/freida.cgi, allows searches for part-time and shared residencies. Many part-time and shared residents have successfully approached residency programs directly to negotiate positions.

5

ON DOCTORING

*Let us allow ourselves to become a part of the
case history — a part of the stories in which we may
play many roles — stories about that moment of
sharing, when all defenses are down, when nothing else
matters, when the lines of priority are drawn. That is
where the greatest reward in medicine can be found.*
— Michael A. LaCombe[1]

In Between Before and After[2]

It takes only five seconds to irrevocably change a life.

It takes only five seconds to tell someone that the person they love
most in life is dead.

As an emergency medicine physician, being the bearer of this
devastating news is a part of my profession. It isn't on any job
description or list of credentialed procedures, like emergency
cricothyrotomy or chest tube thoracostomy. Unlike those hard
skills—lauded and heralded as life saving—delivering the news of the
sudden death of a loved one is rarely acknowledged or encouraged.

It was a week before Christmas, and the Philadelphia emergency
room in which I was training was decked with howling PCP-addled

teenage twins, one miscarriage, a pneumonia, two weak-and-dizzies, a chicken bone in the esophagus, and a gunshot wound to the testicles. Charts of patients waiting to be seen spilled off the counter of the nurses' station. The waiting room was Standing Room Only, and the vending machine was out of Cheetos, causing three different mothers, each with an irritable, ear-infected child, to file complaints with the administration. The television was tuned to a rerun of *Three's Company*; everyone watched, transfixed. Someone was vomiting on the floor.

The call crackled over the radio at 7:48 p.m. "Thirty-two-year-old male, full cardiac arrest, asystole. CPR in progress. ETA, three minutes." Everyone's jaws reflexively tightened upon hearing the age. Nurses pushed patients out of the Big Room. Joking subsided.

He arrived cold, wet, and without hope. He had been celebrating at his office Christmas party when he literally keeled over. The paramedics had arrived in five minutes. They had made multiple useless attempts to electrify his fibrillating heart back to a sensible rhythm. On his arrival to the ER, a well-orchestrated chaos ensued: needles inserted, drugs pushed, monitors read, chest compressed, clothes cut away, trachea tubed, orders shouted. This was continued until the physician in charge "called the code." It was 9:38 p.m., and we still didn't know his name.

The paramedics, in their hurry, hadn't written it down; no one came with him; and when his clothes were cut away, his wallet was lost. His chart said "John Doe." The chief resident told me to go find "Mrs. Doe" and tell her that her husband was dead. He and the other residents drifted back to the sick, the wounded-but-alive patients, as I, the intern, was sent to do the task with the least priority.

It was assumed in my training that notifying the next of kin of the suddenly dead was an innate skill. Unprepared for the task, we were thrown at the to-be-bereaved with the sink-or-swim tradition of most medical training. Besides, the dead were dead, what more harm could one intern do? As emergency medicine docs, much like cowboys in lab coats, we notched our professional belts with lives saved. An unsuccessful resuscitation made us acutely aware of our limitations. Telling the families was confessing failure.

There was no Mrs. Doe in the waiting room, so I returned to the ER and started picking up charts, hoping that she wouldn't show up until my shift was over. The hallucinating twins were beginning to harmonize.

At 10:34 p.m. a short, disheveled woman, wearing a sweater buttoned randomly over a nightgown, was asking for her husband, David. She was 26 years old; one year younger than me. The nurses directed the unknowing widow toward me; their voices casual and expressions flat, carefully not betraying any hint of her future.

"David Baker, he was at his office Christmas party, and someone just called and told me that he got sick and had to be brought to the Emergency Room. Did they bring him here?" The words rushed out of her.

"Was he wearing a gray suit and a tie with Santas on it?" I asked.

Her face fell.

She knew.

Mrs. Baker began backing away from me, away from the crushing news. The terrible fear that had been her front-seat passenger all the way to the emergency room had suddenly leapt up. Shaking her head, she began her chant of denial, softly at first. "No, no, no, no," then louder as I tried to approach her.

She was against the door when I reached her. "I'm sorry Mrs. Baker, but they brought in a man dressed like that from a Christmas Party in full cardiac arrest, and he didn't make it." The facts were finally delivered.

Her faced brightened. Unprepared to handle tragedy, she jumped at the slimmest hope. "If he didn't make it here, where is he? What hospital did they take him to?" She lunged at me, begging me to tell her.

"No, I mean—," I struggled to say it, hating the taste of the words, hating her for making it so difficult. "What I'm trying to tell you, I mean, he's dead."

And there I saw it for the first time; the moment that would define her "before and after." She tried to cry out, but it was stuck in her throat. The buzz of the ER swarmed around both of us.

During my fifteen years of practicing emergency medicine I have come to accept that sometimes death demands immediate capitulation:

the accident too massive, the bullet too on-target, the coronary artery too choked. I am also grateful to have learned, since Mrs. Baker, that as I walk toward a huddled family or a frightened spouse, I am treading on the last few seconds of their *before* to bring to them the painful *after*. The time in between is only five seconds.

— *Katherine Uraneck*
Freelance medical journalist and emergency physician

Heartsick[3]

"Hello, Miz Lucy," I would say as my father led me into the patient exam room. Miz Lucy, a diminutive retired schoolteacher, would be sitting in the chair, gussied up to the nines, with gnarled hands and feet shod in heavy stockings and thick orthopedic shoes. My father, a general internist in a small southern town, would have me touch her swollen hands as he injected the gold that would help her pain. She would exclaim about my growth, my successes in school, and would mention how the good doctor had saved her life more than once. Later, she would drive by our house in her ancient green Cadillac to make sure that he was home in case she needed him or to drop off her special cookies. At Christmas time, our kitchen counter was always covered with cakes, pies, or crocheted afghans made by grateful patients like Miz Lucy.

I remember making a house call with my father on a wintry Sunday afternoon. We drove up to a small house in which a sad, weathered-looking man with slumped shoulders sat in a wheelchair.

"Arthur," my dad would say as he took off his coat and opened up his massive black bag, "how are you?" And the murmuring would start. I would sit on the sofa in the quiet, empty house and watch as my father talked with Arthur. Later, on the drive home, my father would tell me how, as a young man, Arthur had dived into a quarry pond and severed his spinal cord.

And then there was Margaret. Struck down by polio at the age of 9 in a tiny farm town up in the county, Margaret survived in an iron lung; her brother had died. Her mother had cared for her all her life, even moving to a major university town long enough to help Margaret get a college degree. Margaret, only her head visible while her wasted body was encased in the huge tubular machine, would ask me about my latest book while my father inspected her mother's diabetic foot ulcer or assessed Margaret's recurrent parotitis. Margaret's mother eventually developed dementia and, before she died, cursed the daughter whom she had cared for all her life. To this day, my now-retired father still visits weekly, to discuss books, to bring medicines. I still visit at Christmas with my father, taking my children along with me.

These memories are my most enduring and are at the heart of why I became a physician. Now, after nearly 15 years in various practices, having raised my children and finally settled down in a group practice of dedicated, like-minded colleagues, I am glad that I kept the name that connects me to my father and to his legacy of doctoring. I have a dream and the guts to begin to fulfill it, a dream of building a practice with my Miz Lucys and Arthurs and Margarets. My dream is to provide superb medical care as I get to know them over time, to be their physician in my sense of the word, and to grow old with them.

But managed care is threatening that dream. "Growth and profit," the business executive writes on the blackboard as he explains that the practice of assigning patients to individual physicians has been abolished and that patients may sign up with any physician, regardless of known waits for routine or urgent care.

"For a panel size of 4000, we will pay you x more dollars in salary than for the current 2000 patients you are managing," he intones. Our protests are not acknowledged, and our reluctance to add more patients to already jammed practices is seen as "slothful and needy."

As the months go by, my established patients become more unhappy as it becomes more difficult for them to see me. My new patients are enraged at the more than 3 months' wait for a physical. They feel betrayed by the slick advertisements and come-ons. In the office, they sit with lists written on the backs of envelopes to remind them to discuss their headaches, constipation, elevated cholesterol and hormone levels. There just doesn't seem to be enough time for them to begin to trust me nor for me to understand the person behind the list. I dread looking at my daily schedule and long for the short, uncomplicated medical encounter. My face no longer lights up in anticipation of opening the handwritten letter in my mailbox. Nowadays, these are much less likely to be testimonies to my care and much more likely to be complaints about the referral, the waits, or the most recent visit.

My Middle Eastern patient comes to see me. As always, she wears traditional Muslim clothing, her round face peering out of her headdress. Widowed and alone, she is suing her employer for sexual harassment in a long, arduous battle that will determine whether she can continue in the research career that she loves. I have been so impressed with the pluck and courage of this shy, lonely woman fighting to survive in a radically different culture. Our visits usually move quickly through the hypertension and the knee pain to the real reason for her visit: my support, my affirmation, and my reassurance that she will be all right. I see the hurt in her eyes as I am pushed for time one day and brusquely cut short our discussion.

A new patient calls me on the phone. She has menstrual irregularities, insomnia, and mood swings, and the suspicion that she is menopausal has added the stress of a major life transition to her already present difficulties. The wait for an appointment with me is unacceptably long to her. Although I have never seen her, on paper I am already her physician, and she is angry and irritated. I call her back, having already added extra patients to my session that day. Sitting in my office with my elbows on a stack of charts that all bear notes asking me to call patients, I am overwhelmed and vaguely realize that our conversation hasn't gone well. Many weeks later, when we finally meet, my new patient forcefully condemns my lack of compassion on the phone and is uninterested in both my abject apologies and my explanations about "HMO panel sizes" and "time pressures." I know that she has labeled me arrogant and insensitive, and the sense of failure on my part is enormous. Although I spend time rationalizing and working through the experience, her diatribe against me remains one of the most painful moments in my 15 years of doctoring.

I begin to feel as if I am in a war. I speak out at meetings but feel small and unheard. I want to ask the managers and my bosses, "Where do you get your health care, and if your elderly mother is ill, do you want her to see the kind of physician you are attempting to create?" It is the practitioners and patients who will reap what these corporatized leaders have sown.

What about my dream? It has nothing to do with income, with status, or with having built a more cost-effective medical machine but is about the deep satisfaction that my interpersonal relationships and skills with my patients over the years will bring. Above all else, the physician-patient relationship must be preserved. I do not see this happening, despite my dedication to it and my efforts to sound an alarm and rouse my colleagues to action. I feel a helplessness as I face this inexorable attack. I am simply heartsick.

— *Julia E. McMurray*
Associate Professor of Medicine, University of Wisconsin, Madison

My Patient, the Doctor, and Me

I had graduated from residency, finished my fellowship, and was practicing in a high-profile, academic practice at a tertiary medical center. In a sea of eminent colleagues, I saw myself as an imposter, a pip-squeak. I wanted to be as respected as they, the balding, gray-haired, bespectacled, and very well published men. They invariably sat in the front during grand rounds, rows upon rows of polished, gleaming, erudite crania. Instead, I was a young woman who loved to (gulp!) shop and was in search of happiness. As a doctor in training, these traits had all been excusable. But as an attending physician, how would I ever fit in?

I wore glasses and put my hair up in a bun to look older. I published. I maintained a serious expression at all times, going around with furrowed brow and secretly worrying that the furrows would set. My statements became more measured and delivered with long-winded decorum. A friend who had known me in my carefree, resident days asked in bewilderment, "What are you trying to do? Imitate Gandhi?"

My patients were mostly born in the decades before the second world war and ran the gamut from physicists to artists to socialites. Would these men and women, from an era dressed in dapper suits, bowler hats, and elegant shoes, respect me? I was sure their notion of a doctor was more along the lines of *Marcus Welby, MD* than *Dr. Quinn, Medicine Woman.* While mostly articulate and courteous, some were obstreperous and impatient. I was concerned. Would these more difficult patients have behaved better with Dr. Welby? I tried out my stereotype formula on them all, in bun and white coat, somber clothes and manner. Overall, it was a success. The majority responded well enough and things seemed to go along just fine.

But I found that my act was wearing me down. My relationship with patients seemed sterile and unfulfilling. I was too busy trying to conform to the image of who I thought I should be rather than be who I was. I longed to respond to a joke with a loud and hearty laugh rather than a measured, "professional" smile. I wanted to hug a defeated old woman good-bye but merely shook her hand. I wanted to ask questions such as, "How does it feel to be married for sixty-five years?" but it wasn't relevant to the parietal stroke.

I am not quite sure what made me decide to make the change. Perhaps it was the realization that I was so desperately unhappy with the physician I had become. Perhaps it was the rebel within me. Perhaps I was just being self-destructive. Whatever the reason, I had had enough. And so, one day, I took off my glasses and threw my white coat to the winds. I kept the bun. I made my sentences shorter. I drank tea with my patients. I felt as though I had leaped off a cliff, free-falling into a scary space, where it was just me with my patients—no coat for me to slip into, no professional mannerisms to hide behind. I felt strangely vulnerable, exposed, and open to criticism. Naked, without white coat, eyes uncovered. And I found myself swept up into a magical world, strangely enchanted and uncharted. For in giving me permission to be myself, I gave my patients permission to be themselves as well.

Now, when I am trying to check their gait, my patients teach me to waltz. They bake cakes and share recipes. They chuckle with delight when I compliment them on their outfits and scold me if they find out I have not had lunch. They buss my cheeks, and it is contagious. An old sailor from Ireland sings mournful ballads in a rich and soaring voice. I have learned not to care what the others might think.

I get free advice on matters all and sundry from experts. On marriage: "Always tell them what they want to hear, dear, and then do whatever you want." On child rearing: "Tuck them in bed and kiss them goodnight. Let them know you love them and tell them often. Answer all their questions or else they will ask someone else." On fashion: "You should know better than to wear heels that high, Doc. It's murder on your feet." Of the ineffable pain of irrevocable loss: "My mother died when I was five, and that was eighty years ago," the voice dissolving into sobs.

I learned about the great regrets in many folks' lives: "I should've had children" or, alternatively, "I should never have had children." Regrets most always seem to center around family themes. I heard of the fear of losing dignity, like the retired chancellor who told me, "I don't want to end up being turned around like meat on a spit." And about a certain kind of generosity of spirit. How could I agree to have my patient's grandchild named after me, when I was doing so little to cure her, only holding her hand as she got worse?

I learned about death, that it is important to send a card to the family and to call if it feels right. That it is not unprofessional to attend funerals. I learned that it is important to let loved ones know that they did everything they could, because they need to hear it, and to hear it from you. Your words echo long in their minds and bring them comfort. I learned about hope—how it springs exuberant, no matter how dire the illness, and that I had no right to dampen it.

I learned that it is a hard thing to be ill-tempered, because you only get meaner as the years go by. I learned that happy people stay happy, so it is a good thing to work on. That it is important to have friends. That the best things in life are left said. That family is more important than career. I would never have believed I would come to this.

I tried on many gloves before I found the one that fit. I find I can use the tools of my trade so much the better for it. The fabric of my life is richer for my not fitting into a stereotype and, instead, accentuating those individual characteristics about me that are important for my profession. So I've chosen the road less traveled and oh, the difference to me!

— Gayatri Devi

Attending Physician, Lenox Hill Hospital, New York City
Director, New York Memory Services
Author of Estrogen, Memory, and Menopause *(2000)*

Heart Doctor

My CCU attending accosts
me with thistle-laden words that prickle near
my upper trunk. I choke, "The patients appreciate my care."

He retorts, "This is a hospital, not a hospice." Over years
I convince myself I am hospital. Then in practice

the clinging handshake takes seed, in row with
the lingering patient, the family seeking
soothing expression and word, and my helpless
laying on of hands, helping.

And the hospice within, buried in fertile soil,
germinates and flowers tubular fruit
drawn out as if by sun-warmth, feeding
on bracts of gratitude,
to meet the immense need.

— Stephanie Nagy-Agren

Assistant Professor of Internal Medicine, University of Virginia
Chief, Infectious Diseases Section,
Veterans Affairs Medical Center, Salem, Virginia

Common Ground

"We are a Catholic medical center, Dr. Ofri." The medical director leaned back in his chair across from my desk. "Do you have any issues with that?"

His gray hair was severely parted on the right, and I could trace the individual strands that were tethered down on the side by hair grease. He had just finished his long introductory speech with me, enumerating the vast array of services and the selling points of his medical group, clearly trying to impress me with his institution. After all, the reason I was doing a temp assignment here was because they were short-handed and looking to hire.

I was caught off balance by the question. What could he be driving at? Was my Jewish background an issue here? Was my last name too ethnic? I paused and then slowly asked back, "Should I have issues?"

"Well," he replied, in his careful New England lilt, "we do not promote birth control. If a patient requests it, we will provide it. But we do not offer it, promote it, or condone it."

Before my superego could grab control, my New York sassiness spilled out. "So, I don't suppose you perform abortions, do you?"

I could not believe I had just said that.

The older physician did not appear fazed. "No, we do not terminate pregnancies. Nor do we permit referrals to physicians who do. If a patient requests that service, we have them call their own insurance company for referrals.

He stood up and put out his hand. "We are glad to have you aboard, Dr. Ofri. We hope you enjoy your six weeks with us. And," he paused with a smile, "we hope you consider staying longer."

I remained in my office after he left, a little confused about what I had just heard and very embarrassed about the sauciness of my retort. I finally brushed it off, attributing it to high-level politics that I was not a part of.

The staff members welcomed me warmly, giving me a large office and a nurse, Karen, to work exclusively with me. At the beginning of each appointment she took a brief history from the patient, checked their vital signs, and jotted down their medications. When I entered into the room afterward to see the patient, I found all the supplies that I might need for that particular patient neatly laid out. The walls of the examining rooms must have been fairly thin because when I was finished with the patient, Karen was waiting outside with whatever vaccines or medications I had discussed with the patient. Between patients we shared stories of her life in New England and my experiences at Bellevue. And I loved that she kept a picture of her golden retriever, Sam, on her desk.

This was nothing like Bellevue Hospital—the city hospital in New York where I did my residency. Practicing medicine had never been so easy. I noticed that, along with the antihypertensives and cholesterol medications, the medicine cabinet was stocked with free samples of birth control pills. Apparently, no one took the contraception rule too seriously.

Three weeks into my assignment, I met Diana Makower, a young computer programmer at a local financial firm. She was wearing a gray suit with a purple silk blouse. A single strand of pearls hung around her neck. Her carefully applied makeup had started to smudge from the tears slipping down her cheeks. "I think I'm pregnant," she spilled out, almost before I could introduce myself. "I did one of those home pregnancy tests, and it was positive. All I need from you is a blood test."

I put down my stethoscope and pulled up a chair.

"It's a complicated situation," she wept. "I am ending a relationship with my boyfriend, but it wasn't him. I have an old friend, it's never been more than that, but I think he and I might be developing a romantic relationship. We slept together just once, three weeks ago. I really think we could have a serious relationship, but it is not ready for this. I can't believe this is happening,"

"If you do turn out to be pregnant," I asked, "what do you think you would do?"

"I need to have an abortion. I can't have a kid now; I'm single, I don't have a stable relationship yet. I'm not ready for it now."

"Are you sure that's what you want to do? Have you considered other options, like adoption?"

"Absolutely," she said. "I have made my decision. I just need to know where to go."

I suddenly thought of the medical director with his slicked-down gray hair. According to the rules, I was supposed to tell Diana to call her insurance company. Her insurance company? I had visions of a bored bureaucrat slurping on his coffee while dispensing advice on a delicate matter to my distraught patient. How could I send Diana into a situation like that? I excused myself and went to consult Karen.

Karen did not know which local doctors performed abortions. "I stay out of that mess," she said. She sympathized with my predicament but warned me not to let the office manager know what I was doing. "Someone else gave out a phone number once," she said. "Just a phone number. It wasn't even documented in the chart, but somehow it got out, and they got into trouble."

I stared out the window and could see my rental car parked in front of a clapboard house across the street. This Catholic medical institution might choose not to perform abortions, but what about *my* ethical duty to provide the care my patient needed? Sending a distressed patient to an 800 telephone number would not hold water under the Hippocratic oath. It seemed clear to me that my duty was first to my patient and only secondarily to some faceless institution. Unfortunately, as a stranger to this small town, I did not know the local resources.

Grinding my teeth, I reentered the exam room. "As you may know, this medical practice is Catholic," I told Diana, "so we cannot provide referrals for abortion. The truth is, I wouldn't know where to send you even if I could. The rule is that you are supposed to call your insurance company and get the referral yourself. If you get a list of possible referrals, I will call around to find out which is the best."

Diana nodded, and then asked if she could be alone. I left her with a box of tissues and told her she could stay as long as she liked.

I called Diana the next day to let her know that the repeat pregnancy test was positive. When I called, I got her voice mail at work. She had told me that it was a private line, but suddenly I felt paranoid. I did not indicate that I was a physician and left a cryptic message about results being "confirmatory of our original data."

Diana returned my call a few hours later. Her insurance company had given her two phone numbers in the next state over. Her health plan had no gynecologists in this state who performed abortions. Nobody in the state? My patient couldn't get the care that she needed in her home state? I was horrified. I felt like we were back in the 1950s, sneaking around with code words and having to go out of state for an abortion.

I plowed through my roster of patients for the day, but I couldn't focus on the coughs, rashes, and shoulder pains. All I could think about was Diana. I imagined her driving over the state line, tears pressing at her lid margins. The lonesomeness in the car, the bitter highway, the directions scribbled on the back of a used envelope. I imagined her squinting at the scrawled directions, the car slipping ever so slightly out of the lane as her mind diffused focus from the highway to the enormity of what lay ahead.

Between patients I paced around my office, too irritated to sit still. What kind of place was this where some administrative rule could interfere with patient care? When was the last time these bureaucrats sat face-to-face with a patient, watching the tension lines around the mouth quiver, accepting the burden and the honor of tender secrets? I fumed all afternoon, cursing the insurance companies and the politicians whose ideologies and business concerns were elbowing into my office, into the sacred space that my patient and I shared.

Then Karen told me that the wife of one of the doctors used to work at a teen clinic. Grateful for this information, I called immediately. She knew of the two out-of-state facilities and told me they had reputations for treating patients like cattle. There was, however, a private women's clinic two hours north that was professional and reliable. But most insurance companies would not cover the cost of the procedure.

I called Diana at home that evening. She had already made an appointment at one of the out-of-state clinics and was very appreciative of my "insider information."

"Have you told him?" I asked.

"No. No, I can't tell him. Not yet, at least. Maybe afterward."

"Is there anyone that you'd feel comfortable talking to, a friend, a family member? Is there someone who could come with you?"

"No, not really," she replied. "I mean, I have good friends, but I couldn't tell them about this. They wouldn't understand."

I winced at the thought of her going alone. There was a sense of something shameful, something to hide. "Bring your own bathrobe," I added, before we hung up. "It's more comfortable than a hospital gown."

I called her again the following day just to make sure she was okay. I somehow found a pretext to call her almost every day. We chatted a bit, and it turned out that she had grown up in New York.

"Really?" I asked, excited to uncover a fellow New Yorker here in the wilds of New England. We reminisced about our nostalgia for Manhattan and the familiar local hangouts.

I left work that evening and drove home to my hotel. As I sat in my rental car, idling at a traffic light, I felt confined. I pined for the freedom of the foot-based culture of New York, in which everything I needed was in walking distance. Some people feel nervous in big cities; I feel nervous in small towns. No pedestrians on the streets. No one to make eye contact with. No one to negotiate personal space on a sidewalk with. No mass of actual human beings on the street to remind you that you are alive and part of a species. Only cars.

And so I sat in my car, isolated in a metal box with diesel heat rumbling beneath my feet. As the light languished on red, I thought about Diana. I realized that I was probably the only person she'd spoken to about this pregnancy. The burden of her secret bound me to her, as both a woman and a doctor.

I ached to share my own experience, but professionalism, and I suppose some lingering shame, prevented me. I'd been only seventeen at the time and just returning home from my first year in college. I was about to go off to be a counselor at summer camp when I discovered that I was pregnant.

I'd had a steady boyfriend the entire year. Before we got involved I had gone to Planned Parenthood because I didn't want to be irresponsible. I remembered the long talk with the counselor in the windowless room with the overly cheery posters. We'd decided together on the diaphragm for birth control. The package insert listed a 95% effectiveness rate. No one ever spoke about the other 5%.

I lived in New York, the most liberal city in the most liberal state. My friends and parents were all liberal and pro-choice. But I was too scared to tell anyone.

After the pregnancy test, I sat in a park and cried alone. It was a park where my family used to have picnics when I was little. Our dog Kushi would run around in the free open space. Sitting in that park, I longed for the smell of her soft black fur and her warm, all-accepting "dogness." She was someone to whom I wouldn't have to explain all the complicated human confusions. But she'd died the previous year, just before I'd left for college.

I arranged an appointment at a local women's clinic. That night I made a long-distance call to my boyfriend. The geographical and personal gaps were apparently too vast to bridge—he couldn't quite accept what I was telling him over the phone. And he didn't offer to help me pay for it.

The next day I lied to my parents about having a party to go to so I could borrow the car. The clinic had said to bring a comfortable bathrobe. I snuck my mother's out of her closet.

The drive was eerily dissociated. The yellow lines in the road didn't seem parallel to the outer curbs. They listed and buckled, slighting the rules of Cartesian geometry. They drifted to other planes, to the odd dimensions of irrational numbers. Then they'd swing back with a jolt, clobbering into my focus. As the car shuffled closer and closer to the clinic, I felt my body shrinking. It dwindled within itself until there was nothing left but a little girl who desperately wanted her dog.

I lugged myself, or what little was left of myself, up the steps. The room was filled with eight or so women in different colored bathrobes. We could have been at a slumber party, except that no one was smiling.

I pulled my mother's flannel robe around me and concentrated on the orange industrial carpeting.

They gave me a choice of general or local anesthesia. The budding college-educated scientist wanted local, wanted to know everything that was going on, wanted to control the whole biology experiment. But the little girl who yearned for her dog immediately chose general. I didn't want to know. I didn't want to remember.

I awoke crying in another room. It was overly bright, and the sheets were stiff. My stomach pulsed with an alien ache. The nurse said to stop acting like a baby, it didn't really hurt that much. I checked out and went back to the same park to cry some more.

A week later, a letter arrived from my boyfriend. He told me that he felt terribly guilty. As "penance" for himself, he said he could never be with me again. That summer was long and lonely.

In the years that have gone by I have told almost no one. Part of me feels that I should be contributing to the destigmatization of abortion by being open about my own experience. Yet another part of me feels it is something personal. Worse yet, something to hide. I feel guilty and hypocritical.

Sometimes I think about the child that might have been. At seventeen, I had precious few resources to raise a child. I would never have finished college, much less gone to medical school. I might have faced a lifetime of minimum-wage jobs and food stamps. What would my child's life have been like?

I called Diana after her abortion. She told me that the staff members at the clinic were extremely kind and supportive, and that it didn't hurt too much. I breathed a sigh of relief. We spoke a few more times after that. Each time I felt the urge to share my story, but I couldn't.

I am not a politically active person. So much of what transpires in the government seems to have no bearing on my life. But when I see teenage mothers in my clinic barely mature enough to take care of themselves let alone the two or three babies on their laps, I am viscerally aware that my life was at the mercy of laws that permitted access to safe abortion. A different time or a different place and the outcome could have been vastly different.

Doctors often unconsciously separate themselves from patients—*they* are the sick ones and *we*, in our white coats, are different from them. It is humbling, and also relieving, to know that we are all made of the same stuff.

— *Danielle Ofri*
Attending Physician, Bellevue Hospital
New York University School of Medicine
Editor-in-Chief of Bellevue Literary Review

Dawn

Yesterday? Have twenty years gone by?
Your tiny body lying in that hard metal cage they called a crib.

You honored me by asking if I would lie next to you,

Inhibited doctor—too embarrassed about what my attendings, fellow residents, nurses, visitors . . . any and all would think.

But you asked; your love cut through the layers of my protective mental shield and professional white coat like a sharp, accurate laser, an invisible scalpel.

The chair came close to the cage, the side came down, my head next to yours on the pillow and stayed 'til you drifted off in slumber.

I went home that night pondering what happened but not realizing how you touched my spirit . . . Still, two decades later you inspire me.
You instilled in me the wish to feel connected.
You shared the God within.

— *Kathleen Franco*
Psychiatrist, Cleveland Clinic Foundation
Adjunct Professor of Psychiatry, Medical College of Ohio

Life Force[4]

Coherent, elegant, mysterious, aesthetic. When I first earned my degree in medicine I would not have described life in this way. But I was not on intimate terms with life then. I had not seen the power of the life force in everyone, met the will to live in all its varied and subtle forms, recognized the irrepressible love of life buried in the heart of every living thing. I had not been used by life to fulfill itself or been caught unaware by its strength in the midst of the most profound weakness. I had no sense of awe. I had thought that life was broken and that I, armed with the powerful tools of modern science, would fix it. I had thought then that I was broken also. But life has shown me otherwise.

Many of the people who come to my office now as counseling clients have come because modern medicine has failed them in some way, or they have used up its power to help them and they do not know what else to do. They hope to find a way to heal, to cooperate with or even strengthen the life in them. After listening to hundreds and hundreds of their stories over the last twenty years, I think I would have to say that most people do not recognize the strength of the life force in them or the many ways that it shows itself to them. Yet every one of us has felt its power. We who doubt are covered with the scars of our many healings.

So when people first come, this is the place we usually start—talking about life itself, our attitude toward it, our experience of it, our trust or distrust of it. Developing an eye to see it, in others and in ourselves. In the beginning is the life force. After more than fifty years of living, I have learned it can be trusted.

— Rachel Naomi Remen

Clinical Professor, University of California San Francisco
Founding Director, Institute for the Study of Health and Illness
Author of Kitchen Table Wisdom *(1996),* My Grandfather's Blessing *(2000)*

A Doctor Alone With Her Decision[5]

When physicians grab a few moments together for lunch or before meetings, assorted conversational themes surface. We often talk about new techniques, puzzling patients, frustrating restrictions, damnable paperwork. We may make comments about hospital administration, relate news about colleagues, mention plans for the future or children's achievements. Current events, politics, sports, books, and movies can be yeasty matters for discussion.

Every now and then, we discuss what it is like to be a doctor. This happens rarely, only when we have some quiet time and are with people we trust. We acknowledge our tensions, mistakes, burdens, and responsibilities. We muse on the lifelong struggle to satisfy our patients, family, friends, and ourselves.

And seldom, seldom, we talk about being alone.

Who would guess it? Physicians, alone? Physicians are quite public figures. We have many professional relationships and, depending on how our lives play out, we have a family and a few friends. But at core, physicians are alone with their decisions.

I heard a story recently about a surgeon who was alone with guilt. One of the surgeon's patients, a woman in her 80s, had had abdominal pain for a year and had lost 30 pounds. Her gallstones and huge umbilical hernia could readily explain the symptoms. The surgeon decided to operate, although the patient's age was a concern. On the other hand, she was living at home and enjoying life. Both she and her family concurred that the possibility of relieving her discomfort was worth the risk. Surgery went well, as did the immediate recovery.

By the time the patient was readmitted to the hospital a few days later, however, the circulation in her legs had deteriorated. Her toes were gangrenous. Things went from bad to worse. The patient did not respond to several days of care in the Intensive Care Unit. On a Sunday, the family and the intensive care physician felt it was time to stop unavailing efforts and let the patient continue her life's journey gently to its end. The surgeon was called at home. She said she would come. The family awaited her arrival.

After the surgeon changed into hospital greens in the physicians' locker room, she started up the steps to the ICU. About half way up, she turned around, and went back down. She could not face the family or say good-bye. She believed that if she had not operated, the patient might be at home, enjoying a sunny afternoon.

The surgeon had to live with the certain knowledge that her action—performing the operation—had precipitated the patient's decline. On the other hand, abdominal pain and a 30-pound weight loss over a year require intervention. Everyone had agreed.

The surgeon started up the stairs again, paused after a few steps, and went back down. She went to the on-call room. As she tried to collect her feelings—criticizing herself yet trying to find some comfort, giving reasons and rationales, thinking about failure and inevitability—another surgeon came into the lounge.

They chatted. Then he said, "What's up? What's really up?" She told him about the dying patient and how she needed to go to the Intensive Care Unit but had been unable to go up the stairs. They talked some more about how difficult it was, sometimes, to be the doctor, to try hard, to feel defeat so deeply, and to be so alone. Then he said. "I'll go with you." And they walked all the way up the stairs together.

The family was happy to see her. She learned later that they had been waiting for her. They hugged. They cried. They said good-bye. The family thanked the doctor for her skill and wisdom.

Physicians are expected to make sound recommendations and tough decisions. We are expected to be strong, unwavering, to be able to stand it. Caring for patients is not just time-consuming, but energy and spirit-consuming.

Relationships are pleasant, of course, and satisfaction flows back in warm ways. In the end, however, final accountability is ours, and we are alone. We are alone with our caring and our feelings, alone with making the best decisions we can. When bad things happen, and we know we played a part in them, it is much harder than usual to be alone.

This story is uncommon because physicians rarely admit they are having tough times, especially to each other. Here, a surgeon grappled with and acknowledged her burden, and a colleague reached out a kind hand. They walked up the stairs together.

— Linda Hawes Clever
Chief of Occupational Health at California Pacific Medical Center
Clinical Professor of Medicine, University of California, San Francisco

Through the Eyes of a Physician

One of the essential qualities of the clinician
is interest in humanity, for the secret of the care
of the patient is in caring for the patient.
— Francis Weld Peabody, 1881–1927

It was early fall during my internship year when I first met Eileen. A 29-year-old mother of two, she had spent more time in shelters and detox centers than she had at home. Worn down by years of hardship, her face reminded me of youthful promise abandoned long ago in the search for heroin and cocaine. Eileen's life was a roller coaster soaring down at times, inching up the climb to a brighter future at other times. Along the way, she had also battled hepatitis B and C, liver failure, pelvic inflammatory disease, multiple overdoses, and half a dozen suicide attempts, narrowly escaping death on more than one occasion. Often she would simply disappear from sight, only to be found weeks later in jail for theft or drug use or at an outside hospital, recovering from sepsis or an overdose. Each time, Eileen would emerge, usually ill and requiring hospitalization or urgent outpatient care. Through all the fear, stress, and uncertainty, we forged a special patient-physician bond.

Once after a series of hospitalizations for recurrent complications of drug use, my primary care preceptor advised me to set limits with Eileen. If Eileen did not comply, it would become increasingly difficult to deliver the type of care I desired for her.

"You mean I'd have to find another doctor? Don't you believe I can change?"

I saw myself at a fork in the road of our relationship: Should I follow the easier path and let her go? Or should I guide her along the arduous path to sobriety?

"Eileen, people say addiction is for life. Some change, but most become trapped in a vicious cycle. You're too young to die. Think of your family, your kids."

She began to cry, nodding her head in agreement.

I thought back to my medical school days and remembered another woman with sadness. Sandra, an IV drug user, had tried desperately to break her addictions. She was just beginning to learn the joys of being a wife and mother, passions that competed with her cravings for drugs. Her husband and one-year-old daughter reached out to save her—but too late. A shower of emboli from an infected valve left her half paralyzed and unable to speak. Stunned by her tragedy, the image of the young woman never left me.

I was brought back to the present with Eileen's words, "I'm ready to change, Doc."

Soon she was discharged to detox, one that included shelter, counseling, and vocational training. Months later, I heard from Eileen. "Six months clean, Doc. Longest I've ever gone." She had reinitiated contacts with her family, though they were tenuous. She came for a visit soon after, neatly clad in a blouse and pants, ready for a class after our appointment. "Thanks Doc, for sticking with me."

Many of the lessons I had learned about doctoring, about life and medicine, were challenged by Eileen's story. Often we judge our performance as physicians by whether a patient lives or dies, whether we cure or not. But the relationship Eileen and I developed reinforced how intensely personal medicine is. We treat people, not infarcts or pneumonias. Each patient's story becomes a tapestry, woven just as much from their life, family, and personal struggles as from their medical history or physical examination. Through her struggles with isolation, illness, and lost dreams, Eileen epitomized the human condition with all its frailty and vulnerability. Though her feet may slip while traveling the difficult path to sobriety, the vision of her ultimate goal is clearer.

In a day when we struggle to keep up with the pressures of managed care, politics, and technology, we should stop and remember why it is we entered medicine. Eileen's story is far from a celebration of the miracles of medicine. It is a testament to life struggles, one woman's will to live, and her love for her children. Ultimately, we see in it the healing power of the physician-patient relationship, which often transcends the tools of medical technology.

— Preetha Basaviah
Assistant Clinical Professor of Medicine,
University of California, San Francisco

References

Peabody, F. W. (1927). The care of the patient. *Journal of the American Medical Association, 88*, 877–882.

Why You Came to Me

I am the quiet one, the one who absorbs and does not speak. I listen silently, watching with quick eyes yet slow mind. My observations I build into a small pile, then churn them round and round inside my head until the secrets to human behavior are mine to understand. I want to know how fate led you to me, here in this hospital, private in name only. I want to know the reasons behind the actions, the paths to our common ends.

I am the silent one, so much happier listening than speaking. I want to know why this young man will not tell his mother that he has AIDS. Why this intelligent man with soft voice and soft hands, short stature and reserved demeanor, only reluctantly lets himself in on the poorly kept secret. He wakes up in the middle of the night unable to breathe. His favorite foods are swallowed like bitter pills because of the fungus stretching down his throat. And still he pretends. But what else can it be? He knows, she knows, I know, and still we dance around the truth.

They come to me individually, mother and son. He insists on absolute secrecy. So many people in the community know him, so many in his church where he is a leader. "When you round in the morning, please don't stand outside my room, and for God's sakes don't use my name!" He does not want to disappoint or be judged or, worse yet, be despised for a part of himself that he has yet to fully accept. She looks to me for a word, a gesture, an inflection that might confirm her suspicions. She is too smart for deceit, having honed her intuition and street smarts raising five kids on a meager income. Her words remain unspoken: *It will be all right, my child. I've watched you for 30 years and will not turn my back on you now.* But how can she tell him when he has yet to tell her? And how can she tell her husband, whom she knows will not understand? Instead, she confides in me, the only connection between her son and this illness. The separate suffering, the agonizing dance of noncommunication brings tears to my eyes. Afterward, I must throw cold water on my face and think about life before internship.

And the others. I take their history, running through the laundry list of symptoms, medications, allergies, and past medical problems. But what I really want to ask is, "What happened to you, that you've lost all your family and friends, that you haven't thought with lucidity for almost as long as you haven't bathed or injected or snorted or imbibed? How did you get to this unenviable position, the betrayals and disappointments heaping up like polished pebbles, collecting like the Legos you wanted so badly in a better lifetime?" My degrees and fancy education do not buy your respect. You answer my questions simply and unenthusiastically. I hear your anger, your curses, welling up from a lifetime of denials. Can I blame you for wanting a shower, clean sheets, or enough food to stop the rumbling? Can I blame you for trying to salvage your self-esteem by taking a break from the streets, if only for one night? If only I could restore the life you abandoned so many years ago.

I care less about the medicine than about the who and the why. I don't want to just patch up wounds and send them back to their semi-homes, semi-families, and semi-lives. I want to look into the gray eyes dulled by years of loneliness, the dangerous eyes flashing with blame and bitterness, the child eyes so scared that the world is going to leave them behind with nothing more than a paper tag in some distant morgue. I cannot stop until the swirling thoughts line up in rows and columns inside my head, and the answer comes to me clear and sparkling.

I want to know who you are and why you came to me.

— *Anju Goel*
Internal medicine resident, Montefiore Medical Center, Bronx, New York

Generations

Yvonne Braun is dying. She is very young, in her early 50s, and she has a widely metastatic adenocarcinoma of unknown primary. She's been through several rounds of chemotherapy with no response. She came in, this time, because the tumor invaded her spinal cord and paralyzed her from the waist down. She was admitted for radiation therapy to her back, a long-shot attempt to briefly restore some function to her legs. After a week, she has had no response.

One day after rounds, as I'm writing notes, Ellen, my attending, comes up behind me.

"You have Mrs. Braun's chart?"

I nod. She leans on the counter beside me, sighing heavily.

"I don't think she understands, really, what's going on here. She and her oncologist had the code-status conversation, but I don't think he talked to her, really, about what was going to happen."

"It's hard," I say. "It's so sad."

"It *is* hard. You don't want to take everything away from her. And yet, we owe it to her to give her the truth, so she can decide what to do with the time she has." She thinks for a minute, staring into space. Her eyes are both fierce and gentle. "Come." She nods to me. I'm surprised; attendings hardly ever invite me in to their conversations with patients, apart from rounds and formal family meetings. I set aside my charts and follow her.

Yvonne looks up as we walk in, surprised; it isn't the usual time for rounds. Ellen pulls a chair to her bedside and gestures for me to get one also. "Is this an okay time to talk?"

Yvonne nods.

Ellen pauses, choosing her words. "I just wanted to see . . . how you were feeling about things."

"Things?"

"Everything. All of this."

Yvonne waves her hand in a vague, helpless gesture. "I don't understand."

Ellen thinks for a moment, then speaks carefully. "As you know, you have a terrible cancer, one that is going to kill you, sooner or later. I don't know if anyone's talked to you about that. I don't know how you feel, what you think about it, what questions you have."

Yvonne stares at her in silence. It is a long time before she speaks.

"I— " She pauses, shakes her head. "I'm not ready," she says finally. "I'm afraid of dying. I don't know what it will be like. Well, I suppose no one does." A ghost of a smile drifts around her lips. "But I don't know . . . well . . . how it happens." She thinks for another minute, looks up with a strange curiosity in her eyes. "I mean, where does the cancer *go*?"

She gestures vaguely toward her chest, looks up at the doctor.

Ellen sighs. "There are different things that happen," she says slowly. "It's— It's not unlikely that you might get an infection. That's most often how people die. Rarely it's something else—the tumor invades into an important blood vessel or a part of the brain that makes you breathe. But infections are more common."

Yvonne nods, slowly. "So that's it," she says.

"What do you mean?" Ellen asks.

"Somehow I . . . I thought there would be more we could do." Her voice is distant, her eyes focused on something far away.

Ellen nods. "How does that make you feel?"

"Angry, I suppose," says Yvonne, a little absently.

"Angry. . . . at the disease? Or the doctors? Or just angry generally?"

"Well, at the doctors, too, I guess. It just seems like you're giving up."

Her word, "you," hangs in the air. She does not meet Ellen's eyes, or mine.

"To have people be sick, and not to be able to do anything to help them—that's not why any of us went to medical school," says Ellen quietly. "We're angry, too."

"I got two rounds of chemo," Yvonne says. "There's a woman I met downstairs, she has breast cancer, and she got ten rounds. Why aren't you doing that with me?"

Ellen sighs. "The kind of cancer you have—it doesn't tend to respond well to chemotherapy."

"It doesn't tend to. But how do you know, with me? Why don't you try?"

"We do know. Those two rounds that you got, that was us trying. And it didn't work."

Yvonne still looks unsatisfied.

"We could give you chemo," Ellen says gently. "We could keep giving it, even if it didn't do any good. But then what would happen is, you'd get sick, and be in pain and throwing up and miserable, and even more likely to get an infection. And then you'd lose your chance to spend the time that you have at home, with the people that you love, feeling as well as you can. Knowing that it wouldn't help, we don't want to take what you have away from you. That's why we're not doing chemo." Ellen's voice is soft at the end, and full of pain.

Yvonne nods, slowly, thoughtfully; this time she seems to understand, to accept. "I see," she says.

There's a long pause. "Well," Yvonne says, resolutely, "why don't you let me just go home now? To take my few days and be there, at least. If there's nothing we can do."

"Oh." Ellen is suddenly almost brusque. "I don't think it will be anything like that. I think you've got a lot more than a few days. Months, maybe."

Yvonne frowns, doubtful.

Ellen goes on. "I'm more worried about—well, I remember when you came in. We talked, and I asked you what you wanted. You told me what you wanted most of all was to get home. You talked about walking through the rooms of your house, about cooking with your husband. I remember how animated you were about that."

I catch myself being surprised, not having known they had a talk like that.

Yvonne nods, sadly. "That was a long time ago."

"We are going to get you home—you understand that?" Ellen's tone is fierce.

Yvonne looks uncertain.

"*You will go home.*" Ellen's voice brooks no uncertainty. "I'm just afraid that you won't be able to do what you'd been planning when you get there. Like—like walking. I don't think you'll be able to walk."

"Oh." Yvonne thinks for a minute. "Well, that doesn't matter so much really. Just to make use of whatever I do have, and to be there, in my own place, and with my husband—"

"You've got a wonderful husband. I'm very much impressed by him."

Listening, I smile at her choice of words: "very much impressed." Yvonne's husband has been here almost all day, every day, since she came in. He sits on her bed and they hold each other's hands, stare into each other's eyes. He rubs her feet. Even when the whole team is in here in the morning, rounding, you can feel the love between them, a palpable presence in the room.

"I know," Yvonne says seriously. "I wish we had more time together," she adds, sadly.

"Many people never have any time with anyone who loves them that much," Ellen says. "Lots of people never experience that at all. Remember that; that you're lucky, too, as well as being unlucky."

Yvonne nods.

Ellen pauses. "Who else do you have that's important to you?"

"Well, there's Mother . . ."

I can hear love in her voice but also some other emotion. Guilt? Fear? I can't exactly place the conflict that I hear, but Ellen's next question shows she does.

"Does she know how sick you are?"

"No. Not yet."

"When are you going to tell her?"

"It's not so simple. She's seventy-nine. She's still in Germany, where I was born." She pauses. "I never envisioned it this way. I always thought it would be me going to her funeral, not the other way around." Her eyes fill with tears. "I can't bear to hurt her," she whispers.

Wiping away the tears that cloud my vision, I look up and see that there are matching tears in Ellen's eyes. She doesn't say anything, just reaches out to squeeze Yvonne's hand.

"I have a daughter, too," Yvonne adds quickly, changing the subject. "How old is she?"

"Thirty-one. She knows everything; she's been here a lot, helping. She's a great strength to me."

Ellen pauses for a long moment. "Having a daughter . . . gives your life continuity."

Yvonne nods. "It's a wonderful thing to have a daughter."

I want desperately to hear what she says next, but I lose the conversation for a second, swept back upon my own life and history. My mother's breast cancer was diagnosed when I was a first-year medical student. She's doing fine now, but the special terror of that experience colors my interaction with cancer patients, especially women close to her age. It's impossible for me to see them and not imagine her in their place. I cannot find the boundaries, the distance that allows you to watch someone's pain and not be consumed by it.

But I'm thinking of something else, too. My mother's mother died suddenly of a heart attack, in her early sixties. She and my mother had, always, a tempestuous relationship; I know it is one of the enduring griefs of my mother's life that so much went unsaid between them. One of the most vivid pieces of family history I carry is the story of my grandmother at my mother's bedside when I was born. They had not known that I would be a girl, and when I emerged, my grandmother whispered: "You'll get to know what it's like to have a daughter." My mother says it was one of the only times that she knew her mother was glad to have had her, glad to have a daughter. I think of that now, listening to Yvonne—"It's a wonderful thing to have a daughter."

My mother and I, at least, have acted on the lessons that she and her mother didn't have a chance to learn. If one of us were to drop dead tomorrow, the other would have no doubt about how much she was loved; there would be no words that needed to be said. What about Yvonne, her mother, her daughter?

With all this in my mind—Yvonne and her family, Ellen and whatever personal history guides her words, my own mother and grandmother— I have one of those moments of strange clarity in which everything seems interconnected, tied into some deeper truth and meaning. I see an endless network of mothers, daughters, granddaughters, playing out the myriad dramas of that connection. I see joy and regret, sickness and health, life and death, linked in their ever-turning cycles. We each come out of our mothers and give birth to our daughters, we are each beloved, we each will die in our time and in our way, we each have our part to play on this stage.

My head spins, my own life suddenly confused with my patient's. Yvonne's daughter is barely older than I am—what would it be like to go to my mother's funeral? Worse yet—shifting generations—what would it be like to know that my mother would have to go to mine?

Ellen and Yvonne are still talking.

"This might be a time to say some of these things," Ellen is saying.

"I already have."

"Good." Ellen nods and reaches for her hand.

Looking up, Yvonne studies Ellen's face, her gentle but serious expression, her eyes just a little red with drying tears. "How can you—" she asks suddenly. "I thought you weren't supposed to get emotionally invested in your patients." Her voice is tinged with wonder.

"You have to get emotionally invested," Ellen says. "It's the only way to be a doctor."

Yvonne nods.

We get up to go. I don't know what to say; I reach out and squeeze her hand. "We'll be here—Any time you want to talk, I'm here." I don't know it yet, but she will take me up on this; we will spend many hours talking in the weeks to come.

She presses my hand and nods.

In the hallway Ellen turns to study me. I say nothing, but I see her taking in the raw emotion in my eyes. "Are you okay?"

I nod. If I try to speak I'll start crying.

"Here. Let's go to the lounge."

She takes me by the arm and I, soundless, let myself be guided to the patient lounge, a pleasant half-enclosed space with a few sofas and a large window overlooking the water.

"Let me tell you a story."

I nod again.

"When I was an intern, on my oncology rotation, we had a patient—actually she was the other intern's patient, but she somehow gravitated more to me, I think because the other intern was a man, and she wanted a woman to talk to. Anyway, she attached herself more to me, and we talked a lot. She was very young—thirty-two—and she had breast cancer and she was dying. And it was terribly, terribly sad. She had two young children, and she had been engaged to be married. And her fiancé, when he heard about the cancer—he just flipped out, he couldn't deal with it. He disappeared."

I take a deep breath.

"So it was awful."

I nod, and she continues.

"It was Christmas time. And on Christmas morning, I go into her room; and she has this diamond necklace, in the shape of a snowflake—it's gorgeous. She pulls it out from around her neck to show to me; 'Look what I have—'"

"And I say, 'It's beautiful; where did it come from?' She says, 'My fiancé gave it to me.' So—you know he's back."

I smile, brushing away the tears that keep fighting toward my eyes, and she pauses a long moment.

"And then she says: 'Do you think I'll be well enough in March to have the wedding?' March was when they had been supposed to get married. Before all this happened." She takes a deep breath. "It's December. You have no idea how terminal she was— I mean, really. Just slipping away. I have no idea what I said. Whatever I could think of to get through the moment somehow. And I went back to the residents' room and just lost it. The rest of the team came in and there I was sobbing, and they were like, what, what? I told them, and you know what they said? They said, 'If you're that thin-skinned, if you're going to let things get to you like that, you shouldn't be in medicine.' That's what they said. And I spun on them, and I said: 'If I ever stop letting things get to me, that's when I'll quit medicine.' It turned out that the Chief Resident of Psychiatry was sitting there, listening to all this—I hadn't even seen him—and he stood up and said, 'That's the sanest thing I've heard all week.'"

I smile through the tears that are rolling down my cheeks again.

"It's not a bad thing to cry, okay? More than that: it's the right thing. It's what you need to do—for yourself, and for your patients, too. Don't give that up, okay? Don't let anybody talk you out of it."

I nod.

"Sit here for a bit, if you need to, all right?"

I nod again. "Thank you . . . " The words come out scratchy and faint.

She nods and walks away.

All at once I see another line running alongside the first. A line of women patients and women doctors, women students and teachers, running down from Ellen and her patient to me and Yvonne to the students I will someday teach and the patients they will love and care for. Encompassing, somehow, my mother and the wonderful gynecologist who found the lump in her breast, my grandmother who wanted to be a doctor but wasn't allowed to study medicine, who calls me now with questions about her health and says it's good to finally have a doctor she can trust. A network, not excluding men, but based in women's values; doctors and patients sharing each other's stories, laughing and weeping together, sharing difficult truths and happy ones. A network of joy and sadness and healing.

I sit on the sofa silently for a minute, letting this feeling run through me, feeling it strengthen me even as I continue aching for Yvonne. Then I reach for the telephone, to call my mother and tell her that I love her— even though I know she already knows.

— *Emily R. Transue*
General internist
Adjunct clinical faculty, University of Washington School of Medicine

Finding Beauty in Annie[6]

Annie walked into our clinic with her new insurance card.

She was short and funny looking with coke-bottom glasses. She was not a pretty child.

One look by the pediatrician gave her the diagnosis she would carry the rest of her life: Turner's syndrome. He performed a complete workup and referred her to an endocrinologist. Unfortunately, the growth hormone shots didn't really help since she was diagnosed so late.

But Annie wanted a "girl doctor" and insisted on becoming my patient. She wanted someone to talk with about her hopes, her dreams. One day, she ended up on my schedule. We talked for a long time about the future of a Turner's patient, about the sadness she felt when told that she could never bear children. We talked about why depth perception and mathematics were so hard for her, about why she would not likely drive in the future. We talked about tutoring programs and, last but not least, about getting her on DSHS and SSI. She belonged to a managed care plan, and I was sick of doing referrals.

I told Annie that if at 63 years of age, an old Italian woman can bear a child after menopause with the help of hormonal intervention, no miracle was impossible. God only knew that in 20 years technology might enable her to carry an implanted fetus. In the meantime, we would work on getting her contact lenses and a pair of twins (our joke for getting breasts). When Annie left, I dictated a three-page letter summarizing her entire past medical history and future prognosis. We applied for SSI and incredibly for me, got it on the first try. Her first goal was to get contacts.

Months later, Annie came in. She wore contacts and a little makeup. Now an acceptable date, she had gone to her high school prom and had actually danced with a boy. She was so excited. We joked that being short actually gave her one advantage: she could dance with all of the boys since they were all taller than her.

Annie recently turned 18. She has SSI and Medicare. I wanted to continue caring for her, so I applied to become a Medicare provider. After the sixth of approximately 40 blue pages, being asked yet again whether I had committed a felony or fraud, I pitched the partially filled out application into the trash. It was insulting and degrading.

I see Annie for free now. On her last physical, I praised her for her grades, her grooming, her dental hygiene, her personal appearance. She was beaming. She has joined a Turner's club and went camping for the first time in her entire life.

Her mother paid me with the only thing that she could. A tiny little African violet blossoming under a thick bush of ugly leaves. It seemed it was a little Annie in itself.

— *Teresa Clabots*
Assistant Clinical Professor of Pediatrics,
University of Washington School of Medicine

A Visit to the Doctor[7]

The door opened without resistance, and I entered. The doctor's waiting room was decorated with the popular industrial plums, blues, and grays, but there was enough mahogany to impart a sense of reverence. The room was tasteful yet warm, and it reassured me. I was surprised to be greeted there by a patient of my own, a doctor himself. It was like looking into a mirror, with doctor doctoring doctor, doctoring doctor, receding into infinity. My patient was an elderly man, a retired army physician, refined and gentle, with a keen if fading intellect. I sat one chair away from him and leaned toward him, close, but not too close.

He immediately began his own story of two episodes that occurred after I saw him in the office just a month before: eating dinner at a restaurant, hearing fading away, then, plop, on the floor. Same thing a few days later. I did a quick neurologic review of systems: no aphasia or dysarthria, no weakness, no numbness or diplopia. Simple syncope. Stokes-Adams. Pacer malfunction. Still he talked, needing me to know the details, more than once, of his experience. He was 85, alone, and falling down. I listened. Then the door opened, "Doctor?"

My heart beat faster as I passed through the inner door. I was there to reveal myself, to tell my tale of suffering, and I was embarrassed. Immediately upon entering, I looked up to see my doctor's face. She shot me a look of subtle chagrin, a shared confidence. "This way, Doctor." I sat and waited alone in the examining room for just a moment, heart still beating with anticipation. She came to me immediately. She knew the reason for my visit. My daughters had contracted head lice, and I had been doing battle with them for weeks. The lone adult in my household, I had no one to check me for the loathsome pests and, of course, my head itched constantly. I was mortified at having to seek her help with this problem. That I needed her for this intimate task made me keenly aware of my isolation. She spared me further history taking. She touched my head with sure, gloved hands, beginning the examination without delay, all amid a stream of confidences about how this happened to her once and how awful it was. My doctor's touch, her steady hands, her unmeasured understanding filled me with gratitude and relief. She completed her exam. "Nothing. You are fine."

The business at hand disposed of, she crossed the small room and sat informally on the examination table. (Now let's talk like colleagues. You really are OK, this said to me.) And suddenly it was clear to me that I was not OK. Slowly, I began to tell the real story, not the pretext or the first level of concern. I was sad, very sad. I was struggling at work. I was alone and heartbroken, having just ended an important relationship. There was no one to help me. My children and my patients needed me to be full and overflowing. Instead, I was a well gone dry.

The time allotted for our interview had long since passed. Still this good person, this kind and wise person, looked at me and listened. I felt like a fallen autumn leaf. My voice seemed far away and thin, quite empty of meaning. Still she regarded me. Still she listened and prodded me for more. She saw me clearly, more clearly than I saw myself, and then she very gently told me something painful to hear: "Deb, I think you're depressed." It embarrassed me. I felt exposed and weak. My competence was in question. I recoiled at first, but somehow the courage she showed was like the reach of a firm hand. I took it and was grateful.

The door opened and a nurse poked her head in apologetically. "The architect needs to see this room for renovations." My doctor looked up and said with an edge, "He'll have to wait." Again she turned to me, intent on completing our time together, putting the finishing touches on the creation. "He'll have to wait." I was amazed. Do my patients feel this flood of relief and gratitude? Are my patients healed by kindness in this way? We talked about treatment and I agreed to it "for the children." She refused this self-abrogation. "That doesn't make any sense," she said. "You don't deserve to suffer like this." At the time, I didn't believe her.

We finished, and it was time to leave. As we walked to the waiting room, the nurse mentioned again that the architect had waited for us. "That's the way the cookie crumbles," said my doctor. At that moment, she was a wall for me against the crush of life, a stronghold and safe haven. I was awash in gratitude. My business finished, I returned at last to the waiting room. My patient was not there. I felt alone briefly, but the subtlety of the place reassured me, and I gathered myself to face the day.

Outside was a gloomy March morning. The pewter clouds hung oppressively low. Their cold breath penetrated me, but I made no attempt to secure my jacket. I set out across the parking lot toward the hospital, my heart growing steadily lighter. As I walked, a rich collage of understanding began to dawn on me. Something had just happened. I had been blind. Now my eyes were opened. I had been deaf, and now I could hear. I, the doctor, had been struck low by my human frailty, subject to the same feelings of loneliness, isolation, and overwhelming responsibility that belong to other parents, teachers, professionals. I, the doctor, had experienced the great vulnerability of the patient. I needed help badly, so badly that I did not know how to ask for it. Had my doctor brushed me off or quickly written a prescription, I would have come away injured, not healed. I, the doctor, saw with new eyes my huge power as healer, power that wounds if it is not wielded with compassion. At yet another level, I recognized that what had happened in that examination room was simply an act of love. Love in any relationship, including that between doctor and patient, requires the courage to risk revealing oneself unedited, the willingness to notice and to listen, the willingness to surrender one's own ease or comfort, the willingness to share the suffering of another and the courage to risk and accept gentle confrontation. In this way, any loving relationship can heal. Any relationship hoping to heal without love falls short.

That day, I learned what it is to be in need and be taken care of. That day, I felt healing hands upon me and was left breathless with new awareness of the awesome gift and profound responsibility I had been given as a physician.

— *Deborah Young Bradshaw*
Clinical Associate Professor of Neurology,
State University of New York Upstate Medical University

Job Description

Looking down on the stretcher at Mark's seemingly perfect 23-year-old body, it was obvious to me that something was wrong. From his waist to his toes he didn't flinch when I poked his lower extremities with a 22-gauge needle. He had been traveling 45 mph when the snowmobile he was riding struck the telephone pole. The impact snapped his back. Even without a CT scan, I knew his spinal cord was transected.

In a well-run emergency room department, trauma care can be routine. As I finished my examination and took Mark's history, the nurses started intravenous lines, ordered X-rays, drew lab tests, and documented vital signs. I was calling for the Life Flight helicopter to fly him to Albany Medical, our closest trauma center, when I recognized Donna's voice coming from outside the curtain to Trauma Bay 10.

"Where is he? I was told to come here. Where's Mark? Is he alive?" Her terror rushed ahead of her.

My chest tightened as I pulled back the curtain. Donna was my friend. She had been my realtor when I came to Vermont, and we had bonded as we drove around the back roads trying to find that perfect country home. Mark was her son; I hadn't recognized him. In the face of his devastating spinal injury, I knew I had little hope to offer as a physician. As Donna's friend, hope was all I had to give.

This is my job. I have worked in a rural Vermont community as an emergency physician for the past decade. Prior to this, I trained and practiced in emergency rooms in Philadelphia and Albany, New York. Urban emergency medicine trained me for gunshot wounds, craziness, unexpected violence and bad coffee. The day-to-day chaos was dealt with an impersonal anonymity. In Bennington, Vermont, it is impossible to be indifferent.

In this town, population 23,000, if I haven't treated someone personally, I have at least tended one of their relatives or someone they know. Gunshot wounds are rare, usually occurring during hunting season. Chaos occasionally prevails, but there isn't a sense of inevitability associated with it as there is in inner-city ER's. The coffee is still bad.

What connects me with everyone else in this community are but one or two degrees of separation. I have been doctor to my friends, plumbers, city councilmen, and local CEOs. I know which attorney has an alcoholic brother and which store clerk tried to commit suicide. I sit on a board of directors with someone I treated for a bad case of diverticulitis. I had to tell my state's representative that he was having a heart attack. When my house contractor's mother died unexpectedly during my shift in the ER, I was the one who met him in the waiting room. Even at the repair shop, the mechanic updates me on his wife's health since my colleague had treated her for a GI bleed. I rarely wait in line without someone asking me, "Do you remember me?" As my groceries are rung up, my mind races through the thousands of faces hoping one will register and praying that I didn't make any mistakes.

My training had prepared me for the care of the injured and ill, but it had done little to prepare me for the care of a small-town community: how to mind its secrets, tend its worries, and assuage its grief. Those skills I had to learn on the job.

At 42, I still consider myself a young physician. I may not be on the cutting edge of academic medicine, but I am at least close to the blade. Since entering medical school 20 years ago, I have witnessed transformations within health care that seemed inconceivable. The first reported case of AIDS occurred during my medical training. Wearing gloves when examining a bleeding patient wasn't mandated when I first worked a shift in the ER. Managed care, once thought only to be a California anomaly, has left no corner of health care untouched. Almost every decision I make in the emergency department is being regulated, scrutinized, or digitized, and the paperwork seems to grow exponentially.

I deal with these issues, their benefits and defects, on a daily basis, overwhelmed at times with frustration at what seem the Sisyphean complications of medicine. Yet there are still the Donnas and Marks—tragedies immediate and exacting—that transcend this tediousness. And there is the fulfillment of caring for my community.

When I finished my shift on the night of Mark's accident, I drove the 45 minutes to Albany to be with Donna and her son at the trauma center.

I knew they would be alone, the residents and attendings too busy to spend time with them. My shift was over, but my job wasn't finished.

— *Katherine Uraneck*
Freelance medical journalist and emergency physician

Notes

1. From LaCombe, M. A. (1990). Living the patient's story. *Annals of Internal Medicine, 113*(11), 890–891. Reprinted by permission of the American College of Physicians-American Society of Internal Medicine.

2. A version of this article first appeared in *Salon*, a Web site at http://www.salon.com.

3. From McMurray, J. E. (1998). Heartsick. *Annals of Internal Medicine, 128,* 315–316. Reprinted by permission of American College of Physicians-American Society of Internal Medicine.

4. Excerpted from Remen, R. N. (1996). *Kitchen table wisdom: Stories that heal* (p. 3). New York: Riverhead. "Life Force" from *Kitchen Table Wisdom* by Rachel Naomi Remen, MD, copyright © 1996 by Rachel Naomi Remen, MD. Used by permission of Riverhead Books, a division of Penguin Putnam, Inc.

5. From Clever, L. H. (1999, July 6). A doctor alone with her decision. *San Francisco Examiner*, p. A-17. Reprinted with minor editorial changes by permission of the author and publisher.

6. This first appeared in the Pierce County Medical Bulletin. Reprinted with permission.

7. From Bradshaw, D. Y. (1999). A visit to the doctor. *Annals of Internal Medicine, 131*(8), 627–628. Reprinted by permission of American College of Physicians-American Society of Internal Medicine.

6

MOTHERING AND DOCTORING

Erik Erikson once reminded me that, for any mother,
the most difficult thing about having a second baby is
her feeling that she can't split herself in two, that she
doesn't have enough to give to both babies. Mothers who
try to work and mother at the same time feel that way, too.
They ask, Have I enough to go around? Just as mothers learn
they can love two children, however, so, too, does a genuine
concern for both baby and job bring out in them new energy
and abilities. This very upheaval, present in parents who try to
split themselves in two, is a striking reminder of how much
motivation and drive are really available for these two tasks.

— T. Berry Brazelton[1]

Mutual Benefits[2]

I am a better physician because I am a mother, and I know because of my
experiences as a physician that I am a better mother.

— Rebekah Wang-Cheng
Professor of Medicine, Medical College of Wisconsin
Columnist for the Milwaukee Journal-Sentinel *newspaper ("Dear Dr. Becky")*

Doctor's Daughter[3]

As a small child, I often stood on the stairway in my home, looking up at the pictures of my mother. O.U. School of Medicine, class of 1945. I counted the 69 sepia-toned faces many times, always coming back to my mother's in the oval composite photograph. My mother is one of only three women, and her countenance is serious and composed; the hair in a long, wavy cut typical of the period. In an old picture from the local newspaper, written the year before my birth, my mother is sitting at a desk, wearing a white lab coat, staring out at the camera from her desk at the sexually transmitted diseases clinic where she worked. "Young Doctor Works in Town," reads the headline.

"How come you never worked as a doctor, Mama?" I asked frequently. I often went on rounds with my physician-father in the early morning at the community hospital in the small southern town where we lived. In one minute flat, he could tap a chest, letting the straw-colored liquid rush through the brown rubber tubing to puddle in the glass vacuum bottle on the bed. The nurses stood by at attention, in their starched white dresses and peaked caps. In the small emergency area, my father would casually flip his tie over his shoulder and insert the needle for the lumbar puncture that would diagnose the subarachnoid bleeding in his patient. Afterward, we would drive home to the house, where my mother would be standing in front of the stove, scrambling eggs for my three brothers, who sat watching Saturday morning cartoons. My mother was always home.

"Well, I loved you children and felt you needed me at home. You would start sucking your thumbs or the babysitter would quit." On the day I was born in an army barracks hospital, a psychotic WAC ran amok in the maternity area brandishing a butcher knife. My mother hid me behind her body next to the wall and called my father to come take us home. Later on, a German war bride would sometimes baby-sit for my brother and me in a pinch so my mother could work. After the war, while my father was in fellowship training, there was a job for her at the public health department. The syphilis patients would sit on a long row of stools with their hospital gowns open in the back while she went from one to the other, performing the lumbar punctures for diagnosis or test of cure. It was the last clinical job she ever had.

Such were the stories of my childhood. In the small town near the mountains, my father worked first in solo practice, then with a gradually increasing number of partners. He was on call every second or third night for most of my childhood and was rarely home. The special office phone at home, one that we were never to answer, rang off the hook each call night. Ventricular tachycardia, acute myocardial infarctions, diabetic ketoacidosis, and acute leukemia were never discussed at the dinner table but were nonetheless an integral part of the household. His cotton shirts were ironed every afternoon, and a sandwich was always waiting on the table for the 20-minute lunch break he took every day as he read his mail. On Sunday afternoons, I would go into the office with him while he saw patients. Using his secret name for me, I would pick up the phone and say gleefully, "Doctor McMurray's office, Miss Bird speaking," to neighbors and patients who knew me only as a quiet, well-behaved child.

My mother, on the other hand, was at home for us every day after school, cooking dinner in the evenings when my father walked in after rounds. She kept the family in clothes, helped with homework, played music to dance to on rainy afternoons, ferried us all to swimming and music lessons, met with the teacher when my brothers got into trouble at school, and always made it to recitals. She was president of the local mental health society, gave the embarrassing sex talks in schools, and thrilled us all once with a hole-in-one on the golf course. A gifted amateur naturalist, she admonished me not to be squeamish while helping me dissect fish eyes at the lake in the summers. Almost none of the other women in her circle of friends worked; most had never been to college. In the evenings she read all the "Great Books," and she loved nonfiction on almost any subject. I would crawl around her under the covers as she lay reading in bed, feeling the safety and security of her body.

The first crack in her armor of stoicism came when Betty Friedan"s *The Feminine Mystique* was published. After reading the book, she refused to cook dinner for 3 days. She looked at me that afternoon and said, "I was smart; I could have done some things." I urged her to work out a way to drive the 3 hours to the nearest medical school in the state in order to get back into practice. But there were four children at home and one demanding, full-time private practice to support. Secretly, I chided my father for what I took to be his inflexibility in this regard; my mother simply said it couldn't be done.

I grew up, did well in school, and was a pre-medicine major in college. My father was emphatic in his support and unambivalent in his enthusiasm for medicine. "It's a great job. Easy, really. You just hang up your shingle and do things any way you like. People will come to see a woman physician. I wish your mother could have done it."

My mother was more cautious. "Whatever you want to do is fine; don't do it for me."

"How did you decide to become a doctor?" I once asked.

She responded in her typical low-key way, "I grew up in dust-bowl Oklahoma in the middle of the Depression. We had no money whatsoever. My father ran a garage, but I went to the state university. I was a chemistry major planning on going to pharmacy school, when a local couple urged me to go on to medical school. It was pretty simple, really. I just did it."

When my letter of acceptance came from medical school, she sent me a medical dictionary inscribed, "From one to another." Once in my clinical years, I began using her battered brown medical bag. Medical school was overwhelming, but memories of time spent with my father on house calls and in his office sustained me. I fell in and out of love a half dozen times, married during my residency, and ultimately started a family. My first job was exciting and utterly absorbing. Before the baby came, I was in every morning at 7:00 a.m., staying until late at night. No part-time work for me! Child care would be easy in the city where I lived, and my physician-husband was deeply committed to being involved as a father. It would all work out so easily. Why couldn't my mother have done this? I emulated my father at this point. My profession came first.

When my 4-month-old began reaching for his child care person instead of me and started sucking his thumb, I felt he needed me, as we had needed my mother. I cut back to part-time. Sitting with my child on my lap, I asked my mother, "Couldn't you have worked part-time?" This time, the stories were about the refusal of all the practices in town to hire anyone less than full-time. In fact, the only acceptable full-time jobs for women in her social strata were those of teacher or nurse. It wasn't considered acceptable otherwise.

My second child was born, and life got more complex. I would feel crazed with worry and guilt when a waiting room full of patients were waiting for me at the hospital while I sat helplessly in the pediatrician's office with a sick child. The nannies didn't want to work more than 8 to 10 hours a day, and the consultants always seemed to page me in the late afternoon while I was swinging the children out in the back yard. It was difficult to discuss the cardiac ejection fractions of patients receiving chemotherapy with the children squabbling in the background.

As I contemplated my own difficulties, I seemed to be headed down the same road as my mother and began to think more and more about the mystery of her lost medicine. I couldn't believe things had been so cut and dried, so matter of fact. How could she have avoided the gut-wrenching feelings of guilt, love, and inadequacy that I myself so often felt? And so I became instantly alert one hot summer day, as I sat by a pool with my mother and watched my two small children swim.

The question was innocent enough. "So, Mom, just how far did you get in residency exactly? What kind of doctor were you planning to be?"

At her answer I felt a sudden stillness, the sounds of the summer cicadas buzzing loudly in my ears. "I wanted to be a pediatrician, but I got sick."

Sick? My mother was robustly healthy and had not been sick a day in her life. "What do you mean sick, Mother? What kind of sick?"

She answered, "It was stress, I guess." And for the first time she told me the story of how she started in a pediatric residency during the war. Four men, one woman. All the men were married and lived with their families. My mother was given a small room for living quarters on the tuberculosis ward. Being skin-test negative, she was terrified of contracting tuberculosis and asked to be moved. She was then put in a room at the end of the hall in the nurses' quarters. "It was just too much," my mother said in a voice devoid of emotion. She moved to the town where her sister lived, met my father, and married. There it was. A shaky start in the profession: scared, unsupported, possibly unwanted in medicine. The other answer had been in front of me all my life: the demands of mothering, needs of a busy physician-husband, a reluctant profession, and small-town social mores that made employment difficult for a woman physician who wanted a home in addition to a career.

My father retired at the age of 62. After 40 years of working, he told me that he hadn't had a summer off since the third grade. A poem came from him once that said, "I wish I had picked more daisies." Although he would say that he had been more successful than he had ever dreamed, in other moments he would speak of "being sucked dry" by patients or mention fears and anxieties that kept him awake at night, shared with no one. My mother would bask in the glories of her grandchildren and never once mention her lost medicine.

As for me, I have come through. I am fortunate to have been able to work part-time and to have a physician-husband willing and able to be fully engaged as a partner in our enterprise of work and home. But the challenges have been formidable and not simply a matter of more child care, more housecleaning help, or take-out food. Children's needs are not always so easily postponed until after hours, and relationships need constant tending. More equal measures of love and work sustain me, options that were not available to my mother.

Indeed, my mother "could have done some things." She earned her career, working hard in difficult times. Because she was one of only three women in a medical school class, there is a temptation to say she was obligated to continue, no matter what. But as this doctors' daughter, I benefited from her choices and her sacrifices. "From one to another," she passed on to me a legacy of competence and a courage tempered with love, a battered brown medical bag and a dictionary. I understand what I did not see before.

— *Julia E. McMurray*
Associate Professor of Medicine,
University of Wisconsin, Madison

Conversation Hearts

It was not a lesson in nutrition. It was, instead, a moment with a bag of Valentine candy. Preteen girls in this world are vulnerable and fragile—and what they believe about themselves now will shape their lives for decades.

She did not care that I had been on call the night before and then made rounds on 11 complex patients before arriving at her game in the late morning. She knew, rather, that she was 11 years old, caught somewhere between childhood and something else that feels frightening at times. She was not interested that, while she was going for rebounds on the court, I was fielding pages from my cell phone in the stands. It was not relevant to her that I had 27 charts to dictate or that, in the next four days, I had to deliver two lectures and a children's sermon, none of which was written yet.

All she knew was that she has many questions about herself and the world, and sometimes she feels very alone. And she wondered how "conversation hearts" fit into it all. So I built her a message: "HI CUTIE - IT'S TRUE - YOU ROCK - FOR KEEPS - AWESOME - I HOPE - FOR YOU - REAL LOVE - HOW SWEET - NICE GIRL - BE GOOD - I'M SURE - URA 10." We giggled and ate the ones that said "KISS ME - ROMEO - MY GUY." Then the phone rang again and the moment was gone.

When many of us began as women in medicine years ago, we thought that we could be excellent physicians and outstanding mothers. We were right—and we were wrong. We have our 10-hour workdays. Then we come home and try to find out what we missed that day in the lives of our families, who will not long remember what important task we were accomplishing, but only that we were not with them.

It is not just about quality time. It is about being there to help them find answers to their questions, believing that they are important enough to deserve our presence. It is also about time for individual reflection, to nurture our own growth and maturity as persons, lest we lose the joy within each thing we do. We may do great deeds as physicians. Yet if in healing others, we generate brokenness in those who rely most on us, have we really done our best?

It might have been a lesson in nutrition. The teacher in me says it should have been. But that day we remembered what little girls need—the one in her and the one in me. May they not have to wait until next year's conversation hearts to get together again.

— *Janice E. Daugherty*
Director of Predoctoral Education,
Department of Family Medicine,
East Carolina University, Brody School of Medicine

Monday Morning[4]

In the prelight
A heavy sound from upstairs
I turn from the front door
    to investigate.

My three-year-old son stands
        naked
  in the soft penumbra of dimmed hallway light
Clutching his favorite blanket
    picture book and well-rubbed panther
      to his chest.
His toes curl on the wooden floor.

I am dressed and beepered—
No snuggling in the warm water bed this morning
    floating back to sleep till sunlight wakens.
Instead, we hug.
I kiss
     his thin neck.
I feel his small breaths.

His bedroom door stands closed,
    heavy in shadows.

At the operating suite,
The residents still at lecture
The patient not yet here,
I enjoy the rote motions—
  follow the green snake tubing to the ceiling
  barbotage dissolving drugs into syringes
  snap open the laryngoscope.

Around me all is bright   pristine   ordered
Primed.
Sterile instruments attend in precise, metallic rows.

I try to recall his just awakened warmth
  in that brief moment
    before

The patient arrives
Naked under hospital issue
Ready to sleep.

— *Audrey Shafer*
Associate Professor of Anesthesia, Stanford University School of Medicine
Author of Sleep Talker: Poems by a Doctor/Mother *(2001)*

"mommydoc"

One Saturday several years ago, I paid a courtesy hospital visit to Jessica Galvez, a five-year-old patient with severe juvenile rheumatoid arthritis. Jessica had just been admitted to the intensive care unit with a gastrointestinal bleed caused by her medication. Being a second-year family practice resident, I wanted to use my precious free Saturday efficiently. So I brought my visiting parents and three-year-old daughter, Arlen, along with the plan to visit the ICU en route to the playground.

I left my parents and Arlen to wait in the hallway while I visited with Jessica and her mother, Angela. Angela looked like she was barely holding on. She had not slept in two days and was frightened that her daughter would never get out of the ICU. I tried to reassure her, but as I looked at Jessica, my words sounded false. Intravenous lines trailed out of every limb, a nasogastric tube caked with dried blood stretched her right nostril, and her face was swollen from prednisone and too much rehydration fluid. This could hardly be the same girl I had seen several weeks earlier, laughing and running around the clinic room.

As Angela and I talked, I heard "Mama" whispered from across the room. I looked over assuming that it was Jessica's voice. To my surprise, it was Arlen, escaped from her magazine-reading grandparents. She had managed to slip into the room and was now standing at Jessica's bedside. Eyes wide, her fuscia sundress and bouncy pigtails made one bright spot in an otherwise somber scene. Apologizing profusely to Angela, I shooed Arlen back into the hallway.

In that moment I felt like I had broken a golden rule of doctoring. A rule that had been taught to me through example by the senior doctors whom I had shadowed in the early years of my medical training: Good doctors keep clear boundaries between the personal and the professional. These mentors were by and large kind men from an older generation who subscribed to the Marcus Welby school of doctor-patient relationships: Intimacy in the doctor-patient exchange is not a two-way street. Be friendly and solicitous, ask about details from a patient's life but never share details from your own.

By allowing my two worlds to converge, I now felt that I wronged everyone. It did not seem right that Angela, in her time of despair over her critically ill daughter, should experience the rude intrusion of her physician's vibrant three-year-old. At the same time, it seemed wrong that Arlen, in her preschool innocence, should see such unmistakable suffering—especially in another child.

Until Arlen walked into that ICU room, I had managed to convince myself that I kept my home and work lives in two tidy compartments. I changed out of my stained scrubs and shoes before I entered my house and rarely talked about my medical adventures at home. On those rare occasions when my family visited me at the hospital or clinic, I confined them to the cafeteria or a back room. On the other side, I never divulged details of my personal life to my patients. Yes, I just had a vacation but never mind where I went. Yes, I have a three-year-old daughter, but I won't share my parenting challenges, much less her name.

After that Saturday, Jessica moved into our home in the form of an imaginary playmate. She was sometimes Arlen's patient but more often her shopping companion, bus driver, or sister. I had expected Jessica's tubes and swollen face to be the source of nightmares, but that did not seem to be the case. Instead Arlen asked me many thoughtful questions about what it meant to be sick and in the hospital. For better or for worse, Jessica and her half-lit ICU room had opened Arlen up to another world and given her an entirely new perspective on her mother.

Fortunately, Jessica made a rapid recovery and was back at home within a week. I saw her with her mother several weeks later in my clinic. It was immediately obvious to me that my relationship with Angela had undergone a complete change. She spent as much time giving me unsolicited mothering advice as she did updating me on Jessica's progress. We commiserated about the challenges of balancing work and home. During that visit, she saw little of the persona I had worked hard to cultivate: the smiling doctor who asked probing questions of her patients but revealed nothing of herself. With considerable unease, I acknowledged that I was being a doctor and a friend at the same time.

My experience with the Galvezes made me take a fresh look at how I fulfilled my roles at work and in my personal life. I realized that, while that incident was more flagrant than most, the boundaries had never been clear. So much of me flows from home to work and back again. By attempting to establish clear divisions, I was fooling no one but myself.

As a nursing mother, it was not uncommon for my breasts to leak toward the end of a long clinic. I would look down during a patient encounter to see two wet bull's-eyes on my blouse. Usually, I would ignore patients' inquisitive stares and push on to finish the visit as fast as possible. Occasionally, I would be asked if I was nursing. "I don't know how you manage to do all this," they would say. I usually smiled, shook my head, and refocused on their problem. Not once did I say, " It is really hard. I never get a chance to pump my breasts because my practice is so busy. I find pumping to be incredibly difficult, and yet I am committed to

nursing my baby. As a matter of fact, I really miss my baby right now
. . ."

Never did my worlds merge as completely as when I was on call.
Two a.m. phone calls from mothers whose children would not sleep often
coincided with my children's wakeful hour. I would listen to mothers
describe their child's nasal congestion, cough, and restless sleep while
trying to stifle my own child's fussy shrieks. Sometimes mothers would
pause and say, "Sounds like you have a sick child too. Poor thing, you
are on call and have to deal with that at home." In response, I would
often shut the door to my daughter's room so as not to distract the caller
with her screams. Other times, my children would be laughing and
singing while I was trying to calm a worried parent. Then, too, I would
always shut myself in the closet to talk so that the caller would not be
subjected to my household's festive atmosphere.

By the same token, my work life was constantly making appearances
at home. The "hostible pager" was a permanent fixture on my waist;
always getting in the way during wrestling matches or buzzing during
story time. And then, of course, there was often my distracted state as
my thoughts were pulled away to a particularly troublesome patient.

Why then was I making such a concerted effort to keep my two
worlds apart? Keeping work out of the home seemed important to protect
my family from the sadness and suffering that I encountered on a daily
basis and, to a lesser degree, to maintain patient confidentiality. My
motivation for keeping home out of work was less clear. Was it to
maintain an air of professionalism so that patients would feel that they
were getting good care? Was it to not undermine their own suffering or
distract them from their problems? Was it to be as time-efficient as
possible in my busy clinic? Was it to avoid becoming too emotionally
invested in patients and vice versa? Or was it just to maintain a sense of
superiority and control? I am super doc-mom. What is overwhelming for
the average person is a cakewalk for me.

Whatever my reasons were for drawing these rigid boundaries, I now
see that the effort is futile. At work, I never stop being a mother, and at
home, I am still a caregiver to people other than my family. Since that
experience in the ICU, I have learned that acknowledging, rather than

squelching, these intersections can be good for all parties. I now find myself sharing many of my own experiences with sleep-deprived new parents, pregnant women, tortured teenagers, and others. I have realized that I am not distracting them from the purpose of their visit but rather reaffirming their choices and abilities. An anecdote from my own experience seems, in many cases, to prove much more useful than spouting off statistics or the latest research finding. Pictures of my two children are now slipped into the plastic sleeve of my identification tag. I happily introduce them by name and favorite antic-of-the-moment to anyone who is interested. Rather than silently accepting patients' compliments about my ability to balance so many roles, I will now talk about the challenges and conflicts that I face and even solicit advice. These moments have helped me become a wiser doctor and mother and have bolstered the confidence of my patients in their ability to care for themselves and others. Never, to my knowledge, have these exchanges lowered me in a patient's estimation or made her feel that her care was being compromised.

Sharing my work experiences around the dinner table (patient names withheld, of course) has also proved to be a good thing. I have found that explaining to my husband and children why I had a bad day, rather than silently mulling it over, does wonders to ease the problem. I am then able to focus on my family and our household activities. I never cease to be amazed at how much my now five-year-old can understand and how supportive she can be. When I come home in the evening, it is not uncommon for Arlen to say, "Mama, tell me about the kids you saw today." Recently, she asked me to be a special guest in her preschool class. I came armed with stethoscope, ophthalmoscope, and stickers and showed these to the children while Arlen sat like a puffed peacock on my lap. She explained to her classmates: "My mom is a doctor *and* a mommy."

This is not to say that there shouldn't still be boundaries. But in my view, the boundaries have become less rigid. While the Hippocratic oath and the California Medical Board give me some basic rules about how to interact with patients and how to integrate my profession into other parts of my life, the rest is up to me. I need to discover my own boundaries and my own persona rather than accepting that which has been laid out for me. The person (and doctor) that I am expected to be and that I want to be is very different from those older men who taught me. Of course, this is inevitable because I am a young woman and a mom—a far cry from Marcus Welby.

Epilogue

Several months after the ICU incident, Arlen and I were spending the day at the San Francisco zoo. There, in front of the African elephant cage, were Jessica, Angela, and Jessica's two sisters.

Arlen recognized Jessica immediately as one recognizes a much idolized celebrity. "Look Mama, there is Jessica Galvez."

Angela and I sat on a bench and ate popcorn while the girls climbed all over the bronze hippo statue and each other. For Arlen, seeing Jessica was more exciting than anything else the zoo could offer. Angela took a picture of the two girls on the statue, both with outrageous grins. This photo, which I keep on my desk, serves as a daily affirmation of my choice to connect my two worlds.

— Daphne Miller
Assistant Clinical Professor, University of California, San Francisco
Solo family practice, San Francisco

A Mother's Prayer[5]

Our children (reportedly ages 7 and 8) are refugees from Sierra Leone, West Africa. The country and its people have been ravaged by a brutal civil war for more than a decade, but we know nothing of the particular circumstances of our girls. To the best of our knowledge, both children arrived at the Child Survival Center in Makeni, Sierra Leone, in 1997. I remember when we learned that their orphanage was burned down in a rebel attack, and then there was no word of the 17 children or the orphanage staff for several months. We had all but given up the children for dead. Imagine our elation when we learned they had arrived at a refugee camp in Guinea after a 90-mile trek through their war-torn country. All 17 children with their caretakers had escaped into the bush with only the clothing on their backs.

I know nothing of the girls' medical or family histories. I know they experienced the sorrow of losing their families, felt the pain of starvation, and lived in fear for their lives. I couldn't even begin to imagine the horrors they have witnessed, more so after reading further news of that brutal war, including accounts of mutilation and limb amputations of women and children. I'm not sure I want to know what their eyes have seen.

I knew these circumstances in advance and was convinced I could cope with them. After all, I am a physician and I work in the inner city. I treat patients with parasitic diseases, hepatitis, HIV, and posttraumatic stress, as well as those who have experienced domestic and street violence. I take care of many refugees, some of whom have survived torture. I had read about older-child adoption issues. But what I failed to understand was simply how to be a mother and how to share and experience my girls' pain in a very personal way, in addition to balancing work, child care, and marriage.

The emotional burden has been heavy, starting from the moment we met the girls in Africa. I immediately realized that all of the medical reports we had received in advance were fictitious; it was clear that the necessary resources for HIV testing and hepatitis serologies were simply not available. (Later, my daughters confirmed they had never had blood drawn.) My older girl had fevers and diffuse lymphadenopathy. Performing a physical examination on my child immediately after meeting her was heart-wrenching. I was in a state of terror so cold I couldn't bring myself to share my feelings with anyone, not even my husband. I could not leave her, but what consequences would caring for an HIV-positive child have for our family? When another mother in our group asked me to examine her own sick girl (there were 10 children adopted in our group), who she said had not eaten in two days nor urinated in more than 24 hours, my cursory evaluation frightened me.

The child was lethargic with a fever and a pulse rate of 150. She needed to be in the hospital and I didn't know what to do. Where was a hospital? Was there even a hospital in the city? After talking to a physician at the U.S. embassy, and a subsequent middle-of-the-night trans-Atlantic telephone call to a pediatrician in Boston, we brought the girl by taxi to a nearby hospital. There, blood work, chest films, and lumbar puncture were not available. We had to settle for fluids, antibiotics, and a lot of prayer. Miraculously she recovered.

Once we arrived home and our daughters were in the process of their medical evaluations, I experienced firsthand the trauma of phlebotomy. Each girl had to be restrained, screaming and fighting; one soiled her clothing. Both were tested for HIV, hepatitis, sickle cell anemia, malaria, syphilis, and lead, tests recommended for all adoptees from that part of the world. It was even more traumatic when the blood work had to be repeated after a specimen was improperly processed. How many times has this occurred in my own practice? Thankfully, both girls are HIV-negative, although waiting for these results cost me weeks of lost sleep. I wonder about my own past indifference to patients awaiting diagnostic test results.

My younger daughter has had a difficult time with parasites and has horrible teeth and skin. Her age is still unknown. Results from her bone (3.5 years) and dental (6–8 years) radiographs and developmental assessments (4–5 years) are discordant. She has undergone colonoscopy for persistent rectal bleeding, which revealed previously undiagnosed schistosomiasis. Next she faces oral surgery because of poor jawbone development resulting in excessive decay. These are all things I can't let worry me or I would go crazy. We have seen so many specialists that faces, names, and waiting rooms have all blurred together. What has stuck in my mind, however, is that now-familiar look of either outright or incompletely disguised anxiety in mothers' faces as they wait their turn.

My head often spins from receiving so much information. Because I am a physician, other medical professionals seem to assume I have a complete understanding of all of our girls' medical conditions and am therefore capable of making informed decisions. This clearly isn't the case. Objectivity is blinded by parenthood, and I often leave a physician's office feeling confused and scared, trying to remember what was said and always questioning whether I am making the right decisions.

But the major afflictions that plague my children cannot be seen on the skin or measured by stool samples or blood tests. After reciting the story of a fire drill at her new school, my younger daughter added, "Dead people burned look icky." My oldest girl describes people being killed in front of her and of being forced to strip naked and held at gunpoint. One of their friends from the orphanage is covered with scars from cigarette burns. One night during dinner my oldest daughter suddenly became catatonic, overcome with fear at the sound of bass vibrations from a stereo in a car out on the street, which she had mistaken for impending bombing. She was afraid to go into her room to bed, and clutched me inconsolably all night. "I scare, Mama! Bad people!" is all she said. This experience cannot be reconciled with all of the medical information in the world available to me. Now the possibility of sexual abuse has surfaced, although I may never know for sure if the girls experienced this. My younger daughter arrived with the provocative behavior of kissing males on the mouth (even men she doesn't know). Both girls, through description and play, have demonstrated they are familiar with the act of sexual intercourse. When explaining to my younger daughter about the required enema prior to her colonoscopy she was terrified, not naïve to the concept of rectal penetration. She was surprised and relieved that the procedure didn't hurt.

The week our house turned into a no-sleep zone because of the girls' recurring nightmares was also the week our pediatrician happened to be on vacation. My oldest daughter dreamed that rebels from Sierra Leone came into our house and cut out her throat so she couldn't call mama for help. She tearfully nodded when I asked if she had seen something like this before. This was followed by a casual revelation during dinner that the children were forced to participate in beating a captured rebel child-soldier with sticks while he was tied up. They were told that he was a bad boy and that beating him would make him a good boy in heaven. I have never before felt so helpless or out of control. In my sleep-deprived state, I was on the verge of falling apart when a colleague intervened. The next thing I remember is talking to a pediatric psychiatrist from my own institution, who saw us immediately. What if I hadn't received special treatment because I was an employee on the medical staff? In addition, I never would have imagined how vulnerable I felt as the only white person in a waiting room filled mostly with minority families from the inner city. Although I care for this population in my own practice, it is somehow different sitting in the same waiting room, and this unease just added to my feelings of inadequacy, both as a professional and as a person. When a clerk called out the girls' names (mispronouncing them), I directed her attention to us. All eyes in the waiting room turned toward us. "Where is their mother? I need a parent to fill out these forms," the clerk's voice boomed across the room. The insensitive handling of this encounter was an attack on my already vulnerable relationship with my daughters.

Navigating through "the system" in my own profession has been extraordinarily difficult, and the experience has been a wake-up call to how oblivious I had become in my own practice and to how impersonal the practice of medicine has become. With the constraints of 15-minute visits and productivity quotas, I can't remember the last time I asked a patient "How are you, really?" and meant it. I don't have time to get beyond the last mammogram, Pap smear, cholesterol, or viral load results. I had never even thought to consider patients' experiences in the waiting room or what happens to them when I go on vacation. How do they get through the impossibly complicated medical maze—especially those who are illiterate or don't speak English? My insight has certainly changed in the past few months, hopefully to the benefit of my patients. I am suddenly finding out things about their lives I never knew, but should have known. I am much more liberal about giving out my beeper number for emergencies and for those times when patients fail to negotiate the cumbersome telephone system. I now know what it is like to feel alone and helpless.

I was completely unprepared for the drastic change in my life and sometimes feel I have taken on too much. My husband and I haven't had time to think about the challenges ahead, such as how to incorporate cultural diversity into our family or how to deal with and teach our children about prejudice, which is already occurring. I was naïve enough to think we would not meet resistance to raising a multiracial family in the Boston area, on the dawn of the new century. It has been a painful lesson to learn that violence and illness affect not only individuals but whole families, and some days I feel that we are all under siege. Getting through one day at a time is currently my only goal.

Parenting support and career counseling in the academic medical arena are difficult to come by, and there is little time to seek help elsewhere. I feel guilty about conflicting priorities—how does one not compromise one's career and remain sane?

But I know somehow I'll make it through.

International adoption, especially of refugee children, is more complicated than I expected, and although for us it has been infinitely rewarding, there are also stark realities for which I was not prepared. But these children and their past are now part of me. I love them unconditionally. My body aches with unspoken wishes that my daughters will develop a full sense of trust and feel the stability of a family. It brings tears of joy to my eyes to hear them say, "Mama, I love you."

Although I want to erase the past my children have lived and the terrible burdens they carry, I know I cannot. Even so, knowing them has helped to redirect my approach to life and to establish new priorities. They have thankfully influenced what had become a business-like approach to my own medical practice: I am reminded why I went into medicine in the first place. I must remain optimistic that I will find a new balance to my life.

And I pray for the night when I don't cry myself to sleep with worry about these two wonderful girls who are my daughters.

— *Sondra S. Crosby*
Assistant Professor of Medicine,
Boston University School of Medicine

On Being a Medical Mom

Being a medical mom is . . .

Walking into your medical school interview 8 months pregnant and feeling your chances evaporate when the interviewer says, "Mazel-tov."

Being chagrined when your own mother says "But, I thought you'd gotten over wanting to do that."

Having 2 weeks to find day care and hoping it's good.

Leaving with your infant at 6:30 a.m. every morning for the 90-minute commute to daycare and the 8 o'clock class.

Having your baby develop a temperature of 102° every time you have an exam.

Being a medical mom is . . .

Trying to look alert on rounds as a pregnant medical student.

Knowing what sleep deprivation is about before starting internship.

Hearing your kids cheer as you receive your medical school diploma.

Being greeted after the last call of residency by scotch-taped crayon banners proclaiming "No more night call—Yea!"

Being a medical mom is . . .

Begging for the morning car-pool duty so your kids have a ride home from school.

Providing transportation for the after-school program supervisor so you won't be charged an arm-and-a-leg late fee on your house officer income because you are late and the last parent to pick up every day.

Being the lady doctor at grade school career day.

Making Valentine cookies for three classrooms at midnight because it's important.

Hoping your kids will play quietly at the nursing station when they accompany you on your weekend rounds.

Insisting that the family eat dinner together every night — dinner is at eight.

Being a medical mom is . . .

    Managing the house by cell phone.

    Listening to the jokes *they* turn out based on *your* dinnertime medical conversation.

    Gearing up to edit/type term papers at 10 p.m., when you'd really rather close your eyes.

    Worrying all day that there might be a late emergency when you have to leave on time for the play/recital/soccer game/awards ceremony.

    Being amazed and proud of honors received, speeches given, and scholarships awarded them at their graduation ceremonies.

    Being relieved that your professional life didn't ruin them after all.

Being a medical mom is . . .

    Feeling immense pride and elation when your son, who began medical school with you, receives his diploma from medical school.

    Being grateful to have shared this experience with a loving and supportive medical dad.

— *Cynthia Gail Leichman*
Professor of Medicine, Albany Medical College
Director, Multidisciplinary Gastrointestinal Oncology Program

Tsunami Baby

It's 2:55 a.m. My neighbors' windows are all dark, in keeping with the night. It seems that I alone stare out at the few faint stars, as though they will tell me that what I am doing is all right. I am a worrier and, worse for those who love me and hence are stuck with me, a compulsive planner. I am also a doctor and a wife, not necessarily in that order. Sleepless nights have been part of my life for as long as I can remember. That is not what's new. What is new is that, in seven hours, I will lock the door behind me and leave my first-born child on the other side when I go back to work. Almost everything I've done for the last six months has been with her, for her, or about her. This curly-topped, rosy-cheeked, sweet cuddle of a child has been my life.

I have never felt so torn. No one could have made me understand the fierceness of the longing and the wonder and joy of a baby or the depth of the exhaustion from round-the-clock nursing and the helplessness when nothing seems to soothe her. My daughter will not take the bottle and merely mouths at baby food. The times that she does wrap her tongue around the applesauce are still warm-ups: She just turns around and spits it out again. This baby wants nothing but the real thing, her mama's milk directly from the source.

My friends and colleagues did their best to prepare me. "Get a pump. Medela works the best and Kaiser has a great deal." "Work two hour blocks so you're not gushing like an Italian fountain." "Cabbage leaves." *Cabbage leaves?* "Eases the engorgement and they tuck right into your nursing bra." "Nurse lying down—you'll both be better rested for it." *Back to work.* "No more than three days a week, ten to twelve hours if you can swing it financially after a good long maternity leave." *How long a leave?* "At least three months, no six, well, a year, okay five years." And for the final chorus, "It will go by fast. Oh, and find a nanny. A good one."

The pump did the job. So did the cabbage leaves and nursing lying down.

But back to work. I'm fortunate enough to have a solo psycho-therapeutic practice. After ten years of being "out in the world," I can set my office hours to suit my own needs and select for patients who can tolerate a part-time practice. While I was on leave, every patient had a doctor they could see. There was even a backup for my backups set in place. I had a plan.

Having our baby was planned. My husband and I had seven years together, two analyses—one for each of us—and two whole lifetimes of yearning for a happy family in anticipation for this baby. We weren't completely naïve. During my pregnancy, my husband would joke about the tsunami that would overtake us. He always got a good laugh, especially from our other friends who were expecting around the same time as we were. When my water broke, our tsunami baby was let loose, creating a landscape of emotions with heights and depths no plan could map out for the two of us.

In just five hours of contractions and two hours of pushing, our lives were transformed by this 7 pound, 14 ounces of a beginning. She came into the world blood-orange red, coated by sticky strands of white vernix. Her little mouth pursed forward, suckling at the air. I tried to hold her off until the nurse was free to ensure that she latched on properly, but she decided that wasn't necessary. She had her own ideas and knew exactly what she needed. Me.

My husband sometimes asks me if I remember life before our tsunami baby because he cannot. I answer yes, that was when there seemed to be a point to making plans.

Now, it's the little one with the soft spots on her head who calls the shots. She cries, I hold her. She yells, I feed her. She whines, I check her diaper. When she is sad or angry, I am anxious and frustrated. When she is happy or relieved, I am overjoyed. She's staked her claim, and I belong to her. The first time I left the house without her to go Christmas shopping, it seemed as if the world was tilting on its side and I had lost my sense of balance. I missed the press of her against my body. In 45 minutes I was back home breathing in her damp milk smell, delighting in her coos and trills and bubbling raspberries.

I had not planned for this. This awful sense that if I leave her I am lost. The thought of her calling for me and my not coming to her sends me into a kind of panic I have not felt since my first broken heart. I do not want to go. It's almost 5 a.m.

One of my patients had confronted me before I left. He was sure I wouldn't come back from my leave, thinking that I would stay home with my baby. Openly, we discussed his pain over good-byes and his fear of being cast aside, and in the end, he demanded my assurance that I would, indeed, be back. Assurance was easy to give then. I love practicing psychotherapy to help people change and grow. I still do. It's just that now I've got another love who also needs me, and she comes first. I am her mother.

I hope she will understand the choice that I am making. Besides being her mother, and a planner and a worrier, I want to be a person on whom she and others can depend. In this millennial world of excessive choice, there are few vows to make. I have made two, one as a wife—to love and cherish and be a helpmate; the other as a doctor—to do no harm. So I will return to work for my patients, who have tolerated the disruption of their therapy, and for my husband, who has toughed it out as a sole provider in a city where the cost of living has tripled in the last two years.

I won't be taking on any new patients for awhile. I need to find my balance in the wake of my tsunami baby. The only plan I have right now, before I leave, is to walk upstairs and kiss my sleeping daughter on that soft spot of her head to reassure the both of us—Mama will be back.

— *Kathleen Dong*
Former Associate Clinical Professor of Psychiatry, Stanford Universaity
Now full-time mother

A Patient's Wife

"Women endure more," she said,
"Like the death of my son
suddenly, from a heart attack.
I—a mother—thought it would be impossible.
Then I looked into my husband's eyes
and saw the suffering that had no words.
To express myself meant everything."

Is it so? Perhaps.
But I am a mother and a psychiatrist
Not that one precludes the other.
I only quote Aunt Ethel
Who said to me, as I say to my son,
"I love you more than my life."

— *Ruth Cohen*
Assistant Clinical Professor of Psychiatry, Cornell University
Private practice

The Transition Game

In basketball, they call it the transition game: that time when the defense switches to an offensive stance, the transition between rebounding and going toward your own basket. Mothers, too, play the transition game, and it is as tricky and skillful as any move on a hardwood court. The transition is between work and home—more specifically, turning off your job persona and becoming that simple yet all encompassing character, Mom.

I am an emergency physician at a busy hospital and trauma center. After 10 hours of taking care of unstable and critical patients, I come home to find my three-year-old snuggled up to his dad, watching a Barney tape. *He was waiting up for you,* my husband says. I scoop my son in my arms and take him straight upstairs.

I'm playing the transition game. Just moments before, I was managing patients, supervising residents, calling technicians, ordering labs—in short, running an ER. Now I'm teasing a three-year-old in "feetsy" pajamas to brush his teeth. I'm still in my hospital scrubs, looking like I'm ready to perform surgery. Into bed he goes, and of course, I must lay with him and read him a story. Tonight it's *Make Way For Ducklings,* a gift for his third birthday. While I read the tale of Mr. and Mrs. Mallard, my pager is digging into my left hip. As we discuss the future of the eight ducklings, my son lays his head on my chest and is so quiet I know he'll be asleep soon.

The transition is pretty much over by then. I'm completely Mom now. My doctor role is finished, my shift is becoming a distant memory, and my son is going to sleep. Victory. Now I can go eat myself into oblivion, since I haven't eaten all day.

Do men feel this strange duality, I wonder. When one of my colleagues returns from a busy shift, is it also odd to turn into Dad and put away the trappings of the job?

There is redemption in the transition game, though. After a day when I watched a man die of a ruptured aorta and another almost hemorrhage to death from an ulcer, it makes perfect sense to read about the Mallards' search for a home for their ducklings. The end of life, and preventing the end of life, is a mad preoccupation. A child reminds you of the beginning, that there are always beginnings, and they are ripe for exploration. Phone calls, computer readouts, lab values are just white noise. The symmetry of life saves me. When I get to be Mom again, I'm back to beginnings. And where there is a beginning, there is hope.

— *Bonnie Salomon*
Emergency physician, Lake Forest Hospital, Lake Forest, Illinois
Freelance writer

Interview for Clinician-Educator Position

While attending an epidemiology course, I am invited to dinner by a group including three physicians from the university at which I'm to interview for a faculty position the next month. It is an impromptu, informal interview. In tow is my 10-month old, whom I'm still breast-feeding.

"What are your interests outside work?"

> *Well*
> *I like to bake from the A-B-C cookbook*
> *I like to prepare arts and crafts*
> *We take walks in the neighborhood*
> *We play billy-goats-gruff on the school play equipment*
> *Play kick-ball*
> *Play chase*
> *Play dress-up*
> *Read board books*
> *Sing and dance to children's songs.*

"I enjoy cooking, painting, hiking," I say,
"And I'm really into my kids."

— *Stephanie Nagy-Agren*
Assistant Professor of Internal Medicine, University of Virginia
Chief, Infectious Diseases Section,
Veterans Affairs Medical Center, Salem, Virginia

Spiderlings

As I take care of chronically ill patients everyday who have end-stage renal disease and are on dialysis, I am reminded that this is it. This is the main show. Every day must count. I write in part to capture those moments that go by so fast never to return. For instance, at our house now with two children, every sentence begins with *Mama*.

> *Mama-Mama where are my shoes?*
> *Mama-Mama did you sign my homework folder?*
> *Mama-Mama what happened to the dinosaurs?*
> *Mama-Mama how come they let that big guy skate in the Olympics if he keeps falling down?*
> *Mama-Mama how do they make those tires that can run over nails and not go flat?*
> *Mama-Mama what are we having for dinner?*

I answer all clothing and food questions, but I sometimes pass on those that involve Olympic Committee policy or polymer chemistry. I'm not above expounding on creative theories about the extinction of the dinosaurs with something like, "Tyrannosaurus rex refused to bathe for a week and all the dinosaurs around him keeled over dead. Now go take your bath."

Mama-Mama has reinforced my sense of being at the center of the universe for my children. I am their pivot point. They send out the Mama ping and when my reply bounces back to them, they feel secure in their location in life. Mama-Mama can answer all questions, perform all tasks, meet all needs. Mama-Mama is the center of knowledge, the hero of the planet.

I knew that my children would eventually mature enough to see beyond the Mama-Mama universe, but it had been our accepted world for so long that I was not prepared when my seven-year-old slipped out of the Mama-Mama orbit. It was near Martin Luther King's birthday, and he and I were driving home from an evening celebration of music and dance in honor of the civil rights leader. From the back seat, Cabell was planning his future as either a soccer player or professional football star.

"I like football," he said, "but I cannot decide which position I should play, Mama. Mama, if you played football what position would you play?"

"Well you know, Cabell," came my words of Mama wisdom, "I loved football when I was your age. I thought it was the world's greatest game. I watched college games and professional games and at night I would dream of being a football player. I would dream of being a quarterback in charge of calling the plays, taking the snap, and rolling back to pass the perfect spiral. I would dream of being a tight end sprinting out long for the pass and making the perfect catch with my fingertips. I would dream of being a linebacker, agile and quick, breaking through the line and sacking the quarterback with awesome power."

There was silence for a moment in the back seat. Then Cabell said, "That's not the same dream Martin Luther King had."

In that moment, he was out of the Mama-Mama universe, and I knew it. It was bound to happen, but who would have thought I would get ousted over football. Of course, at bedtime Dr. King wasn't there to scratch his back and Mama-Mama worked a little gravitational magic.

Sometimes raising children is like knowing the natural history of diabetic nephropathy. You can see that the renal function is normal, but once the proteinuria is there, what can you do? You pull out all your tricks, like tight blood sugar control, blood pressure control, ACE inhibitors, but you know the future. Raising children is like that for me, too. You know the prognosis, but you do whatever it takes to slow it down.

Last September on a Saturday afternoon off, my husband and I were hauling rocks from a pile near my garden to the road bed by the pond. These were the same smooth pebbles that, two years before, we had moved from a pile near our house out to cover the walking paths of my garden. We have a long tradition of doing the same work time and again.

As sometimes it happens in Southside Virginia, the September air was still summertime warm. Frank and I worked in tandem shoveling the rocks onto the tractor lift. We wore shorts and tee shirts, and Frank had begun to drip sweat from his brow. We were ready for a rest when Cabell called us to come see what he had found in the backyard. As we walked over to where he was crouched in the grass, he said, "Look at this spider."

Actually, in the previous two weeks we had looked at a lot of spiders. Cabell's second-grade class had finished the unit on frogs and toads several weeks before, and since then, we had switched from hopping after amphibians to peering at arachnids. We had identified sheet webs on the windowsills and found a funnel web in the privet hedge. We had observed the spider that lived in the giant web outside his bedroom window to catch bugs attracted by his light at night. We could identify the spider cephalothorax, and we knew that the sticky silk was dispensed from the spider's abdomen by the spinnerets.

That day, Cabell had a new spider lesson for us. We hunkered down beside him and followed the beam of his index finger to the tan and black spider making her way among the stalks of grass. At first, she looked like an ordinary spider, and then Cabell pointed out the cargo of tiny spiders she carted on her back. "See," he said, "she's a mother spider. Maybe she's a wood spider or a jumping spider, but she's carrying all of her babies. They are called spiderlings."

I loved that word, *spiderlings*, and sure enough, there must have been a hundred very tiny baby spiders clinging to the back of the mother spider. We watched her labor along, and Cabell continued, "She'll carry them until they get big enough to be on their own. Then one day they'll leave her back and crawl to the top of a blade of grass. Then they'll send out a string of silk." Cabell swept his hand from the top of the grass out into the open air. "The wind will catch the strand and send them flying off. It's called ballooning." The three of us sat for a moment gazing over the field imagining the troops of spiderlings sailing off into the world away from the mother who had carried them on her back.

My husband looked at Cabell and asked, "Will you ever go ballooning away from us?" "Nope, never," Cabell replied with an honest heart, and he grabbed his soccer ball and ran off to play leaving us there in the grass.

Frank and I stood and watched Cabell dribble the soccer ball in the
far yard. I crossed my arms, squinted my eyes, and leaned toward my
husband, "I don't believe him," I grumbled. "He'll be ballooning off before
we know it. With no warning, one day he'll just leave. I say we stock up
on scissors, and any sign of a silk strand, we snip it at the abdomen."

"It's a deal," Frank nodded. "His cephalothorax is grounded."

— *Dugan Wiess Maddux*
Private practice nephrology, Danville Urologic Clinic

Teeter-Totter

There is no way to plan ahead to integrate family and career. If you are
not yet a parent, you have no idea how incredibly in love you will fall
with your baby. If you are not yet in practice, you have no idea how
much you will belong to your patients. What you can do is learn to be
flexible, to set priorities, to accept help, and to make amends. You can
never do full justice to both realms.

In my experience, there was more flexibility in academic, urban
medicine than in suburban private practice. Salvation is finding a niche.
For me, it was developmental pediatrics, a fascinating, time-limited field,
suited to my particular talents. I limited myself to this focus after
discovering that I could not bear to leave my own sick children at night to
go see someone else's.

The two arenas, family and medicine, enrich each other. You will be
a much better doctor for having been a parent. You will be a much better
parent for having been privy to the human drama of medicine. What your
children lose in time with you, they gain in pride and inspiration in
having a professional role model.

When feeling torn between family and work, it is important to
remember that you suffer from an abundance of blessings. The privilege
of doing work that you love and having a family you cherish are causes
for rejoicing in spite of your fatigue and strain. There is no steady state.
You will never achieve a durable balance between career and home. Flux

is the norm, the only constant. You will always be giving more in one area or another. You are astride a teeter-totter. Don't be frozen in the middle, trying to keep it perfectly level. Learn to prance, slide, skip, skid, and skitter from one end of the see-saw to the other.

— *Marcia Quereau McCrae*
Developmental pediatrics

Breast-Feeding: Straddling the Fence Between Work and Home

Like many, I often feel myself pulled between the competing demands of family and career. For years, I have struggled to keep the two worlds of home and work separate and in balance, ever fearful that the demands of one will overwhelm the other. There is some truth to the old adage, "good fences make good neighbors." But the artificial fence that I've erected between home and work has been challenged by the birth of each of my children—in particular, the question of breast-feeding after the maternity leave is over.

My first child was born eight years ago. I nursed solidly for five weeks, toughing it through the pain of sore nipples and blocked milk ducts—definitely not the blissful mother-child bonding experience that I had fantasized about. Just when I finally got the hang of it, I had to start planning the return to work. I tried using a small electric breast pump but had little success and great discomfort. This pumping business, I decided, was not for me. At that time, given the long hours and stress of my job as an emergency room attending, it seemed to be a good choice. Besides, my first child was a hypervigilant, easily distractible baby who seemed to prefer the speed of a bottle to the process of nursing. I weaned him gradually; when he was about three months old, I stopped altogether.

With my second child, I was reluctant to stop nursing. She was a cuddly baby who nursed easily, and rather than pummeling my chest or pulling off to look around, would gaze up at me and smile. I made no special preparations, however, when I went back to work and, as a result, spent one or two horrible ER shifts with breast engorgement. After one particularly frenzied week in the midst of flu season, my milk supply dried up. I was sad to lose that special connection with my baby but felt that the decision not to pump was right, given the unique demands of my unpredictable work environment. I also felt strongly about getting back to my old self and pursuing my career, ostensibly unfettered by the demands of home. Running off to pump in the middle of a busy ER shift seemed unprofessional, not the kind of message that I wanted to send to my colleagues, patients, nursing staff, or residents.

With my third child just this past year, I was again challenged by the "nursing-mom-returns-to-work" issue. To wean or not to wean. To pump or not to pump. This time, I was returning to an office environment where I had control over the pace of my schedule and the privacy to close a door if necessary. Yet I still worried about how I would fit yet another activity into my hectic schedule. Would it interfere with my ability to care for my patients? Was it unseemly, unprofessional?

When my baby was five weeks old, I rented a hospital-grade breast pump and tried pumping between feedings—only two ounces in 10 minutes. It was awful. With all the pressures of a busy office practice and academic commitments, did I really want to add this to my daily routine? I returned the rental machine and, appalled at the $250.00 price of the portable hospital-grade pump, decided to wean. But after one or two formula feedings, the baby cried inconsolably for a 24-hour period. Fearing that she would become colicky with formula, I rushed out and bought the expensive portable breast pump and decided to just do it. Five months later, to my surprise, I am still nursing.

I have learned many valuable things from this third experience. Using a hospital-grade machine takes less than 15 minutes and is not uncomfortable or painful. Amazingly, I can eat lunch, return phone calls, and pump at the same time. The carrying case looks enough like a computer case to fool most of my colleagues who are not "in the club." Most important, I love being able to maintain that special nursing relationship with my baby and to think that I am doing something for her in the midst of a busy working day.

Apart from the personal and practical things that I've learned for myself, carrying around the pump and integrating this task into my day has made me more aware of the limitations of the hospital work environment. I am fortunate to have my own private office and some flexibility in my schedule that allows me to take a 15-minute break if necessary. I often wonder what accommodations are made for residents, nurses, and hospital employees who wish to continue nursing when they return to work. Are these women standing in bathroom stalls, using manual pumps? Or are they abandoning breast feeding earlier than they would otherwise because of work constraints? Walking around with the pump has made me feel more connected to people with special needs and has given me a new appreciation of the challenges they face in caring for their health in the midst of busy, demanding schedules.

At hospital and medical school meetings, rather than tuck the pump discreetly under the table and pretend it isn't there, I leave it out in the open to remind me that there is nothing embarrassing, unseemly, or unprofessional about integrating breast-feeding into the workday. The pump is a visual reminder to me of my family responsibilities and the real constraints that I have on my day. Far from making me less of a professional, they have made me a more mature, balanced, and integrated person.

— *Rebecca J. Kurth*
Assistant Clinical Professor of Medicine, Columbia University

A Reminiscence

I remember one time at the park when the children had runny noses and wet diapers—and all I had in my purse was a stethoscope! Other mothers gave me a little scolding but thankfully rescued me.

— *Patricia Collins Temple*
Professor of Pediatrics, Vanderbilt University Medical Center

The Second Road

Yellowed scrapbook pages
With neatly pasted memories

of carefree days and slumber nights,
when girls still dreamed of life to come.
Knowing then that most of all,
I longed to be a mother.

of crowded halls and musty labs,
a student's quiet search begins.
Beneath the dim of midnight lamps
I hoped to be a doctor.

How many years
since that day

of orchids, lace, and sacred vows,
no longer one but two.
Months filled with wonder, joyful growth
'til you arrived, a sudden burst of love.

of cap and gown, Hippocratic oath,
suddenly my life transformed
by beepers, codes and sleepless nights
amidst an endless sea of patients.

Only now
do I understand
the privilege yet vulnerability
of being

a mother.
This love from depths I never knew,
the patter of your feet still echoes
past days of laughter and simplicity.

a doctor.
Work bound by neither time nor place
I catch a glimpse into your soul,
burdens others could not share.

Two paths intertwined,
One existing for the other.
Life richer for the second road
—I journey forth.

— *Eliza Lo Chin*

Former Assistant Clinical Professor of Medicine, Columbia University
Currently at home, planning a return to clinical practice

Patients as Patron Saints

In my experience, female doctors have so many advantages, it's almost embarrassing. You need to take a slightly countercultural viewpoint to appreciate some of these factors, but they're more enduring than many of the traditional fruits of medical practice. True, during training you may notice a general perception that women are, in some sense, pretenders, wannabees. Most of that vanishes instantly in the light of private practice. There, it's all in a woman's favor. Not, of course, if you look from the traditional male perspective: comparing hours worked, income, publications, and measuring productivity in terms of number of patients seen. The rewards that really matter—trust, meaning, delight in the small details of existence—simply flow out of the experience of primary care.

I found, a little to my surprise, that not only my patients but other women in the community were rooting for me. Just because I was a woman doing health care, they somehow shared in any success I had. People of both sexes seemed prejudiced in my favor. They expected me to listen, to be compassionate. And because I met those expectations, they cheerfully put up with my being argumentative and opinionated as well.

It took me too many years to realize that I didn't have to practice in the traditional way. As long as I paid stringent attention to current medical information, patients actually appreciated a slightly offbeat approach. They seemed to value a clear explanation more than being handed a prescription. I came to understand that the principal commodity I had to offer was my careful attention.

My patients led me to trust my own lights. I began to see myself in much the same role as the teachers, craftsmen, and parents I worked with. My job was to listen, observe, and interpret.

I spent too many years squelching my impulses because someone might think me unprofessional or even merely unconventional. If I were starting to practice today, I'd take time to tell jokes to both patients and colleagues. I'd treat my staff as valued partners in our work. I'd never hesitate to take needlework to meetings. I'd sing while suturing or sigmoidoscoping. I wouldn't hesitate to interrupt a patient visit to greet my children after school.

If I were starting over, I would not let my motherly guilt make me apologetic to my patients about having a family or to my family about having patients. Doctoring has informed my mothering and vice versa. Medicine taught me to be "on," fully present and functioning, all the time. My patients respected my commitment to my family, and my kids knew that during certain times I was available to serve patients. I don't regret having modeled responsibility and service.

Perhaps the hardest challenge of medical practice has been the knowledge that someone was always waiting for me. My schedule inevitably created pileups: meetings, visits, and telephone calls jammed into too little time. The only way to survive this without succumbing to hurry sickness is to pour oneself utterly into the present. When each patient or friend or loved one has your full attention, you enjoy the interaction as much as is possible, and it's worth waiting for.

The key is never to promise what you can't deliver. Don't allow scheduling of more people than you can serve. If you commit to a soccer game, you'd better not end up at the hospital instead. "Mommy's on call" means the patients have first dibs that weekend. Someone will take the kids to the game—you've got to have a backup plan—but you can't promise it'll be Mommy. If you don't arrange coverage for the day of your tenth anniversary or your child's fifth birthday party, your megalomania or workaholism has got the better of your good sense. And if you can't arrange coverage, you're in the wrong practice. Of course, you've got to be willing to cover for someone else's big events as well.

It's much harder with the two-physician family, of course. We discovered this most vividly when my husband and I failed to drive two cars to the neighborhood grocery store one blizzardy day. He was called to an emergency Caesarian section while I stood in the checkout line with two toddlers and a cart full of groceries, wondering how many phone calls it would take for me to locate a sympathetic person to drive us home.

The logistics of a physician's life are so crazy that it's vital to suit one's choices to one's needs. In our case, this meant a modest house one block from the hospital and three blocks from my office. I could run home at lunchtime and nurse a baby or carry her to a noon meeting at the hospital. I found one could nurse quite discreetly underneath a blouse or sweater, and I rather enjoyed the look of surprise on my colleagues' faces when I suddenly produced and burped a baby.

It's been great fun to encourage my patients' self-confidence and freedom. If we doctors see each patient as a delight, we usher them into the sanctuary of self-acceptance. They've got to get there before they can go on to improving their health.

My advice? Listen, listen, listen. Never repeat something a patient has told you in confidence. Find something in common with each patient. Go out on a limb. Sing. Hug. Dance. (I had a beloved Alzheimer's patient with whom I'd waltz each time I went to see her. I couldn't examine her until we'd danced a few turns singing "Somewhere, My Love" together.)

Argue, as long as you think it'll increase someone's understanding. Do whatever you need to do to wake your patients up. Dare them to try things. Use metaphors, poems, stories. Pray with patients. Role-play.

You don't need to belong to the medical establishment or accept the party line. Visit a Third World country to get a sense of people's real needs and your own priorities. Nourish a healthy skepticism toward whatever's being sold. Think about whether it will profit the patient.

The two practices my patients appreciate most are these: my annual review of "Are there any medications we can get rid of?" and my dictating the note in their presence. The latter gives patients a new and clear idea of what I've heard and how I've processed it. It also gives them a chance to correct me if I've got any of it wrong. It keeps me scrupulously honest. And ah, the psychological high: I walk out of the room with my dictation *finished.*

Only after I began this practice did I discover how few patients understood their visits in terms of gathering data, forming hypotheses, and making plans. Letting them in on this is like recruiting them as members of the team. And as faulty as my memory is, it's a luxury to be able to say, "What was that third thing we discussed?" and not to have to come up with it myself.

Having patients is a tremendous privilege. It's a chance to do things we all need to do: to stay in touch with marginalized people, to plumb the depths of human experience. Especially in family practice, our patients become a cloud of witnesses—patron saints, supporters. People who recognize a connection to you as their doctor. We make this connection by treating each client, as in the old monastic story, as the Messiah. By being 100% percent present. By recognizing the essential worth of ourselves and every other, and by admitting that, in spite of the frustration and vulnerability inherent in it, doctoring is just plain fun. Not easy, but fun. It's of a piece with mothering. What compares with a life of envisioning, encouraging, and supporting people's growth?

— Alison Moll
Preceptor at York Hospital's Family Practice Residency Program
Author of Miracles Like Breathing *(1997)*

Mother's Day

In celebration of Mother's Day, the local newspaper had invited young children to submit drawings that described their mothers. Encouraged by my husband, our six-year-old daughter entered this contest. To my great surprise, she drew me as a "Supermom," replete with white coat and stethoscope standing next to the car; all around on the periphery were the school, playground, A&P grocery store, kitchen, and hospital. She won first prize and at the same time, taught me a valuable lesson—a wonderful mother's day gift. Though proud to be a "Supermom," I was surprised to see just how much I was doing in her crowded drawing. Yet I had never explored how many of those activities could be shared with my husband. Certainly, he was willing and even enjoyed participating in what I had traditionally considered my responsibilities. My own mother had done all these, but she was not a physician, nor did she work outside the home.

We need to break through our cultural traditions and share with our spouses the many tasks of the day. We don't have to be supermoms. Raising children together is a wonderful, fulfilling experience. And we should allow fathers their own style of parenting, accepting the fact that they might have a different way of accomplishing the same job.

— Nalini Juthani
Professor of Clinical Psychiatry, Albert Einstein College of Medicine

"To Love and to Work"[6]

Society has much to learn from our feminine values and ability to function within a relational context. Instead, women are often co-opted by the traditional male assumptions as we struggle to speak in their voices and to work their hours. Too frequently we simply add in the expectations of career to the responsibilities of family without questioning why it's so difficult, even for the superwomen. Socialized to make life easier for others, we avoid the negotiations necessary to make life easier for ourselves.

Understanding the developmental unfolding tells us there is time for women to lead rich and full lives without trying to do it all at once. The early years of parenting are precious and should not be given away too cavalierly to meet corporate and academic demands. Women in mid-life bring a talent and energy to the professions that society cannot afford to ignore. However, the creative possibilities of a sequenced life are often stymied by the rigid stairsteps of the workplace.

. . . This is not a trip to be taken without considerable forethought and as good a guide to the shifting terrain as you can find. "To love and to work" will always create periods of conflict and tension for women, but in hindsight, the journey seems worth the investment. In both the family and the workplace, our male peers and partners have something to learn from the essential humanness of the quest. Perhaps together we can find ways to make the road less daunting for the next generation.

— *Nancy B. Kaltreider*
Professor of Psychiatry Emerita, University of California San Francisco
Editor of Dilemmas of a Double Life *(1997)*

Balance

Growing up in a household where medicine was god, I vowed before entering medical school to lead a more balanced life. Yet as I progressed through training, that balance seemed ever more elusive. Multiple moves separated me geographically from supportive friends. I tried to stay involved with dance and music, but sleep generally won out when free time was available. My spiritual life was unraveling; my quest to find a life partner, a disaster. I arrived in San Francisco a wreck on every level. Welcome to fellowship.

That was nine years ago. Much has happened since then. I write now as mother and wife, as physician and individual.

Perhaps because marriage and motherhood seemed unattainable for so long, my appreciation for them is enormous. And yet, the sheer determination that helped get me through medical training has proven quite useless in my family life. I have found instead that intuition, patience, and a form of noneffort are required. While I sensed this first in my marriage, it wasn't until pregnancy that I realized my approach to life really had to change. I was cruising through the second trimester, frantically trying to get all my work done before the delivery. A growing sense of fatigue was at odds with demands at work, but to cut back seemed so unprofessional, so stereotypically— well, *female*. On a routine prenatal visit at 29 weeks, though, I was stunned when the obstetrician told me my cervix was dilating. An hour later, I was in the hospital, hooked up to all sorts of monitors that told me what I hadn't been willing to acknowledge: I was in preterm labor. I knew all the statistics about physicians being at higher risk for pregnancy complications, but it never occurred to me that *I* could actually be one of those people. Yet here I was, patient instead of physician, with the healthy baby for which I had longed so much now at risk of becoming like those I had cared for in the newborn intensive care unit.

Such an event really does get you to sit up and take notice. After three weeks in the hospital, infusions of mind-altering drugs, and a fair amount of introspection, labor stopped, and I was sent home to continue bed rest for another four weeks. I thought a lot about myself, my baby, and how I had ignored my body's attempt to tell me what it needed for a healthy pregnancy. My own denial of physical needs reflected what I felt was expected of a professional woman. Although I was grateful to be in a stimulating, challenging profession, there seemed little room to acknowledge or embrace my personal needs as a woman. After my abrupt exit from the work world, I became enveloped by a cocoon of thoughts and emotions, as though by concentrating all my energy on this growing life, I might convince it to stay.

It worked—perhaps a little too well. Jasper eventually came into the world a week and a half postdate. I was delighted and exhausted. He was like a beautiful, fragile visitor from another world. Learning to care for him was an excursion into the unknown. My efforts to soothe him frequently missed the mark. Gradually, I found myself guided by inner resources I never even knew existed.

As a pediatrician, I understood the basic tenets of child development. Perhaps a little hands-on experience was lacking, but surely that would quickly be acquired. Things began to run amok, however, whenever I tried to implement one of my knowledge-based interventions. I soon found myself up against a mounting wave of motherly intuition that ran contrary to much of what I had learned about child care.

Things came to a climax when we found ourselves faced with a baby who, over time, seemed to be having more problems with sleep instead of less. My husband and I read Ferber's classic, *Solve Your Child's Sleep Problems*, planning to carry out its instructions with firm resolve. But at the end of four nights, I found myself sobbing in my pediatrician's office. It had sounded so reasonable on paper, yet it felt so wrong inside. I decided then that I simply had to follow my instincts or motherhood would become for me an intolerable contradiction between mind and heart. We threw the book away and forged ahead. Jasper eventually migrated into our bed on a regular basis, comforted to sleep by our presence. His breast-feeding schedule never did become "reasonable," but his strong, thriving body continually reassured me that there must be something right about my approach. At two years of age, he is a warm, affectionate, playful, observant child, who at least so far doesn't seem particularly damaged by my deviations from the norm.

Over time, I have come to view much of what is taught to pediatric residents about child care as highly politically based rather than the pinnacle of knowledge I once considered it to be. It amazes me what few studies we have to support what is taught as the correct approach to child rearing. Even these studies are often misinterpreted to support mainstream cultural values, such as independence and convenience.

I find now that affection, spontaneity, reverence, trust, and joy play a far more valuable role in child development.

Being with my son has encouraged me to embrace those characteristics in myself that are nonlinear and nonutilitarian and that emanate from the heart, drawing me closer to my own humanity. It has made me aware of the simple yet profound effect that accommodating the needs of children has on our lives, enriching us all as we create space for their true selves to unfold.

Parenthood has profoundly altered my sense of self. I feel as though every molecule in me has been affected. The balance I had always sought intellectually, I now realize in a physical sense. I can't help but feel that this has made me a better, more insightful physician. It certainly has made me a happier one. I feel blessed to work in an environment that allows me to balance both work and family. My hope for all men and women is that this balance becomes an expectation rather than the exception it is today.

— Cynthia J. Kapphahn
Clinical Assistant Professor of Pediatrics,
Stanford University School of Medicine

Numbing Down

Arriving home after a 12-hour night shift, I passed my husband and three-year old son on the front walk, just as they were leaving for preschool.

"Mommy's home!" my son yelped. I knelt down to kiss him hello-good-bye and told him to wake me up as soon as he came back home.

I was a second-year resident in family practice and 12 weeks pregnant with our second child. I felt on top of the world. I was doing and having it all: work that I loved and a beautiful thriving family. Not only was being Superwoman possible, but it wasn't even all that hard.

My first trimester had been effortless, fortunately, as I had no time for morning sickness or fatigue while keeping up with the busy pace of residency. But changing out of my clothes that morning, I was surprised to see some light spotting. I automatically called my midwife but without much emotion, as if I were calling a consult for a patient. She recommended that I return to the hospital for an ultrasound.

The technician methodically scanned my belly as I lay in the darkened radiology room. Her blank expression and minimal conversation, in retrospect, should have alerted me that something was not right. The radiologist was summoned to confirm and then tell me: there was no heartbeat. The fetus measured only eight weeks old, having died four weeks prior. I was shell-shocked and devastated. How could this be, and why was my body so slow in recognizing a no longer viable pregnancy?

I was given a week off from work to grieve and recover, during which time I underwent a D&C. I had wanted the remnants out of my body as soon as possible so that I would no longer feel pregnant, could mourn the loss, and try to move on. What I didn't expect was that the procedure was far more emotional and gut-wrenching than the miscarriage itself. I felt as if I was betraying my own body's rhythm, not honoring some instinctive hold on the little embryo until my body was ready to let go. I felt confused and violated as the aspirator scraped the insides of my womb, forcing my uterus into violent contractions of resistance.

My grief was profound. How could my body be capable of delivering death as well as life? I felt as if something had invaded me and devoured the life within. My belief that I could do it all—be a wife and mother and doctor—was suddenly being eroded. I felt incapable of doing any part of it well.

In the beginning of residency, my dual identities of both mother and doctor had enhanced each other. Now they seemed in constant conflict, each role diminishing the other. How was I to reconcile this? I wasn't willing to give lesser care to my patients, nor could I neglect my family more than I already had. Unprepared for these ambivalent feelings, I brushed them aside and carried on.

Remarkably, I was pregnant again one month later. This helped alleviate my unresolved grief, and I was able, cautiously, to become excited with this new pregnancy.

I had just begun a new obstetrics rotation at a large county hospital. My days consisted of running from one healthy delivery to another, and in between, doing exams and sonograms on the numerous patients that we served. The temptation to sneak a peek at my own belly was too much to withstand. So I recruited a colleague one afternoon, and squirting some of the cold blue gel on my abdomen, we peered at the monitor.

"There's the sac. Is that the fetus? I'm not sure. I'm not used to doing first trimester sonos. Are you sure about your dates?" my colleague asked.

"Um, yeah, I'm very sure."

"Well, I'm not very good at this. You probably should have one of the senior residents do this for you." She touched my tummy with her hand, then turned the machine off and went to see a patient.

I knew it already—in my heart, in my head, in my bones; this was another nonviable pregnancy. But I had 20 more hours of being on call and laboring patients to care for. And so I delivered four babies that night, all of them beautiful and miraculous births with ecstatic mothers and families. I became completely immersed in their stories, not allowing myself to think about my own pregnancy until the next morning when it was time to go home. After sign-out rounds, I curbsided a senior resident; she confirmed that it was a blighted ovum, a false pregnancy, a sac with nothing in it. I was numb. I drove home. I told my husband and I went to bed.

I did not stop after that and went back to work, continuing to deliver babies and surrounding myself with women and mothers and life and birth. Not only did I not have time for another D&C, but I couldn't bear the thought of reliving that experience again. I chose instead to allow my body's natural resolution this time.

Four weeks later, at the busy start of a 24-hour shift, I admitted a young woman in labor. Her labor progressed beautifully over the course of the night. At 5 a.m., she was dilated and ready. The delivery room was filled with a sense of excitement, almost giddy with anticipation. As I began to coach her to push with her contractions, I felt an odd sensation in my own belly, almost like a contraction itself. Briefly excusing myself,

I ran to the bathroom and discovered my underwear soaked with blood. I quickly changed scrubs and returned to the delivery room, just as the baby's head was beginning to descend. I discreetly pulled the nurse aside to brief her about my situation.

"I just thought you should know that I am actually having a miscarriage myself right now. I've known for a while, so it's not too upsetting, and I should be fine to continue with the delivery."

She looked at me with disbelief. "Are you sure you are okay? Maybe you should give the OB residents the heads-up just in case," she said.

I paused. And as I stood there, a spreading dampness ran down my legs. I ran to the bathroom where I passed two tennis ball size clots. The bleeding was brisk and bright red—signs that would immediately raise alarms if I were examining a patient. I changed scrubs again, checked my pulse which was stable, and returned to the delivery room. The patient's labor was booming along. The nurse asked me again to call the OB residents. This time, I agreed. They came within minutes and ushered me into the delivery room next door.

"But my patient is about to deliver. I need to be there!"

"Stephanie is covering. You are hemorrhaging and we need to take care of you."

So there I was, in stirrups myself, my mind still in the adjacent room, wanting so much to help deliver a life. This body of mine—both woman and doctor—draped in its white coat, trying to create life yet weeping from the inside out.

Afterward, I drove myself home. My husband and son were waiting for me. They tucked me into bed.

"You take a nap, mommy," my son told me, "and when you wake up, we'll play." He kissed me and pushed back the hair on my forehead; just as I had always done for him. Then he tiptoed out and closed the door. I wept for a long time—for my son and husband who have learned so often to manage without a mommy, for the babies that never were, and finally just for me.

— *Rebecca Tennant*
Stay-at-home mom and writer

Maternity and Medicine[7]

Having had three of my four children while in medical school, during internship or residency training, I have always had a very personal interest in maternity and medicine. Even now, I can vividly recall the agony and ecstasy of returning to work three days postpartum because there was no maternity leave. I was grateful to my son, who, while he did not have the good grace to wait to be born in the delivery room, did appear on a Tuesday night before the Thanksgiving weekend, thus giving me two extra days off. There was a physical brutality in having to return to work before episiotomies or pelvic diatheses were healed. Yet there was a kind of heady triumph in doing what "couldn't be done"—having a family without losing the pace of the fast track.

— *Anne E. Bernstein*
Clinical Professor of Psychiatry, Columbia University
Private practice
Co-editor of Psychodynamic Treatment of Women *(1993)*

Parenting Without Pregnancy

Just today in the office I met Ruth, a delightful 37-year-old woman, herself a physician. She had just changed insurance plans and simply needed a referral. My day had already been hectic, so I was especially relieved that this would not be a long, complicated visit. I eased back in my chair to begin the interview.

Slowly, her story tumbled out—the unexplained infertility followed by a barrage of tests, invasive procedures, hormone injections, and plans now for one more try with a newly developed technique. The endless attempts at conception had evolved into a cyclical pattern around which the routine of everyday life had been arranged. As a resident, she began to realize that the inflexible demands of medical training and the clockwork precision of infertility treatment were simply incompatible. Now six years later, she continues to forego her medical career to pursue unsuccessfully the higher reproductive technologies that have not yet created a child.

I thought back to those achingly barren years in my own life, a distant yet ever-present memory despite my now being the mother of two wonderful teenage sons. Even my deep love for them has not completely erased the agony of that earlier experience. Like Ruth, I had come to medicine late, having first pursued a career in speech pathology. So while most of my classmates worried about the dating scene—or lack thereof—my husband and I began trying to conceive our first child. But when time passed, I became anxious. And so began our journey into the infertility maze of basal body temperature charts, hormone pills, pelvic ultrasounds, and scheduled sex.

Infertility was a lonely, painful time. Those who have not experienced it cannot possibly fathom the terrible loss that a woman feels— the loss of control, loss of bearing a genetic child, loss of feeling a human being grow inside of you. These feelings may lessen with time, but they never fully go away. They come back in different ways over one's life span.

I found little support within the medical establishment. The rigid timetable of medical training just does not allow for the unpredictable demands of pregnancy, childbirth, or infertility. My erratic schedule as a resident only compounded the frustration. How could I possibly get accurate basal body temperatures when I never got to sleep at night! Though surrounded by medical people, I felt lost and alone in my chosen profession. There were very few colleagues and practically no mentors in whom I could confide.

Month after month passed, turning into years. Still no baby. After two and a half years, we began to consider adoption. Discouraged by domestic waiting lists of at least seven years, we actively sought out international agencies and orphanages. By coincidence, one of my intern colleagues was from Bogota, Columbia, the site of one of the orphanages. Even more fortunate, his family was actually related to the director of the orphanage. They were great catalysts in helping us create our wonderful family. We received our son, Gabe, on April 28, 1986, and our son, David, on August 8, 1988.

When one door closes, God opens another. I consider my children among His greatest blessings. So although we lost many things to infertility, we have not missed out on the bountiful joy, trials, and tribulations of parenting.

— Toby Jacobowitz
Associate Medical Director for Hospice of Washtenaw
Private practice, internal medicine/pediatrics

Body Snatcher

Medical training with its infinite demands and inhumane work hours teaches us, as physicians, to be strong. As we learn to adapt, we may begin to believe that we can survive anything. Occasionally, however, a challenge arises to remind us that we are, after all, only human. The takeover of my body by an initially two-celled invader (later called Vincent) proved to be the most humbling experience of my medical career.

I became pregnant during my last month of internship at Vanderbilt. Although they offered congratulations, my fellow residents were not pleased. Schedules had to be rewritten, extra call parceled out in anticipation of my maternity leave, still 8 months away but an unbelievable 6 weeks long. I knew that my colleagues were wondering why I had such colossally bad timing—why couldn't I have waited until the last year of residency when call would be much lighter? I wanted to explain that I was tired of continually deferring family life for medicine and that I had seen too many infertile couples during medical school. Already in my early 30s, I was having nightmares of being alone in a nursing home with no children to take me out to lunch on Sundays.

Getting pregnant, it turned out, was the easy part. Staying pregnant was the real challenge. During the first trimester, I felt like my body had been abducted by aliens. I tried every trick in the book—flat ginger ale, Saltine crackers that I carried around in my pocket only to spray patients with crumbs whenever I took out my reflex hammer, and even an occasional Phenergan if dehydration seemed imminent. Still, I had horrible nausea that seemed to occur at the most inopportune moments—like when I was awakened from sleep by my beeper or when I had to present a patient on rounds or when I was in an area of the VA where none of the toilets worked. One day, I discovered that I could use the bathrooms of the comatose patients, which at least quieted my recurring nightmare (the one that had replaced the nursing home nightmare) of vomiting on my attending's stylish silk tie.

I found a surprising ally in the second-shift charge nurse. Observing my frequent, often abrupt bathroom trips, she concluded that I must be pregnant and immediately became protective. I later learned that she had threatened with bodily harm anyone who tried to disturb me during evenings on call when I could be found snoozing on a cot in the call room. Without her protection, I never could have completed the rotation.

Two months into my pregnancy, I almost lost Vincent. I noticed some light spotting and—after notifying my attending and resident, both mercifully understanding—hurried to the obstetrician's office. She casually informed me that this represented a "threatened abortion," that there was nothing to be done but I should stay home on bed rest for a week anyway. I cried until the bleeding stopped. There really hadn't been much, but I found myself checking for more during the rest of the first trimester.

As with most pregnancies, conditions improved by the second trimester, and I began thinking of Vincent more as a baby and less as an alien usurper. His first kicks startled me during afternoon rounds. The nausea subsided as I began happily eating for two. A sense of purpose and contentment washed over me. For a brief time, I stopped worrying about how I would juggle residency with a baby or how I could find affordable child care or whether he would be born with some horrible birth defect that I had read about during genetics class or if I could even survive labor and delivery to bring him into the world.

My worry-free period ended prematurely when I began having contractions at 28 weeks. I had been on my feet constantly, working hectic 12-hour shifts in the emergency room. At first, I thought they were just Braxton Hicks contractions, but at the insistence of my husband, I went to see my obstetrician. She diagnosed preterm labor and immediately prescribed Terbutaline with complete bed rest for the next 10 weeks. Again, schedules would require radical changes, and I would not be able to finish residency on time.

I remember once hearing an attending scold a young pregnant woman for working too hard and not taking care of herself. "You are with child. This is the most important fact in your life right now. What others expect of you is nothing compared to this." We as physicians would agree with this advice, yet we would never give it to one another. We expect ourselves to be superhuman, never sick or constrained by demands of personal life. Logically, I told myself that pregnancy was not a weakness, that I couldn't help preterm labor, and that my colleagues would eventually understand. But I couldn't help feeling that taking five months off would brand me as weak, inferior, or just plain undependable. I understood my fellow residents' lack of support: You can't blame a hungry animal for not being happy when his already scarce food supply is threatened.

It would be difficult to take away more of the little sustenance, in the form of time off, that my fellow residents had. But I needed to heed my obstetrician's advice instead of trying to handle everything on my own. I could live with my colleagues' disappointment or even their disapproval. I could live with finishing my residency later than planned. I could live with the boredom of spending 10 weeks on the couch after working 12+ hours per day in the ER. I could not live with the risk of jeopardizing my son's health.

And exactly 10 weeks later, as I held Vincent for the first time and he made those incredible newborn sounds, I knew that I had done the right thing.

— *Liza Sharpless Bonanno*
Psychiatrist, South Community Behavioral Healthcare

Redefining Motherhood

I have always sought to do my best in whatever I set out to accomplish. As a medical student, I admired great clinicians, desiring one day to emulate them. That these physicians were almost exclusively men seemed irrelevant at the time. Actually, I thought being a woman gave me a slight advantage over my male colleagues. The nurturing, caring manner often attributed to the female gender helped me to relate more easily to patients.

Both in medical school and residency, I was surrounded by brilliant, competent female colleagues; my career path seemed perfectly clear at the time. But then motherhood intervened, changing my life in ways I had never anticipated. Still, I believed that I could manage it all, not knowing then how unrealistic my expectations were.

I aspired to be like the best clinician I had ever met—my residency program director—and the best mother I had ever known—my own. Not once did it occur to me that each of these role models had devoted their primary focus, energy, and time to that single pursuit. My mother had always been there for me—for piano, Girl Scouts, story hour at the library, games on the living room floor, and homework problems. How could I possibly do all that and still keep up with my male colleagues who spent their extra time at work, writing grants, or networking? It didn't seem fair. They had wives who stayed home to raise the kids. There was a clear division of labor. So was it just a problem of time? Could I be more efficient, lengthen the day to 30 hours, or become more competent at both jobs so that it would be easier? I looked around for some proof that it could be done. Were others out there facing the same issues?

I had no clear concept of what "best" meant in terms of being a physician mother. I felt guilty being the last parent to pick my daughter up from school. I felt guilty arriving 30 minutes late for morning rounds because I had to drop her off at school. I felt guilty not working after I got home most evenings. I felt guilty that someone else was so integral in raising my child.

I finally decided that my definition of "best" would have to come from within. I felt good about finding my daughter quality day care and about the effort I put into my relationship with her provider. I felt good about baking cookies for the class once a month and getting the class a gerbil named "Twinkle." I felt good about spending quality time with my family and planning special excursions for the three of us. I felt good about the care that I rendered my patients, particularly when helping them through difficult situations. I felt good about the contributions I was making through my research. Perhaps I would be better at each individual role if that was all I did, but clearly I was doing my best at being both.

Now, I see myself accomplishing quite a bit. I add to my daughter's life by being fulfilled and productive, and I add to my patients' lives by being a woman. The hardest part of becoming a mother has been adjusting my expectations to match reality and realizing the need to re-create my own definition of what is "best."

— *Karen P. Alexander*
Assistant Professor of Medicine, Duke University School of Medicine

Taking Children Seriously[8]

Sometimes having a child as well as a job seems like living a double life. When I leave home for the adult world, I do a physical and mental inspection to ensure that all vestiges of my life with my daughter are hidden. Are there cereal spills on my skirt? Has toddlerthink spilled into my mind? I have a recurrent fear that I will be caught, that I will be found humming our household's song of the month (currently "Tender Shepherd") or that some adult will round a corner and I will blurt out "Peek-a-Boo," and that this aberrant behavior will reveal me as an impostor in the adult world.

I am fascinated by the gap between the parts of my lives. As a family doctor, I might have thought that some of my work would relate to the lives of children. Yet I never spend my adult time discussing any of the issues that are so compelling when I am discussing the finer points of "One Fish Two Fish Red Fish Blue Fish" or trying to persuade my daughter of the wisdom of wearing shoes.

Even time assumes a different meaning. It is sometimes hard for me to reset my brain to realize that at home time is no longer a medium for checking tasks off a list, the more the better. My daughter may spend the afternoon doing 20 things or one, or use the whole time to decide between possibilities. The process, her interest, and our interaction are all more important than what we have to show for it.

As I reflect on the problems that merit adult attention, I find that many of them have their origins here. Children grapple daily with developing self-esteem, individual identities, trust, and confidence. How many of us wish that our bosses or employees or spouses had mastered these concepts?

If adults took children more seriously, we might find our lives enhanced by the addition of fingerpaints and fairy dust. Better yet, we might provide our children with the skills to make a better world than the one we have given them.

— *Jessica Schorr Saxe*
Family practitioner at CMC-Biddle Point, Charlotte, North Carolina

Notes

1. From Brazelton, T. B. (1997). *Working and caring.* New York: Perseus. Copyright © 1997, 1995 by T. Berry Brazelton, M.D.

2. Excerpted from Wang-Cheng, R. (1996). The echo of my mother's footsteps. In D. Wear (Ed.), *Women in medical education: An anthology of experience* (pp. 127–133). Albany: State University of New York Press. Reprinted with permission.

3. From McMurray, J. E. (1999). Doctor's daughter. *Annals of Internal Medicine, 131,* 222–224. Reprinted by permission of the American College of Physicians-American Society of Internal Medicine.

4. From Shafer, A. (1992). Monday morning. *Annals of Internal Medicine, 117,* 167. Reprinted by permission of the American College of Physicians-American Society of Internal Medicine.

5. From Crosby, S. S. (2000). A mother's prayer. *Journal of the American Medical Association, 283*(9), 1109–1110. Copyrighted (2000), American Medical Association. Reprinted with permission.

6. From Kaltreider, N. B. (1997). "To love and to work": Balancing priorities throughout the life cycle. N. B. Kaltreider (Ed.), *Dilemmas of a double life: Women balancing careers and relationships* (pp. 3–30). Northvale, NJ: Jason Aronson. Reprinted with permission

7. From Bernstein, A. E. (1992). Maternity and medicine. *Journal of the American Medical Women's Association, 47*(3), 77. Copyright © 1992 American Medical Women's Association, Inc. All rights reserved. Reprinted with permission for education use only.

8. Excerpted from Saxe, J. S. (n.d.). Adult world could benefit from taking children seriously. *The Charlotte Observer,* n.p. Reprinted by permission of the author.

7

MAKING CHOICES

*It would be easier to live with a greater clarity of
ambition, to follow goals that beckon toward a single
upward progression. But perhaps what women have to
offer in the world today, in which men and women both
must learn to deal with new orders of complexity and
rapid change, lies in the very rejection of forced choices:
work or home, strength or vulnerability, caring or competition,
trust or questioning. Truth may not be so simple.*
— *Mary Catherine Bateson*[1]

Finding the Balance Point Between
Overdrive and the Mommy Track

As one travels within one's own institution or to national meetings, the
conversation among young female academic physicians inevitably turns
toward personal issues. Common themes quickly emerge.

The single woman looks pensive as she describes how, although she
has managed to become quite competent in clinical, research, and
educational endeavors, she would like to get married and have children
someday. These women acknowledge that, as the second half of their 30s
are upon them, they worry how they'll ever have time to find a mate.

The mothers with small children, looking truly haggard, describe a usual routine of 12-hour workdays, 4 to 5 hours of sleep a night, racing between home, work, and their kids' day care or school, and feeling like a rat on a spinning wheel. They sew Halloween costumes at midnight, worry frequently about what they are missing at home and at work, and can't recall a single thing they've done for themselves lately.

In between these two groups uncomfortably sits the partnered woman who, when asked about kids, responds, "But I have a dog." If pressed for an explanation as to why she chose to pass up the opportunity to be a mother, not infrequently the reply is, "Well, my career requires one hundred fifty percent effort. How can I possibly add children to this picture?"

If these women could hurtle themselves to the end of their lives for just one moment, what would be their response to the question, "Did I make the right choices?" Surely they do have some choices.

These women fear and loathe the label "part-time" to describe any part of their careers. They fear being taken less seriously than their male colleagues; they fear being left behind for promotion, leadership positions, and opportunities; they fear a loss of self-identity as a high-functioning, high-achieving academic physician.

What are their alternatives? First, they could cut *back* to full-time. Yes—just full-time. Not 12 to 14 hours a day, six to seven days a week, month after month. By reorganizing one's group, setting limits, and exploring endeavors outside of medicine, the amorphous career octopus could fit back into a reasonably sized box. Sometimes the sides of this career box will bulge, but the top and the bottom should not be blown off: This is a 30-year marathon, not a five-year sprint.

Women (and men for that matter) could even consider cutting back a little more. Working at 80 to 90% of a full-time equivalent, the physician would have time to volunteer, attend personal appointments, and take care of the details of life. In private practice, physicians call this "my day off" not "I work part-time." Of course, academic productivity may slow down somewhat, but the ultimate goal would still be achieved.

There is no time like the present for people to make critical decisions about how they want to live their lives. As seen everyday in these very same academic institutions, tragedies happen, and life may not be as long as one assumes. Academic physicians need to be brought back from the brink of physical exhaustion, isolation from family, and mental ill health to a balance point where the personal and the professional aspects of one's life are complementary. When combined appropriately, these will lead to a high-functioning, high-achieving, and satisfied individual.

— Mary Lou Schmidt
Associate Professor of Pediatrics
University of Illinois College of Medicine

Between Lawn Cuts

Since the acquisition of a Fisher-Price doctor's kit as a preschooler, my life has followed a fairly straight and unquestioned (some might even say pedestrian) path to becoming a pediatrician. Despite my parents filling the traditional roles of stay-at-home Mom and provider Dad, they encouraged each of their six daughters to pursue education and careers. My mom had seven children in 10 years, abandoning her own professional goals to give each of us the foundation to pursue ours. The irony of it is that, had my mother not made this enormous sacrifice, I doubt that her six daughters would have become what we did—a lawyer, a doctor, an educational consultant, a Wall Street trader, a teacher, and a reading specialist.

So how is it that I'm currently on a leave of absence from my job as an academic pediatrician and at home with my three young children?

To my utter dismay, I have discovered that real life cannot be programmed. My internal Franklin Planner had timed our first child at the end of residency. But after three years of repeatedly negative home pregnancy tests, my husband and I were told that biological children were an unlikely event in our future. I was devastated. I loved my job, but the daily contact with children and incessant questions regarding my lack of them were a source of constant pain. At that time, the question of career versus family was utmost in my mind; the obvious answer was that I would drop it all in a Big Apple minute to be a mother.

While pursuing adoption, the "impossible" happened, and I became pregnant with Charlotte. The daily joy she provided quickly buried the agony of those years of infertility. My husband Harlan and I experienced that universal parental world shrinkage in which we focused on her every detail while boring others with stories of her earth-shattering accomplishments.

Three years later, gentle Ben was born. Working and a quality family life were still possible. Despite being in an academic center, I found ample support. I can remember a lunch meeting with one of my colleagues that resembled a dairy farm—both of us hooked up to our breast pumps, double-pumping away. For me, there was enough self-imposed stress that working would have been intolerable if I was not accepted and encouraged to do the most for my family.

Six years out of residency, I felt the need to improve my skills as an academic physician. I was accepted into a Faculty Development Fellowship at Michigan State University, a program that would entail a cumulative travel time of about five weeks out of the year. My husband, being the good guy that he is, encouraged me to do it. We felt it was necessary for me to grow and advance professionally.

A number of weeks before leaving for Michigan, I discovered I was pregnant with my third child. I was thrilled but stressed about the impact it would have on my work and my colleagues. I know many a woman who has spent more energy worrying about breaking the news to coworkers than rejoicing in this new life event—pretty warped but there you have it. When my first trimester ended and I spread the word, I felt such relief. The world did not end, and reactions to my news were far more supportive than I had expected.

Wild Will arrived on schedule (the only time in his short life that he's ever cooperated) toward the end of my fellowship. After my maternity leave, I returned to work with renewed vigor. I now had the skills and the desire to pursue new projects, to be a better clinician and teacher. However, things began to, if not quite unravel, fray a bit. Life with three under the age of five was hectic. I was still nursing Will, commuting an hour to and from work, and trying to secure grant funding. Although enjoying the swim, I was basically just treading water.

My mother was then diagnosed with a lung nodule. Many have written about encountering the patient perspective of medicine, and my mother's situation began a new, frequently disturbing relationship between our family and the medical world. She had a lobectomy, but later was found to have metastatic colon cancer in her brain, bone, and kidney.

With all that was going on, I began the nightly routine of not sleeping, an area Will had a major talent in facilitating. My anxiety was staggering (this was the only time I found Lamaze breathing to be particularly useful). I couldn't imagine leaving my job, but I also couldn't imagine continuing the status quo. In the light of day, I began to share some of my thoughts with family and friends. Those who knew me well encouraged me to take the plunge and stop working.

One day in the midst of this internal struggle, I arrived home from work and Charlotte, five at the time, came running to greet me. "Mom, I didn't see you all day. You must stop working. We can become poor and then you can go back to work." I was somewhat taken aback—half amused, half guilt ridden. She told me that if I really wanted to work, I should "cut grass." I explained that, even if I chose that career, I would still be away from home. Her reply: "Mommy, just two people's grass while I'm in school."

During my training, there was a professor I very much admired. She seemed to have struck the balance—an accomplished physician and mother as well. Recently, I met this woman's daughter at a cocktail party and gushed out words of praise for her mother. Her simple reply shook me: "It's nice you had that experience with her, but I had to spend all my time at the neighbors."

Possibly just a bitter daughter, but I'm now working on Charlotte's future cocktail talk. Maybe it will go something like this: "When I was a child, I remember seeing my mother between lawn cuts."

The wonderful thing about our profession is the many capacities in which we are able to participate. Although I had always anticipated a well-paved, straight path, I now enjoy the tangents, the off-road experience, the surprise detours. I'm working on being at peace with all those life clichés about enjoying the ride and smelling the roses. Most important is that I make the right personal choices and am here for my family at critical times. If asked, I would definitely choose the same career. I know I will still work as a pediatrician—I need this for myself and do feel that I bring something to the table. Being a mother is numero uno but—and this is sharing more than I let out on the average day—I need more intellectual stimulation. My kids are great fun, yet there are still days when life is monotonous and the word *Mommy* is grating. Despite this, I'm glad to be at home, sharing their daily routines. There's no same answer for all of us—the sharing of collective experiences may help to clarify decisions for some.

Since I've stopped working, things have become clearer, because of both external and internal inputs. I realize that I am unique and fortunate in that financial factors have allowed me to have a choice—not true for many women. I do like having a career and wholeheartedly believe my children will benefit from my continuing to work once the situation is right. The change in my mother's condition and the realization that she won't always be there have caused me to think about the life-shaping role mothers play in their children's lives. We're encouraged to set goals in our professional careers, building up that *curriculum vitae*, but now I'm working on my MV—my *madre vitae*. Charlotte, Benjamin, and Will to provide references upon request.

— *Anne Armstrong-Coben*
Assistant Clinical Professor of Pediatrics
Columbia University, College of Physicians & Surgeons
Medical Director for Covenant House Newark New Jersey

Not Having Children

I am grateful for—if a little apprehensive at—the chance to reflect on my decision not to have had children. This chapter is devoted to achieving balance in our professional lives. Ordinarily, this phrase—at least when applied to women doctors—means reconciling the demands of motherhood with the demands of medicine. The choices that come to mind are starting a family during medical school or during residency, live-in help or day help, attending your child's daytime recital or being a good full-time soldier for your division chief.

Such careful attention to these hard questions ought not imply that all women doctors choose to have children. I think it might round out the discussion in these pages to consider the rightfulness, for some women, of the other choice.

My decision to not bear children was a steadfast one, but it was neither a fully articulated nor an internally uncontested choice. I remember one long conversation with my older sister Louise, talking as sisters do about life and love and dreams and fears. I was a third-year Harvard Medical student, working so hard, feeling so proud of my accomplishments, having finally mastered the knack of staying up all night. As we talked on the phone, I was doodling elaborately, creating endless circles, whorls, and arcs. Years later, I saw in that scribble a very clear drawing of an ovary with well-delineated follicles, corpus lutea, and even an egg being released at the ovary's surface. So I suppose I was thinking with an inner body-mind about fertility and reproduction without releasing such thoughts to absolute consciousness.

By my fourth year of medical school, most of my friends were making decisions about *when* and not *if* to have children. Passionate discussions surrounded me about the merits of taking a year off between medical school and internship, given all the pressure such a decision placed on one's fertility. Being in a long-term relationship with a man who did not want a family, I felt external to such decisions. Only much later did I see how my choice of this man was, no doubt, influenced by his stance vis-à-vis reproduction.

I say this to point out how little support there was, either internally or externally, for a woman to say clearly and audibly, "I do not want to have a child." Perhaps there was support to which I was oblivious, but I remember feeling able to talk about these matters with only one or two very close friends. I even felt a certain pressure to acknowledge that perhaps someday, I might want to have a family, as if there were something wrong with choosing otherwise. How helpful it would have been for me to have had some vocal reassurance—from within medicine and maybe even from women within medicine—condoning my choice to not reproduce.

There seems even now something unduly selfish or solipsistic about such a choice. Why would a woman forego the most powerful act at her disposal? How could a person turn down the biological and spiritual imperative of becoming the medium for another life? Not having a child denies a woman irreplaceable emotional, sensual, and intersubjective experiences—no number of students or mentees or nieces and nephews can (or ought to) stand as surrogates to one's own child. And yet, the choice to reproduce can be seen in part as a demotion of your own life, an admission that anything you can do on your own cannot possibly equal—in importance, in passion, in longevity, in reality—that which your offspring might do.

There was then and is now very little warrant for such a point of view. Those who live through their fertile years without choosing to have children are pitied by some, assumed to have been barren or dismissed as selfish by others, and marginalized by all the family-centered activities of their age-mates. The childless state seems evidence of deep, deep failure. And the extraordinary efforts made by women to have their own biological child—through in-vitro fertilization or surrogacy or any of the increasingly outlandish methods of conceiving or bearing a fetus—enact the culture's governing appraisal that having kids is what women ought to do. Being a woman seems irrevocably tied up with being a mother, and so the childless woman has somehow let herself or her species down.

So there I was, over 30 by now, out of residency, having outlived a relationship that had sustained me through training. Who was I now, on my own, I asked? Was I to continue to live by myself and for myself? Had it not been for psychoanalysis, I might never have resolved these questions. It took many years of hard work to understand, accept, and celebrate my formative choice to remain childless. I finally allowed myself to take as success and not defeat my accomplishment in living without children.

In time, after residency, I started a Ph.D. program in English, a complex scholarly enterprise that ended up taking almost 10 years of extraordinarily hard work. No doubt, I intensified my own professional expectations of myself, measuring my accomplishments against those of women colleagues and expecting myself to have done *more* than did my friends who were also mothers. In some cases, I did, and in others, I didn't, so I eventually learned that having or not having children was not the only factor involved in productivity or scholarly creativity.

By now, I am a grandmother. I married a man considerably older than myself, who had grown children from his first marriage. So at age 44, I became stepmother to a 44-year-old, a 38-year-old, and a 36-year-old. I "inherited" a 13-year-old granddaughter and an 8-year-old grandson. Four years ago, my middle stepchild had a son, the first grandchild born since I joined the family. How extraordinary that, all of a sudden, I am cooking for 14 at Thanksgiving, planning a garden with one child, and renovating a kitchen with another. I feel the responsibility and groundedness of devotion, protection, and unconditional love. I feel blessed to have, as it seems to me now, all the rewards of all possible choices. The combination of accident, foolhardiness, and wisdom that guides all of us in our lives was, in my case, marvelously generative and generous. And when Julian calls me Grandma Rita, I feel fully and inalterably all the richness of fertility and progeny.

I hope that all women at the start of their adult lives can look with equal regard on those two paths in front of them—a life with children and a life without children. Although most women will bear children, this fact ought not obscure the possibility of the other choice. Especially as we women physicians counsel and accompany young women medical students to join us in our great calling, we should remember the many, many possible lives ahead of each young woman. By our attention to the nitty-gritty of live-in help versus day help, we ought not convey the assumption that all successful women doctors must be doctor and mother, too. We can include within our set of professional choices the choice to retain ourselves and those we love at the center of our lives, lives ever generative, ever prodigious.

— *Rita Charon*
Professor of Clinical Medicine and Director, Program in Narrative Medicine
Columbia University College of Physicians & Surgeons

Missed Opportunities

In reflecting back, I have been advancing my career for over 23 years and hopefully have another 20 years ahead of me to practice medicine. In the big picture, there is still time to write papers, network, attend national meetings, and give grand rounds. But if you did not take the afternoon off to go to your child's second-grade play, that opportunity is lost forever.

— *Barbara Cammer Paris*
Clinical Associate Professor of Medicine and Geriatrics,
Mount Sinai School of Medicine
Medical Director of Geriatric Inpatient Services, Mount Sinai Medical Center

Taking Stock

Most people assume that I decided to restructure my life and work because of family pressures: three young children, a professional spouse, an aged and ill mother-in-law. Those people are only partially correct. The reasons for stopping and taking stock of what I was choosing (and not choosing) go well beyond trying to find time to get groceries, do laundry, and drive the kids to soccer, skiing, and baseball. The real reasons get to the very heart of what life is and who gets to decide what is important.

When I took stock over the last year, I found that I was spending too much of my time doing things that were not of value to me, although they were certainly of great value to others and to my academic career. So I rearranged things to be more valuable for me. Now I spend most of my time at work doing things I truly enjoy. I read—novels, poetry, essays, medical, and nonmedical works—almost every day. I spend time just thinking about perplexing issues in medicine, in parenting, and in marriage. I have the luxury of leisurely meetings with residents and students, time to paint and explore with my kids, as well as keep food on the table and clean clothes available. And I have more of myself, a more enriched and happy self, to share with my kids and my husband.

— *Kathy Kirkland*
Assistant Professor of Medicine, Dartmouth Medical School

Life Choices

I think there are few things in life that are irreplaceable or irresistible. These include the people you love, the experiences that make you feel you've reached the heights and the breadths of your being, and time. And these priorities will conflict with each other. But try to keep them foremost in mind as you make your life choices in the face of outside pressures such as family, academic performance, job demands, financial obligations, illness, politics, and other misfortunes, from violence to "acts of God."

— Kathleen Dong
Former Associate Clinical Professor of Psychiatry, Stanford University
Now full-time mother

Composing a Life in Medicine

I entitled this essay after Mary Catherine Bateson's book, *Composing a Life* (Bateson, 1990), which profiles the lives of four extraordinary women. The thesis of her book is that very few successful women follow a straight line to reach their goal. More often, we lead discontinuous lives—lives interrupted personally or professionally as we make minor or major midcourse corrections. At certain times, we transition into new roles: starting or ending medical school or residency, getting married or divorced, having or not having children. We wear many hats, balancing professional lives with our personal lives as wives, mothers, daughters, and friends.

My suggestions for composing a life in medicine follow:

Put first things first. As the organizational consultant Stephen Covey (1990) exhorts us, decide what are the most important things in your life and make time for them. For me, my children and family top the list. School plays, soccer games, and PTA meetings are a priority. Carry one calendar to record these events along with your professional activities. Take an occasional day off work to go on the school field trip. There is no better way to get to know your children, their friends, and their teachers.

Say "no." You will be asked to take on many roles in both your personal and professional life. Match your commitments to your priorities and skills. When you make the transition to a new place in your life, recognize that you cannot continue to do all of the things that you originally did. Step out of roles that may constrain your growth. Last year, I chose to close my research lab. I loved my years in the lab, but something had to go.

Do not aim for perfection. In her commencement speech to the Mt. Holyoke graduates in 1999, Anna Quindlen (2000) exhorted them to give up the punishing quest for perfection, "a quest that causes us to doubt and denigrate our true selves." The cartoon character Sally Forth expressed it another way. Sally was bemoaning to her husband, John, that she couldn't figure out how to work full-time, be a great mom, and keep a clean house. John's answer: "Lower your expectations." While we cannot compromise our standards on patient care, there are other places in life where we can redefine our standards. Take housework. I am now learning to live in harmony with *frahoons*, my Irish great grandmother's word for the cobwebs in the corner of the ceiling.

Pace yourself. Medicine is a marathon, not a sprint. Whether you are in practice, academia, or industry, there are no milestones to reach that are age dependent. Take your birth date off your CV. What matters are your skills, your talents and your goals, not your age.

Contract. Hire out those jobs that you don't want or need to do. For me, that includes housecleaning, yard work, and window washing. One year, I cooked the turkey for Thanksgiving but bought all the vegetables at the local gourmet emporium and took the kids to the movies. Everyone, except the turkey, was very happy. If you have children, pay whatever you can afford to get the best child care. There is enough guilt with parenting, whether you work or not. Don't compound the situation worrying about what is happening with your kids while you are at work.

Volunteer. In the words of Winston Churchill, "We make a living by what we get. We make a life by what we give." When you volunteer, you will get back far more than what you give.

Choose your partner well. For those of us who marry, and studies show that 70% of us will, the single most important factor contributing to our long-term success is selecting the right partner. I feel exceptionally lucky to have found and married an incredibly supportive, insightful, and emotionally stable spouse. He is my best friend and greatest ally. Most important, we share core values and mutual respect—as well as passions for Duke basketball, browsing in bookstores, and Paris.

Each woman must weave together her own threads to create a life in medicine, a life with balance, enriched by our diverse experiences. Sometimes, like an artist weaving a tapestry, we will put down one thread and pick up another. Sometimes threads from earlier pursuits will resurface later in our careers. Like any work of art, no two lives will look the same. The tapestries we are creating as women in medicine are wondrous when viewed both individually and collectively.

— Joyce Rico

Medical Director, Fujisawa Healthcare, Inc., Deerfield, Illinois
Adjunct Clinical Associate Professor of Dermatology, New York University

References

Bateson, M.C. (1990). *Composing a life*. New York: Atlantic Monthly Press.
Covey, S. (1990). *The seven habits of highly effective people*. New York: Simon & Schuster.
Quindlen, A. (2000). Anna Quindlen's Commencement Speech, May 23, 1999. © Mt. Holyoke College www.mtholyoke.edu/offices/comm/oped/Quindlen. shtml

On Packing for the Information Superhighway

After spending several years working in a hospital system, I left clinical practice to start a new adventure. The trip would be fun. It is impossible to describe the anticipation of going to work for an Internet "start up" when you have spent so much time learning about the human body and it's response to illness.

Still, I felt nervous about leaving the familiar trappings of clinical medicine for the virtual space of the Internet world. The decision was simplified, however, by the workings of my hospital's new managed care system, a business model in which doctors had became "providers" and patients, managed care "lives." Besides, the time spent in meetings, paperwork, and referrals left little time for the real needs of doctoring. Unsure of where I would end up, I sought out opportunities that would offer professional satisfaction and time for my family. With a new baby on the way, I was anxious to lead a more reasonable life on evenings and weekends, one not regulated by emergency rooms and beepers. I wanted to enjoy the full experience of motherhood—from breast-feeding to potty training and all those "firsts" that come in between—without the stress of running a busy clinical practice.

So when I was offered a position at Elixis, a physician-owned company that created Internet software, I jumped at the chance to try something new. My background in technology and business was limited, but I was reassured that most skills would be learned on the job. I tried not to feel intimidated by the qualified credentials of those around me. Fortunately, my clinical experience proved valuable, and I soon fit into the marketing and development efforts as the Manager of Medical Affairs. I was thrilled to get my new business cards with the Web address on the back. My old colleagues began calling me "Cyberdoc," though I was not really practicing on the Web. We were developing a novel, Web-based medical data system, an application service provider (ASP) in which physicians could store and access information. I read voraciously on HIPPA (Health Insurance Portability and Accountability Act of 1996) trying to figure out a way of standardizing data formats for the electronic exchange of health information while still maintaining privacy and security requirements. I learned about the intricate process of software creation, Web site maintenance, and the new language of "platforms," "servers," "stored procedures," and "custom tags." Traveling to meet strategic clients and giving demonstrations at national conventions added a new dimension and challenge to the job.

As a physician, I never dreamed of doing anything outside of clinical medicine. But I am forever grateful for the events that brought together this exciting opportunity for personal growth and a look at "the other side of the fence." Meanwhile, my son Jonathan is now cruising and will soon walk. Taking this detour has allowed me to share in his exploration of the world, observing his expressions as they develop, one by one. I love being home with my family every evening and making holiday plans without having to juggle call schedules or vacation coverage. Despite my initial anxiety, it turns out that everything I needed for this trip, I already had.

— *Cynthia Rasch*
Private practice, internal medicine
Former Medical Affairs Manager for Elixis.com

Thoughts on Time Management

My mission is to take the best possible care of my patients and to use wisely the health, talents, and resources given to me. When the results, requests, insurance forms, and phone calls flood in, I put them into four categories—I have to do this as soon as possible; I want to do this; this should be done eventually; I don't need or care to do this—on the basis of their compatibility with my mission. An amazing number of tasks can be dealt with once the priority of each is established.

Most important, I have learned to say "no" when the request would compromise time that I have set aside to care for my patients, my family, or myself.

— *Veronica Piziak*
Chief of Endocrinology, Scott and White Clinic
Professor of Medicine, Texas A&M University
Professor School of Rural Public Health Texas A&M University

Note

1. Bateson, M. C. (1990). *Composing a life* (p. 233). New York: Penguin Putnam.

BARRIERS

As a feminist in a medical academy for over a decade,
I am still and always surprised not only at the relative lack
of a feminist presence in that institution but also at the
scornful associations with the word itself. I wonder how and
why medical education has remained seemingly immune
from a broad-based feminist critique from within, given the
fervent intellectual feminist debate in college and university
settings and in the larger U.S. culture. I look at the energy,
ambition, and intelligence of women students and colleagues
who often face the difficulties of blending demanding career
with other full-time responsibilities of partners, children,
and extended families and friends, not to mention other
interests outside medicine. I see these same women year after
year, not moving in appropriate numbers into positions of
increasing authority and prestige in the academic ranks and
clinical specialties. I know, and they know, that medical
education—indeed the huge and powerful social institution
of U.S. medicine—is controlled by a huge majority of white
men. Yet as I look at these same extraordinary women,
I am aware that not many would name themselves feminist.
— Delese Wear[1]

Glass Ceiling[2]

Almost, it seemed, I smelled
the patch of withered grass, the green of stale,
imbued with glutinous spit, now dried;
as integral a part of his scuffed leather shoe soles
as orange bug-splatters on a windshield.
My nostrils curled. He shifted
so his right shoe angled on the glass topped desk
and the left pointed, like a sword, at my shoulder,
its steel tip awash in smug aplomb.
From my seat, my vision framed
by his shod legs, modern caveman clubs,
I watched the metronome
of his breath, up, down, up, down,
stirring the point of his purple striped tie
on his polyester covered abdominal dune.
I thought of my great-aunt,
the one who did not turn up
at her own wedding, an arranged marriage.
"I'm not chattel," she said, and insisted
on an apology from the groom she dumped.
My interviewer stretched back in his swivel chair
and clasped his hands behind his hunter head.
"I hope you don't plan on getting pregnant,
we have problems with calls then, you know.
The men sure have it hard."
His feet remained lollygagging, eye-to-eye with me.
All I could think of was the story of my grandmother,
about how she died after the birth of my father
with a weak smile of apology,
as if she had failed her husband
with all that hemorrhaging.
"Well," he straightened up at last,
brought his feet back to floor with a thud.

"You've got the job." Jots of loosed dirt
shimmied on the glass.
I hoped he took off his shoes
before his next appointment, scrubbed them hard,
for if not
he would always stink
of saliva, chewed gum, crushed weeds and inferiority.

— *Bhuvana Chandra*
Pediatric psychiatrist and writer

Why Don't You Quit?[3]

I remember assisting at a 2 a.m. delivery on a clerkship, when the obstetrician suddenly asked if I were married. I indicated that I was the wife of another student at the same school, and he loudly responded, "Well, why don't you quit—you got what you came for."

— *Nancy B. Kaltreider*
Professor of Psychiatry Emerita, University of California San Francisco
Editor of Dilemmas of a Double Life *(1997)*

Woman in Orthopedic Surgery Stories

There were eight of us women in a class of 84 at the Yale School of Medicine, class of 1967. Emboldened by our entry onto the wards our third year, we asked the Dean one day, "Eight of us in each class—sure looks like a ten percent quota. Why is that?"

He responded, "Oh no, girls, that's just the percent of our applications that come from women."

But five or so years later came Title IX, and suddenly, the entering medical school classes all over the country were 25 to 30% women.

In our first-year anatomy lab, the professor wandered around the room asking questions. He talked like a Brooklyn truck driver but was one of my best teachers—so I thought—because he really liked to teach. Then one day when we were dissecting the lower back and buttocks, he announced to the class in a loud voice, "Miss Williams, Miss Gluteus Maximus of 1963, is going to demonstrate this lab for us."

I became interested in surgery, particularly orthopedic surgery, during my third year of medical school. After making rounds on the ortho unit one day, I said, "This is really fun—do girls do orthopedics?" (This was 1965 or so—before I was enlightened about the political importance of language.) The Chief Resident responded, "I don't think I know of any, but I don't know why not." Bless him—and the Chief of Orthopedics, who was also very supportive. Later, I found out that some institutions would not even accept an application for a surgical position from a woman.

At the time, trauma was one of the most appealing things about orthopedics to me: putting the broken pieces together again. I remember my interview at Roosevelt Hospital in a large office with three white-coated faculty members (all men) in a semicircle facing me.

They were each looking over copies of my application when one asked, "You're from Yale . . . do you know Dr. _____?"

I said, "Yes, he's the one who suggested I look at Roosevelt."

"He's very good-looking, isn't he?"

My memory is blank from that point on. I think and hope that I said something like, "Yes he is, but I don't see what that has to do with my application." I don't even remember if I was accepted there—it was irrelevant after that.

During my surgical residency at the University of Pittsburgh (Pitt), I was treated like one of the guys and not really singled out. I liked that feeling, but in retrospect, there was a lot of discrimination that I just didn't respond to or let myself remember. I was the first woman in the orthopedic program there and the second woman in the entire surgical program.

I stayed on the faculty at Pitt, and after a few years, Dr. Ferguson, the Chair, sought my advice, "Mary, I have a problem—we've got two women applicants for the residency for next year."

"Gee, Ferg, you always take more than one guy," I answered.

"You think it would be OK, to take two women at a time?"

"Sure," I said and he did, although one of the women eventually chose another program.

Most of the things that happened to me because I was a woman were not too serious. There were some sexual advances that I easily rebuffed. Fortunately, I never felt that my career was threatened. But a few instances made me realize that some men in surgery just couldn't bear to see a woman do what they did—it was too threatening to their egos.

Once while rounding with the residents, a partner of mine told me that he had seen one of my patients. "She's doing very well," he said. Then looking at the rest of the group (all men), he added, "But you know, a woman's just got no right to be able to do a triple arthrodesis."

Fortunately, most of it was more easy going. One of my mentors still enjoys telling this story.

"We'd be doing an intramedullary rodding, and Mary would ask for a step stool. Then she'd ask for another. Then pretty soon she was standing on three or four stools—but she'd never let me help her."

I don't think I ever got to four— three maybe, but I do remember being annoyed that he'd keep asking if I wanted help.

As an examiner for the Orthopedic Board exams, I was riding on the airport shuttle bus with a large bag of books that I'd bought during one of my breaks. The man sitting next to me asked, "Did you spend your time here shopping?" When I didn't quite understand, he repeated the question, adding, "while your husband was examining?"

"No," I said, "I'm the examiner."

He looked a little stunned, and didn't quite know what to say. I think he mumbled, "I'm sorry."

"Did I just raise your consciousness a little?" I asked, but he turned away and looked out the window for the rest of the trip.

— *Mary Williams Clark*
Chief of Pediatric Orthopedics, Sparrow Regional Children's Center
Clinical Professor of Orthopedics, Michigan State University

Life in the Boys' Club

The evolution of my professional being is not dissimilar to what other women surgeons have described. My early professional life as a student and a resident started with the blind enthusiasm and idealism of the young. The length of training (10 years of residency and fellowship) was taken for granted. The long days and nights on call, the emergencies at odd hours were all assumed to be a part of my life, and I expected to spend many a night, weekend, holiday, or missed date dealing with them.

An entire decade passed me by, and only after many years of sacrificing my personal life for my career, did I realize the toll it had taken. At the time, it seemed to be all or nothing, anything less than 100% commitment was unacceptable. I still suspect that was true then. Only in recent years has the concept become acceptable that physicians can have a life.

Throughout my training and early years as a junior faculty member, I strove to be better than the men, working harder without complaint in hopes of at least being considered their peer. The greatest revelation of my more senior years was that, in trying so hard to fit in the male world of surgery, I had been completely blind to issues of sexism and discrimination. It took me 22 years to realize what was *really* going on around me and to start doing something about it.

After over two decades in the medical profession, at a time when everything in my career seemed to be falling nicely into place, I hit the "glass ceiling." My promotion and tenure were opposed on ludicrous grounds, used as a cover for professional jealousy and gender discrimination. The resulting battle for academic survival was an experience I would not wish on anyone. I won, but at great physical and mental costs. I was criticized for wasting too much time with my patients and spending too much time teaching students. Involvement in women's professional organizations and activities was frowned on. The working environment became unreal, with scenes straight out of the movies: The lock on the office door was changed while I was on vacation, documents were altered—I could not continue to work in such a climate.

I was fortunate to meet my current Dean, a wonderful woman firmly committed to doing all she can to change the status quo, who actively recruited me. Accepting the new position was an extremely deliberate choice at a time when I had seriously considered abandoning medicine altogether. My passion for photography was beckoning, but the prospect of working with such an individual, finally having a mentor, and learning from a woman who truly had made it to the top of academic medicine and yet remained first and foremost a caring human being was irresistible. There were other attractions, not the least of which was the challenge of building a new division entirely from scratch.

Now, years later, I am a tenured full professor, Section Chief and Assistant Dean. I am the Women's Liason Officer to the AAMC (Association of American Medical Colleges) for my school and have been appointed to the AAMC's Women in Medicine Coordinating Committee. I landed on my feet but will never be the same again. Those who have not lived through the depression, the unfairness, and the lies cannot possibly understand the emotions and true physical illness that go along with such an experience. Sadly, all too many women *do* understand, because they also have been there.

Has being a woman made a difference in my career? Absolutely. No doubt there are still down sides. Surgery remains a "boys' club." I live with this fact daily, and despite the positive impact of organizations such as the Association of Women Surgeons, I do not expect the atmosphere to change completely during my professional lifetime. On the plus side, I have been blessed with being part of some experiences reserved for women, such as the ELAM (Executive Leadership in Academic Medicine) fellowship. This wonderful, yearlong program has given me not only new knowledge and skills but, perhaps more important, a network of professional acquaintances, friends, and supporters.

My career choice always seemed obvious: I love surgery, I love kids. Pediatric surgery gave me a way to combine these two passions. I made this choice very early in my medical career, worked toward that goal for what seemed like an eternity, and have never regretted it. Repairing a life-threatening congenital anomaly and watching the child grow and thrive into adulthood with a normal life expectancy is an unparalleled pleasure. It is a specialty that constantly keeps you on your toes: There are no cookbook answers—you must be ready to use your ingenuity and improvise. In pediatric surgery, you do not just treat the patient, you treat the family. And to see a happy, healthy family leave the office or hospital is one of the most gratifying sights I can imagine.

I firmly believe that my being a woman enhances the interactions with my young patients and their families. Children seem to feel less threatened. Mothers and grandmothers feel more at ease, often simply (and correctly) assuming that I understand them. I certainly have had patients referred to me for that reason alone. I do not feel the need to maintain a macho, rigid mask of detachment in the face of their emotions. I can do my job properly, yet continue to be the person I have always been. Maybe this has nothing to do with being a woman, but I like to think that my gender brings to my career much more than a firm commitment to succeed: I hope it allows me to retain the sensitive and humanistic qualities we would all like to see in our health care providers.

— *Roberta E. Sonnino*
Professor and Chief, Section of Pediatric Surgery
Assistant Dean for Student Affairs,
University of Kansas School of Medicine

Professionalism

The beautiful, privileged, yet often frustrating part of being a woman physician is the amount of self devoted to the job. Men must also face this, but the emotionality that we as women add to our work seems more intense and, quite honestly, may not always be required.

The challenges along the way have been many, though I find myself constantly facing this dilemma: my assertiveness misinterpreted as abrasiveness, my confidence misconstrued as arrogance, my potential interpreted as ambition. We are expected to be equally competent as the men, yet not advertise our professionalism. As women, we must still bear the soft qualities that make our gender socially appealing. These mixed messages are disconcerting for the young woman professional. If you speak up, you're abrasive; if you're demure, you're not capable. Eventually, one must come to a comfortable acceptance of her own purpose and sense of self-worth. Provided we maintain good rapport with our patients and serve them well, what others perceive is inconsequential.

Problems balancing home life and career are not unique to women physicians. They are also an issue for men who make home life a priority. It truly becomes an issue of priority, and a respectable, giving relationship between caregivers and family is needed. No family is perfect, and no lifestyle devoid of these issues. Life is simply lived too quickly over a very short time. The struggles we face are a factor of that pace.

Being a physician is not glamorous; it is a service—a lifelong devotional endeavor. It is truly a privilege that comes naturally to some, is perfected with time, and stays with us, I hope, long after we take down our shingle.

— *Rosa E. Cuenca*
Assistant Professor of Surgery,
East Carolina University School of Medicine

The Feminization of American Medicine[4]

I am part of the feminization of American medicine, a minuscule player in the changing landscape of a profession whose pulse, until recently, was transfixed by men with women in supporting roles at home, in the office and in the hospital. This type of organization allowed men to focus their efforts single-mindedly on medicine and to build this great field into what it is today. We have inherited a profession whose lifestyle is difficult to reconcile with the basic definition of what it is to be a woman. Women are therefore unlikely to travel the road that many of the men took because the steps they left for us are too narrow for all the roles we live. The medical profession may eventually evolve to accommodate our needs and our biology, but until then it is up to women to create the means to build careers and lives that bring satisfaction.

— *Kathryn Ko*
Chief of Neurosurgery, Brookdale University Hospital
Author of The Survival Bible for Women in Medicine *(1998)*

An Interview Tale

The interviewer, an imposing six-foot-plus, blond-haired, head-and-neck surgeon who brought images of Beowulf to mind, sat approximately 15 feet away from me. Sweat pooled under the arms of my brown wool pantsuit, an outfit that strayed from the traditional navy skirt suit set. This was strike number one against me. The others I had made even prior to sitting down: I was female, a minority, and vertically challenged. "How many siblings do you have?" the interviewer asked, innocently enough.

"None," I replied, not knowing where this line of questioning would lead.

"Was that lonely growing up as an only child?"

"Yes, I would have loved to have siblings, at least two or three."

"So you probably want to have at least a few children to prevent them from having your own fate?"

I answered enthusiastically with a big smile on my face, "Oh, yes, definitely."

"Hmmm . . . ok." The interviewer scribbled something in his file. My heart sank. I had succumbed to his well-disguised illegal question. The rest of the interview was a blur for me and likely meaningless for him. The questions were routine; my answers automatic.

This scenario was not an isolated experience, though, at other times, I managed to play the interview game with more finesse.

I have always liked a challenge. The interview trail for my surgical subspecialty certainly gave that to me. I was constantly reminded of inherent attributes that I had no power to change. Ambivalent comments from acquaintances haunted me at every turn. "No one will marry you if you are a surgeon," or "You should have picked something easier."

It angers me that questions regarding life decisions such as family and marriage can be made grounds for discrimination. Women physicians should be free to embrace their potential as future wives and/or mothers. These are fundamental aspects of our identity, whether or not we choose to fulfill that potential.

I can only hope that, with the rising numbers of women in medicine, these barriers will be overturned and that some day, we can safely wear pantsuits and wedding rings to interviews if we so choose.

— *Priya Krishna*
Otolaryngology resident,
Southern Illinois University School of Medicine

Not Easy to Please[5]

Surely this is a little difficult. We were told that the great objection to women entering professional life was that they would not care to marry, hence the desire to keep them out. Now conditions are reversed and the objection is that they do. Really it is not easy to please.

— *Woman's Medical Journal, 1893*

On Reaching Visible

For Nina and Nancy

Many years they looked through me,
Her story streams warm effusive,
Sans regret, a pioneer decades
In research

They looked right through me, she says
A hopeful novice bound to persevere.
I am, on the edge of my seat,
That person invisible

What power, she says,
plodding among souls unfiltered
No decorum no obsequious doublespeak,
disturbing but Zen nonetheless
To simply *be*

Forging many years brings glory and presence
Faces blur opaque, clouded then obscured
Veils drape and drag pretenses
The blinders of hierarchy

A beacon, a leader enduring,
she stretches out her arms
and moves ahead

— *Susan K. Schultz*
Associate Professor of Psychiatry,
University of Iowa College of Medicine

Triple Jeopardy

They called it a junk ship. A small boat with no motor, only oars. We huddled in it close to my mother for comfort, my brothers and I. We must have been on the river for days. Only five at the time, I can hardly remember. I do know that we were fleeing the Japanese soldiers who had just invaded our province in China. And I remember that one of my brothers became desperately ill, having contracted dysentery from the crowded, unsanitary conditions on the boat. We had no access to medical care while on the river and by the time we reached the nearest town, it was too late. This tragedy left a deep impression on my young mind: From that time on, I wanted to be a doctor.

The war ended, and my family moved to Taiwan. I eventually graduated from the National Taiwan University Medical College in 1958. I chose to specialize in obstetrics and gynecology, but female residents were not permitted in the surgical specialties. Intent on my dream, I came to the United States.

I still remember my interview at Philadelphia General Hospital. We waited together in one room—25 applicants, all Caucasian males, probably all American graduates—and then me. Despite having done well in the interview, I knew there were already three strikes against me: I was a woman, an Asian, and a foreign medical graduate. Two weeks later, I was elated to learn of my acceptance as one of four residents.

Residency was a delightful experience where I learned much, both in the social and medical spheres. I enjoyed the company of my coresidents, many of whom introduced me to their wives and invited me to their homes. They sometimes joked about my pronunciation, especially when I mixed up the consonants R, L, and N.

I had intended to return to Taiwan to teach and practice, but unfortunately, gender discrimination still prevailed within the surgical fields. There were no female residents, let alone female faculty members. So instead, I began a research fellowship at Pennsylvania Hospital, eventually becoming a research associate at the University of Pennsylvania Medical School.

Shortly thereafter, I married and moved to New York. Since 1969, I have been teaching, practicing, and conducting research at New York University School of Medicine. My experiences at NYU have generally been positive, despite some subtle discrimination that exists even today. I can recall a conversation with my chairman about starting salaries back in 1969. When I objected to the exceptionally low figure, he responded, "You don't need much money. You are supported by a husband. The male

faculty need more money because they have to support their families."
Only after strong protests that equal work should merit equal pay did he
finally increase my starting salary. But to this date, I am not convinced
that the increase was truly equitable. Furthermore, it took me longer than
my male Caucasian colleagues to be promoted to the tenure track and
eventually to full professor.

Even with a demanding schedule, I still enjoyed a wonderful family
life. My two children are now grown—my son a music production
manager, my daughter a radiology resident. I feel blessed that they not
only grew up without any major disasters but have both thrived in their
respective fields. We lived a short block from the hospital so that despite
my work, I could be readily available. Fortunately, I had wonderful child
care arrangements and a helpful, supportive husband. My children's
school plays, musical recitals, or athletic events were always a priority,
and I think that meant a lot to them.

Several of my medical school classmates stayed home when their
children were young, later resuming their careers as their children grew
older. Each woman's situation is different. Whether one chooses to work
or stay home depends entirely on the individual. You must follow your
own conscience or you will never be happy. In my experience, it is
definitely possible to pursue an academic career and still maintain a
happy family life but not without some hardship or sacrifice. You may
have to give a little on both sides, because there is simply not enough
time to be perfect at everything. Someone once asked me whether I
would do the same thing if I could start all over again. Absolutely.

— *Livia Shang-yu Wan*
Professor of Obstetrics & Gynecology,
New York University School of Medicine

A Minority Perspective[6]

I think of myself as a physician. Not as a black physician. Not as a female
physician. Nor as a black female physician. These distinctions are

important because as one adds racial, ethnic, or gender modifiers, subconscious or perhaps conscious adjustments are made regarding value, competence, and worth—usually occurring in a negative direction. I am admittedly a product of the socially and politically turbulent '70's; therefore I'm sure that my gender and race as well as my good grades played a part in both my college and medical school admissions. But in real life, many factors come into play during the admissions process for *all* of us. The difference is in the operating word—*factors*. African Americans happen not to have the long legacy of family money, physician relatives, and friends of import or the "good old boys network" operating on their behalf. So how important are the factors that get us to and in the door? Is it not important what happens once you've entered through the proverbial door? Are the curriculum or tests any different for a woman, an African American, or the offspring of a prominent white physician? I don't believe so. Therefore, once a medical diploma has been earned and conferred, racial, ethnic, or gender modifiers serve only to lend a diminutive effect on one's efforts and hard work.

One would expect that in medical education, the playing field would be more level. Not so. Some individuals are placed in "special" tracts educationally, others in "special" tracts conceptually. There seems to be no end to the lowered expectations and opinions of the African American student, resident, and practitioner. I can still recall the morning after our junior medicine orals (which were traditionally perceived as hazardous to one's health). The resident eagerly asked the scores of the two white male students (who received 3.0 and 3.5 of a 4.0 possible score), less eagerly the score of the white female (3.0) and last, almost as an aside, my score (4.0). The message came through loud and clear as to whom he thought would or would not perform well. I was reminded once again not to let the opinion of others affect my self-esteem, performance, or attitude; an additional burden to carry in the midst of an already burdensome experience.

— *Beverly M. Gaines*

President, Beverly M. Gaines, M.D. & Associates PSC
Assistant Clinical Professor of Pediatrics, University of Louisville

My Path Through Medical School

I came from a large, for the most part, supportive family of five brothers, one sister, an electrician dad, and a stay-at-home mom. There were no doctors in my family. I didn't even know one personally. The only successful people in the family were men—most of them engineers. That included my brothers, brothers-in-law, and husband. So naturally, I followed in their footsteps. But when my husband saw my unhappiness with engineering, he said, "Sure, go to medical school."

During that first grueling week, he pleaded daily with me to quit. His was not the only resistance that I encountered. My mother-in-law assured me that, because of my frequent absences from home, my son would grow up to be another Charles Manson. My own parents, also staunch believers that mothers should remain at home, gave me no support in caring for my two children. My brothers and their wives merely stood by, amused. Even my colleagues and friends thought I would never make it.

To be perfectly honest, neither did I. When I got a broken chair on the first day of lab, I didn't bother to ask for a replacement, thinking I would be using it for only a short while. I turned in my drop card once over winter break but by January had retrieved it. Every test I passed seemed like a miracle, but each one caused my husband only more distress. In spite of his initial encouragement, he considered medical school my hobby and demanded that I fulfill all the household responsibilities first. This meant that I sometimes had to clean bathrooms at 5:30 a.m. Many of my grades must have been achieved by divine inspiration, because I simply couldn't start studying until late at night when everyone else was asleep.

Notwithstanding a wounded—but intact—marriage and a struggling family, I somehow made it. We celebrated this bittersweet accomplishment and had our third child, an event that was truly one of life's greatest gifts.

Today, as the mother of five, I am proud to be a physician. Yet my greatest satisfaction comes from being a mother, a role that helps me keep all things in perspective. I have never won any great awards, nor do I claim to be the best mother or the best radiologist. Instead, I carry my experiences from one role to the other, hoping that all those with whom I come into contact will benefit. I may not know the effect of all this on my children until they grow old enough to point out my mistakes, but one of my daughters asks many questions about bones and lungs and says she wants to be a doctor. As they say, imitation is the most sincere form of flattery.

— *Barbara K. Pawley*
Assistant Professor of Radiology,
University of Louisville School of Medicine

The Life of Women in Medicine

*Why are men never asked, "How will you
balance your career and your family?"*

Throughout our marriage of 22 years, my physicist husband and I have traveled a great deal to optimize both our careers and family life. At times, the academic sacrifices seemed large indeed, as my research projects in academic psychiatry often had to be jettisoned in midstream to accommodate the needs of my husband and children. But ultimately, my family was more important than my career. Of course, all the moving around has meant a real loss of continuity. Despite my 47 years, I have the CV of a 30-year-old. So when I come up for promotion, one question will be whether a university can take into account all the moving around and backsliding a woman must sometimes do to keep all family members content. What no institution will directly confront is the subtle but often pervasive lack of seriousness toward women who want to pursue an academic career while still providing a nurturing, loving environment for their families.

— *Barbara R. Sommer*
Assistant Professor and Director of Geriatric Psychiatry,
Stanford University School of Medicine

Leave

During my internal medicine residency in the 1970s, one of the fellows in another division became pregnant. She was the first woman in that division to get pregnant while training. Women behind her were anxious to see how the issue of maternity leave would be handled, since there had been no precedent and certainly no maternity policy. We soon found out: Her Division Chief informed her that if she took more than the allotted two-week vacation time for maternity leave, he would never take another woman into his fellowship program. He also implied that it would affect the strength of his recommendation when she applied for future jobs.

She took only two weeks maternity leave. This had a chilling effect on the women in my residency program. Even I began to question my career choice. Ironically, this same Division Chief is now a high-ranking official in academic medicine. I doubt that anyone has since discussed with him this event or its impact on the women in his division.

Two years later, during my gastroenterology fellowship, I became the second woman in my department to become pregnant while training. Remembering the reception of the other Division Chief, I was nervous about breaking the news to my own Chief. When I did, I told him of my plan to take six weeks of maternity leave, two of which would count as vacation time. His response could not have been more positive. He not only congratulated me soundly but fully supported my decision to start a family, pointing out that a six-week hiatus from a long career was insignificant—and he was right.

Over the past 30 years, women have made impressive gains in medicine. Thankfully, within the hierarchy of men, more individuals have supported women's careers than the Division Chief that my colleague encountered.

— *Grace H. Elta*
Professor of Medicine, University of Michigan

Emotional Conflicts of the Career Woman[7]

For many years, I have been especially interested in problems of career women that result from their increasing participation in what has been considered "a man's world." This pertains not only to women in medicine but to women in many other professions and careers such as law, business, government, and banking, where women now have unprecedented opportunities for high-level commitment and responsibility.

Women have always worked. The stress I am referring to is not derived from hard work—but from other factors. Since the recent women's movement, a definite change has taken place in women's attitude toward their work. They are now choosing to pursue a career as part of their sense of identity. This is the important distinction. What has been called identity work was formerly restricted almost exclusively to men. A woman's identity was traditionally defined by marriage and family, as wife and mother. A man's identity was primarily defined by his work, with marriage and family giving him the necessary nurturance and support. When men pursued a career, the entire family was oriented toward helping him. On those occasions in the past when a woman pursued a career, she usually gave it up when she got married or adapted her career to her husband's and children's needs. It was not uncommon for a woman to drop out of medical school after marriage or drop out of practice for 8 to 10 years to take care of her family.

This is what is now changing. Women who enter professions now do not plan to drop out for marriage and family. They are becoming deeply involved in their work and look forward to further career development plus family. Work outside the home affords an opportunity for a direct process of self-actualization, while marriage and family require that the woman subordinate her own needs to the needs of others; therefore, her validation and sense of worth must come through others. In addition, the culture has always rewarded men for their achievement outside the home and paid only lip service to women's traditional activities in the home.

Men's lives allowed them total, undisturbed concentration on their work, while women's lives consisted of constant interruptions, fragmentation, and demands on their energies by others. Now that women are seeking self-actualization through work, they are confronted with specific conflicts that cause anxiety and that must be resolved.

This struggle is caused by a divided or uncertain sense of identity experienced daily, many, many times at all stages of their professional career. It is not only that a professional woman is impelled to divide her time and energy to cover both home and work, but also that, unlike the male professional, she is constantly beset with divided loyalties and a sense of guilt. As soon as a young man becomes inclined toward a profession, this system is built and maintained for him by the women in his life: first his mother, often his sisters, later his girlfriend, his wife, and his secretary. When a woman becomes a professional, she most often provides her own support system. Many of my patients went into their careers without family support, and sometimes with the family's active disapproval. Amazingly when these same women got married, they *automatically* relegated their own professional needs to those of their husband and family. Their own personal growth went underground without apparent resentment, although it took its toll in depression, unhappiness, and psychosomatic syndromes.[1]

It is not surprising that many men feel threatened by the growth and development of women. Men have always had their dependency needs fulfilled automatically by their wives or other women around them without having to acknowledge this to themselves. Their personal wants such as food, laundry, clothing, warmth, and nurturance at home have been supplied by mother, sisters, girlfriend, wife, or secretary. It takes a very secure man to give this up willingly and without resentment. Some men need reassurance from women that the moves women are making for themselves do not represent rejection. Some see moving away as moving against and have actually said to their wives who are involved in new activities: "You don't care about me anymore." Often they do not verbalize this but feel it and act cold and withdrawn. Most women shrivel up in their emotional climate of passive resistance and often become immobilized with repressed rage. They give up their plans for growth and development without realizing that men need time to adapt to the new changes and that most eventually will do so. It is not all a loss for men, since women's growth and self-fulfillment relieve men of the excessively dependent needs of their wives as well as add interest to the relationship.

If women continue to develop in work or career as an expression of their identity, then certain changes are essential in both men's and women's personalities. This will come about only if men share in the nurturing of infants and toddlers and in the house care associated with family living.[2] Care for the intimate dependency needs of the infants and toddlers must be experienced by the child as coming from both men and women. Men must give up their narcissistic pursuit of work at the expense of their families.

These are points at which a profound resistance develops, preventing any significant change from occurring in the patriarchal society. Yet without this, we achieve only a superficial redistribution of labor and merely the illusion of change. It is my belief that if these changes come about in the personalities of men and women, we will witness a process that will be truly liberating, relieving both men and women from the rigid stereotypic molds that have crippled humankind and caused untold misery.

— *Alexandra Symonds*
Founder and first President of the Association of Women Psychiatrists

Notes

1. Symonds, A. (1978). The psychodynamics of expansiveness in the success-oriented woman. *American Journal of Psychoanalysis, 38*, 195–205.

2. Symonds, A. (1978). Editorial: Psychoanalysis and women's liberation. *Journal of the American Academy of Psychoanalysis, 6*, 429–431.

Kath's Graduation

Growing up in a large family with five brothers, I always felt like one of the guys. But after completing my surgical training, I realized that wasn't the case. I may see only men and think I'm one of them, but they see me—a woman and I'm different.

At first, I thought something was wrong with me. I responded differently than the men. Instead of saying, *I'll fix it*, I'd say, *I'm sorry, I won't do it again*. Instead of being aggressive, bold, and willing to take chances, I was argumentative and dared to question my superiors. While my male coworkers swore on a daily basis, I swore once and was almost kicked out of the program.

After a while, I realized I wasn't wrong. There's more than one way to skin a cat. I was just different. I looked different, responded differently, acted differently. I was a woman and a minority in the field of surgery.

But being a minority did not mean that I wanted to be treated like the men. I didn't miss the locker room scene with jokes about lesbians or boobs. I simply wanted a good education so that I could give the best care to my patients.

And I know I got that.

— *Kathryn A. Carolin*
Assistant Professor of Surgery,
Wayne State University

An American Experience

I had just completed a thorough history and physical on a patient and given her medicine to correct her arrhythmia and eliminate her chest discomfort. Imagine my surprise when, 15 minutes later, she was asking the lab tech if he was the physician. Tony tried to explain that he was there to draw blood for the tests I had requested. That's when she informed him of her preference for a white, Irish male physician. Being an African American woman, I definitely did not meet the requisite criteria. I tried to look as sympathetic as possible when I apologized that there was no white, Irish male physician here to take care of her. "It is good that you know what makes you feel most comfortable," I added.

My thoughts flashed back to residency training. It was 3:00 a.m., and I was running down the hallway with a stretcher full of medications, a defibrillator, and an elderly man in complete heart block. He looked up at me from the stretcher, a veil of concern slowly crossing his face. I introduced myself, hoping to put his mind at ease. I was the doctor who would be taking him to the CCU and caring for him along with the brilliant, award-winning team of cardiology specialists.

The concern on his face deepened as he grimaced, " Oh, great, you're a doctor; that's wonderful, a woman and a doctor?" It seemed at once both a revelation and a question. "Are there other doctors in the cardiac unit who are not women?" he asked, and this time I was sure that I saw hope in his eyes, that there might be "others."

I assured him that we were quite a diverse team of men and women. Then I smiled broadly as I raved about the great care he would receive that night, exclusively from myself and my female resident.

Black, white, Latino, Asian, young, old, male, female—it doesn't matter. I simply don't fit the stereotypical physician image. Given this humble visage, what should I be? Once while I was teaching a team of medical students, interns, and residents, a patient's family member walked across the emergency room and into the doctor's area to hand me a bed pan full of urine. Even with the long white coat, stethoscope, and M.D. name tag, even mid-sentence in my discourse, I was still mistaken for a nurse's aide or a cleaning lady.

— *Dorina Rose Abdulah*
Clinical Instructor of Medicine, Harvard Medical School

A Warm Gesture[8]

My neck was stiff from long hours of tension, muscles aching from pulling against a retractor. The day had been exhausting and I was post-call. Evening rounds were endless with continuous pimping. The attending relentlessly tormented the interns and students. For the umpteenth time I questioned my decision to enter medical school. All day I wore a strained, forced smile. The final straw was the unexpected death of a favorite patient.

The other student on my team was a classmate, a casual acquaintance. We'd had some contact during the preclinical years, volunteering at community clinics and socializing at various school functions. I'd had lunch several times with his wife. Now we were on the ward together. We had quickly developed a camaraderie, covering when the other was late for rounds, feeding answers behind the attending's back, and switching call schedules when necessary.

I survived rounds without falling asleep and we proceeded to the cafeteria to refuel before heading home. Sitting there relaxing, I was overcome by a wave of sorrow remembering the patient just lost. Tears filled my eyes. I should have stopped by her room, but now it was too late. Quietly he listened, offering condolences.

His offer of a neck rub was welcome, a warm gesture of friendship. As his hands began to knead away the stress in my muscles, breaking up the knots of restrained emotion and feigned placidity, a feeling of relaxation displaced the strain and tension. He provided support and strength, one colleague assisting another, as I would have done for him.

I took a deep breath and brushed the tears from my eyes, ready to head home. It was dark so he offered to walk me to the car. I was grateful to have him along and not to have to wait for the police escort. When we reached the car, I squeezed his elbow to reinforce the verbal "thanks." As I fumbled in my pack to find the keys, he reached over, I thought to say, "you're welcome." Instead, with a strange grin on his face, he extended his hand past my shoulder placed it firmly on my breast. Startled, I turned my back to him and opened the car door, forcing his arm while trying to discount it as a directional mistake. As I got into the car, his arm returned, deliberately, to grab my other breast. Forcefully I flung his arm aside. I snapped, "You don't need to be doing that!" I slammed the door and raced out of the parking lot.

Confused and shocked, I drove automatically down the street. I was trembling, fervently gripping the steering wheel for some stability.

Physically I felt ill, as the revulsion of the incident hit: unwanted, deliberate sexual advances from a colleague. Had I somehow given him permission to touch me in that way by accepting the neck rub? I had seen it as a safe, innocent gesture from a friend—nothing more. Had I unconsciously encouraged him? Was it the way I was "seductively" dressed in scrubs?

Brought back to reality by the blaring of a car horn behind me, I focused on the stop sign and began driving. Somehow in my daze I made it home, turned off the phone, and curled up in a corner of the couch. Alone in the dark, I was consumed by disbelief, shame, and anger. Who was going to believe me? It was my word against his. Then I began to remember earlier incidents. He'd made numerous inappropriate personal remarks over the past 2 years that I had shrugged off as crude jokes. I had discounted other, more subtle brushes against my breast as unintentional. I had treated him as a colleague, on a professional level. I felt my trust betrayed.

The next morning on rounds, he acted as though nothing had happened. I stood there with a feigned smile, suppressing an overwhelming desire to escape from him. I had to maintain my professional dignity and keep it intact through rounds. His indifferent behavior made me wonder if I had imagined the entire incident. Then, I caught him staring at me with that same strange grin. I resolved never to be alone with him again.

I sought support and advice from friends. Many male friends implied I had done something to provoke his behavior. Some trivialized the incident. "So he copped a feel? What's the big deal? He shouldn't get kicked out of school or have it affect his career." Women, generally, listened sympathetically and related their own experiences. Much to my outrage and subsequent relief, I discovered that I was not the first woman he had accosted in this manner. Other classmates had previously confronted him without that changing his offensive behavior. The picture was emerging. Mine was not an isolated incident.

For several months I tried to deal with my feelings. I felt sickened if I encountered him. I was on edge, flinching if my closest male friends

THIS SIDE OF DOCTORING

innocently touched me. I was unable to tolerate any sexual humor. Most of all I was angry at how the incident had changed me.

I was tempted to brush the incident aside for the sake of his future and his marriage. After discovering that mine was not an isolated incident, however, I could not. I was concerned that my future interactions with male colleagues and my chances of getting into a good residency program might be affected if charges became public. I finally decided it had to be done.

Three months after the incident, I walked into the Dean's office to report it. As I began relating my experience to the sexual harassment adviser, she responded that I was not the first to report him for his behavior. I had done the right thing. Or had I? Had I stopped him early enough to change his behavior? He will still graduate. The charges will not affect his residency, but he will have a permanent record of the incident, in case it ever happens again. No one can accuse me of having kept silent.

— *Name Withheld*

A Lesbian Voice: What Does It Mean to Be a "Dyke Doctor"?

Our local "Women in Medicine" group had just set out to march in the Gay Freedom Day Parade in San Francisco. A moment of panic gripped me when I saw the T-shirts that had been designed by one of our younger members. "DYKE DOCTORS" was painted across the front in large, bold strokes. *But that's not me,* I reassured myself silently among our group of traditional lesbian physicians. Never one to be that "out" with the lingo, I didn't want my friends to know how many years it had taken for me to even say the "L" word without my heart leaping up into my throat. So I bit my tongue, put on the T-shirt, and grabbed a "Lesbian Physician" sign, chanting with the others as we marched the streets of San Francisco: "Two-four-six-eight, you need a Pap smear even if you're not straight."

I had my first relationship with a woman when I was 16 and then spent the next five years dating men, desperately trying to fall in love so I could get married, have babies, and go to medical school within a traditional lifestyle. But that was not to be. In my senior year at Mount Holyoke, I met Nancy, another pre-med, and fell in love. She followed me to Texas where I began medical school and where she enrolled the following year. We actively hid our relationship, worried that we would be expelled or that our parents would cut off tuition assistance if anyone ever found out. Using code words, we lived a double life off campus and developed "underground" connections with other gay and lesbian colleagues.

In those days, lesbian women typically attended chiropractic or osteopathic schools, not Western medical schools. I was one of 16 women in a class of 125 students and could pass for straight to the point of being felt up during surgery by orthopedic residents for whom I was holding retractors and even being propositioned by a trustee of the medical center. But my emotional ties were to women, although I couldn't quite figure out how motherhood would fit into the picture. Not only did I not know any lesbian mothers in San Antonio, but "Zero Population Growth" was the politically correct stance. Toward the end of medical school, I tried partnering with a gay man who was a pediatrician and who also wanted kids. Unfortunately, that relationship fizzled once I started my residency at UC San Francisco. So I finally accepted the fact that I was a lesbian and that I would have to make my own path.

In 1976, I was the only woman my year in the OB/GYN residency. It was hard enough surviving as a female, let alone surviving as a lesbian. Being on call every third night for four years left little time for the requisite concerts, music festivals, and bar gatherings for meeting other lesbians. But finally, I did meet Lesley, a wonderful woman who was doing her internship. Together we founded the annual "Women in Medicine" conference, which provides a forum for scientific exchange, networking, and peer support among lesbian physicians and their families. Now in its 18th year, conference attendance includes a significant contingent of children. So it is from this perspective I speak.

Being a lesbian physician means the following:

– Being anxious when interviewing for a new position: Will they be hostile if they know I am a lesbian, or will they be more hostile if I accept the position and then "come out?" Is it possible to work here without telling them anything about my personal life?

– Worrying about bringing my partner to a work function that includes partners and wondering if anyone will include her in the conversation or be freaked out and ignore us as a couple

– Not having to worry about being a good wife, since there are no stereotypes for lesbian couples

– Worrying about how to obtain health insurance for my partner

– Being open to alternative treatment modalities

– Having a significant number of lesbian patients, particularly since many of them have had negative experiences with the Western health care system

– Developing a referral list of colleagues who will treat my lesbian patients sensitively

– Usually not having a spouse at home to raise the kids or keep the home front going when I travel to meetings

– Often not sharing details of my personal life when chatting with nurses, not knowing who is homophobic and who is not

– Mentoring lesbian medical students so they will have a better experience than I did when I went to medical school

– Hoping to protect my children from the inevitable name-calling that results from having parents who are different

Since that day of the T-shirt crisis, I have come a long way in accepting myself as a lesbian. I am an out Professor of Clinical Obstetrics and Gynecology at the University of California at San Francisco. Recently,

I was featured on the Learning Channel's "Maternity Ward" as a high-risk obstetrician. I doubt the viewers had any idea they were watching a lesbian physician committed to providing competent and sensitive care. My sexual orientation wasn't relevant at the time. It shouldn't matter. But it does. It matters because of the boundaries and discrimination created by homophobia, precisely those factors that have made mine and my children's lives more difficult. I speak out so that younger lesbian physicians will have an easier time, so that they won't have to worry about their children and discrimination, about health insurance, or about the lack of governmental benefits. And I hope that, in the future, all lesbian patients will find sensitive and caring physicians. We know we cannot bring about these changes ourselves. We need and deserve the help of our colleagues, patients, and families.

— *Patricia A. Robertson*
Professor of Clinical Obstetrics and Gynecology,
University of California San Francisco
Co-Director, Center for Lesbian Health Research

Notes

1. Excerpted from Wear, D. (1997). *Privilege in the medical academy: A feminist examines gender, race, and power* (p. 33). New York: Teachers College Press. Reprinted with permission.
2. Chandra, B. (1999). Glass ceiling. *Annals of Internal Medicine, 131*(6), 437. Reprinted by permission of the American College of Physicians.
3. Excerpted from Kaltreider, N. B. (1975). The hazards of feminine physicianhood. *Harvard Medical Alumni Bulletin, 50*, 10–13. Reprinted by permission.
4. Excerpted from Ko, K. (1998). The feminization of American medicine. In *The survival bible for women in medicine* (p. vii). New York: Parthenon Publishing. Reprinted by permission of the publisher and author.
5. From the *Woman's Medical Journal*, 1893, as quoted in More, E. S. (1999). *Restoring the balance* (p. 23). Cambridge, MA: Harvard University Press. Copyright © 1999 by the President and Fellows of Harvard College.
6. Excerpted from Gaines, B. M. (1991). Minority perspective. *Louisville Medicine: Bulletin of the Jefferson County Medical Society, 39*(4), 13–14. Reprinted with minor editorial changes by permission of the Jefferson County Medical Society.

7. Excerpted from Symonds, A. (1983). Emotional conflicts of the career woman. *American Journal of Psychoanalysis*, *43*(1), 21–37. Kluwer Academic/Plenum Publishers. Reprinted and abridged with permission.

8. From A warm gesture. (1992). *Journal of the American Medical Association*, *267*(5), 743. Copyrighted ©1992, American Medical Association. Reprinted with permission.

9

CONNECTIONS

For to be a woman is to have interests and duties,
raying out in all directions from the central mother-core,
like spokes from the hub of a wheel. The pattern of our
lives is essentially circular. We must be open to all points
of the compass; husband, children, friends, home,
community; stretched out, exposed, sensitive like a spider's
web to each breeze that blows, to each call that comes.
— Anne Morrow Lindbergh[1]

The Doctor in the Family[2]

My nephew died at home this morning.

Sam's mother sat on a soft taupe sofa, holding him in her arms. The May sun streamed through the windows while Sam's father leafed through the mail in a worn armchair nearby. The schoolyard down the street was alive with children's games, including those of Sam's older brother. A brain tumor, now coma, had been blended into the ordinary happenings of daily life for a long time. And then Sam took his final breath.

Sam spent most of his 5 years living a healthy, vibrant life at home with his parents and brother. He dressed as an ice cream cone last

Halloween, and as Doc from *Snow White and the Seven Dwarfs* the year before. He loved his dollhouse, the color yellow, his best friend Lilly, and salty pretzels. But Sam also spent many days in hospitals. He had an astrocytoma, diagnosed when he was 4 months old. Throughout his life, the juxtaposition of apparent health with periods of critical illness obscured the hazy boundary of futility and appropriate medical care. Sam would undergo brain surgery one day and be home swinging in the back yard the next. At 2 years of age, he reported nausea one evening after dinner. Several hours later, he became lethargic. His parents rushed him to the hospital, where he had seizures and was posturing on arrival; his parents were told that the end was near. The following day, he awoke asking for his mother. He was discharged from the intensive care unit 3 days later and went home to bake a cake covered with colored sprinkles in his Easy-Bake Oven, with Lilly at his side. Despite his dire prognosis, Sam attended preschool, grew into a size five banana yellow fleece jacket, and traveled from his home in Massachusetts to the beaches of Maine and Oregon.

Sitting in my office, I was admiring a photograph of Sam dancing on the Oregon coast, with Tillamook Head in the background. My brother had just telephoned with the news of Sam's death—four and a half years later than I had expected it.

When Sam's disease was diagnosed, I immediately framed the issues of his illness in terms of probabilities and asked myself whether treatment of his illness was futile. Most physicians are taught to frame illness in terms of probabilities: of survival, of response to treatment, of complications from treatment. We base such probabilities on the medical literature and on our own experience. As I framed Sam's illness in my mind, I struggled with my role as the doctor in the family. I was a medical resident at the time. The tenets of evidence-based medicine and the realities of good and bad outcomes filled my days. Although I decided to withhold advice and opinion about Sam's care, I repeatedly asked questions about goals and potential outcomes. I offered to explain issues that might be confusing to Sam's parents, to serve as an interpreter of sorts. I offered to help his parents seek other medical opinions through my network of physician friends and colleagues. But my concerns about futility were probably evident. I remember sitting slouched in a chair wearing sweaty scrubs, my refrigerator empty and eyes burning after a night on call, listening to Sam's father describe that first magnetic resonance imaging scan four and a half years ago: "A very large tumor, near the brainstem (is that right?), not operable . . . "

Early in Sam's illness, another physician in the family advised Sam's parents not to pursue treatment. Years later, when Sam was attending preschool, his parents recalled the comment bitterly. The comment seemed glib in retrospect, although I suspect it was born from thoughtful consideration—thoughtful consideration of outcome probabilities. I felt thankful that I had withheld such thoughts, unaware that my beliefs may have been apparent even though I didn't give them full voice. I continued to believe that my medical education gave me some deeper understanding of the complex issues surrounding Sam's illness and treatment. I knew the probable and ultimate outcome of his illness. I continued to see myself as a potential advisor with the ability to guide Sam's family through the maze of the health care system, using my medical training as their light. The physician in me accompanied me everywhere and dominated my conversations with Sam's parents. As Sam's illness unfolded, as treatments succeeded and failed, I channeled new data into my physician construct and formed new probabilities about Sam's future.

But Sam's life taught me a lesson that had otherwise eluded me. In the final analysis, Sam defied all expectations. He defied all probabilities, living longer and healthier than expected. He brought joy, not sadness, to the people he met. When Sam sponsored a hospital blood drive, 100 of his friends came to donate. Not realizing how remarkable it was, he bounced around from donor to donor as though it were a birthday party. He loved a celebration. When Sam was 2 years old, he and his brother disrobed, climbed in the bathtub together with party hats and honkers, and celebrated the removal of his central line—his first real bath. On the day before his last operation, Sam was the master of ceremonies and stood on a chair telling jokes while friends and family laughed, gathered around his kitchen table. The ultimate outcome of Sam's illness became increasingly irrelevant. The possible outcomes of the future gave way to Sam's life, happily lived.

Sam taught me that probabilities play no role in family illnesses. Probabilities guide diagnosis and treatment choices for patients, but they distance us from the individual person. Behaviors and outcomes of populations are not easily applied to individual persons, although most of us become accustomed to doing so in medical practice. After all, for the individual person, the outcome either happens or it doesn't—whether it was probable doesn't really matter. In our medical practice, however, probabilities provide necessary guidance to counsel patients and to help them understand the spectrum of possibilities and make difficult choices. The probabilities derived from populations are the foundation of our medical practice. Thus, in our professional lives, we learn to live with our uncertainties, the fact that we will make mistakes in our estimations, and the fact that patients will defy expectations, just as Sam did.

Applying probabilities to the lives of our loved ones, though, is different. There are risks. We must live with our mistakes in estimation for the duration of our relationships, usually the rest of our lives. Probabilities objectify, and they rely on assumptions. Our families rarely need objectification and assumptions. They need the love of family and friends—sometimes no more, no less. The last thing Sam or his parents needed was another physician. Their lives were filled with expert medical opinion: pediatricians, neurologists, neuro-oncologists, and neuro-surgeons. Sam received extraordinarily good medical care, accompanied by much kindness. He and his parents became sophisticated negotiators of the medical system and knew more about pediatric brain tumors than I will ever know. Sam and his family needed their aunt, their sister, their sister-in-law. They didn't need, or want, a doctor in the family.

Medicine is a humbling profession. The intensity of effort required to become a physician weaves our professional selves deeply into the fabric of our lives and our perceptions of the world. To acknowledge a limited role for our professional abilities in our personal lives is humbling. In the end, though, it may free us to be husband, mother, daughter, grandson, nephew, sister, or aunt. This recognition freed me from concerns about decisions that were never mine to make. Had I been the decision maker, I fear I would have made the wrong decision and denied Sam the life he so richly enjoyed.

— *Marie F. Johnson*
Assistant Professor of Medicine, University of Colorado
Currently on leave of absence to raise three children

Tobacco, Tulips, and Terminal Care[3]

Seventy-two hours was a long time. But soon the conflicts would be resolved. While John's body struggled for breath and his soul struggled for eternity, she considered the internal conflict she faced. What role should she play? Doctor? Daughter? Could she somehow be both? As she contemplated his death, memories of his life and their shared bonds trickled in. She reached across and held his hand and automatically checked a radial pulse for rate and rhythm.

John smoked—a lot. Mostly back when cigarettes and martinis were still fashionable and Ronald Reagan's face adorned Chesterfield posters. Early years on the farm that his immigrant father had dug out of the Pennsylvania countryside were filled with responsibility and love. Childhood dreams were born in a one-room, clapboard schoolhouse with eight grades huddled around a coal stove. The teacher, fresh from the Pennsylvania Normal School, gave John his first taste of books and cigarettes. Neither one seemed dangerous at the time.

With Pearl Harbor, life settled into a happy routine of marriage, postponed dreams, and ration books that doled out cigarettes and sugar. Postwar days saw a good job as a machinist, promotion to shop foreman, a new baby girl, and a sense that some dreams could come true. Then came the angel of sudden death for his beloved wife. Her progressive mitral stenosis from old rheumatic disease brought her to the University hospital for one of the first commissurotomies, but not soon enough. At 46, he was left with his daughter, his books, and his Camels.

His world now centered on this little girl, who was both the remnant of his love and his life. He moved next door to the big white-columned house of his mother-in-law. There she and two widowed daughters, who had returned to the only home they had left, carefully watched over the child. Yes, there were days the little girl missed the presence of a woman she barely knew. But most days she was far too busy growing up in the safety of a father's love to be disturbed by such things.

As she grew, she shared John's passion for books and listened with her heart as he taught her compassion and integrity. School passed quickly and easily. She basked in paternal pride. Then she declared her intention to apply to medical school. The family told her that Marcus Welby was a figment of some television producer's vivid imagination. But her father's piercing blue eyes just smiled. He reassured her that sensitivity and science were not mutually exclusive. Armed with his confidence and the innocent courage of youth, she soon conquered medical school, residency, and fellowship, and returned home to the University. The relationship with her father changed. Although John could never quite relinquish his little-girl picture of her, they now talked as adults. During long hours over coffee, they shared ideas. With her support he had quit smoking during her medical school years. But this decision was to come too late.

Caring for him as a daughter and not a physician, she entrusted him to Dr. Mike, her favorite pulmonologist. This triangle worked well. John continued a restricted but independent life in his own home, enjoying frequent visits from his two young grandsons. During these years, her career matured uneventfully until she was asked to assume the position of Coursemaster for the ethics program in the medical school. Without hesitation, she said yes. She had always been interested in ethics, and she eagerly greeted this challenge. The students met her enthusiasm in kind, and as students always do if allowed, taught her. Soon her work expanded to include housestaff education and often faculty as well. The problems were rarely easy, and often none of the alternatives were pleasing.

Then the tobacco years began to catch up with John. The baseball games with his grandsons were replaced by checkers. The pulmonary function test results and arterial blood gases began their slow downward spiral. Finally, Dr. Mike suggested gently that now was the time for home oxygen. John was skeptical and reluctant to encumber what little freedom he had left, but was soon persuaded by the relentless dyspnea that dogged his every step. He asked her, "What do you think?" She hedged, "That's what we have Dr. Mike for." The Gemini twins of doctor and daughter battled to an uneasy truce. She arranged to be at his home when they delivered the system—a compressor for the house and a large liquid tank to refill the portable canister. She listened closely as they educated father and daughter about how it all worked.

Then one Thanksgiving, John made his first of many journeys to the medical intensive care unit. The careful attention of Dr. Mike and the housestaff paid off and John slid home, bypassing any real consideration of a ventilator. Three months and three hospitalizations later, John and his daughter sat in his room talking when one of her favorite residents came in.

"You know, I think I would like to take a trip," John said.

Not sure where this was leading, the resident replied, "Oh?"

"Yes, to Holland," said John.

The resident shifted his weight on uncomfortable feet and said "That would be nice. I believe the tulips there are really beautiful."

"Maybe," said John. "But mostly I would like Holland because they let you put people to sleep there like we do animals when they're suffering."

The resident's eyes mirrored the apprehension that crept into his soul. He rambled on about how John was a long way from that. The older man just smiled. His daughter, the doctor, thought a long time about what he had said.

John went home, calm and stable again for a time. Then Dr. Mike called: "John has discussed suicide with me and has made specific plans. I think you'd better remove the guns in his house if you can without upsetting him." Her father had collected and rebuilt antique firearms for many years. His finest pieces were displayed in a gun case he had carved by hand. And so, when John was away playing with his grandsons, she arranged to have all the ammunition and firing pins removed and stored at her house. If John ever noticed, he never spoke of their absence.

Another month, another hospitalization. Again he cheated the ventilator and made it to the floor. Then early one morning, her phone rang. John appeared to be in respiratory failure and in imminent danger of arresting. The resident had already called Dr. Mike. Dutifully noting the do-not-resuscitate order on the chart, the resident wanted to verify its accuracy.

"Yes, that's correct," she said. "If he arrests, you are not to begin CPR. You may go with inhaled beta agonists and other meds, but no intubation. I'm on my way." Her calm voice masked the terror she felt in her heart at losing this special person. She drove slowly and deliberately; a selfish part of her wished he would be gone before she arrived, sparing her the inevitable. He was not. The medicines had worked their magic again.

Two more months and two more hospitalizations later, she continued to think. Home was no longer an option. After his last discharge, she had arranged around-the-clock sitters. John stayed at home less than 24 hours. Whether from hypoxia or the blessing of some unseen angel, John became more forgetful and understood fewer details around him. After thoughtful consideration, she chose a hospice program especially known for its respiratory care. It was a hard choice, one made with her memory of his previous wishes and not his mind now. Dr. David, the director, was both geriatrician and a treasured friend of many years. The staff were efficient, caring, and concerned beyond her expectations, but that could not stop the tears as she toured the facility. Her promise of professional detachment withered and died.

The days and weeks stretched into spring and early summer, and she almost believed John could get well and go home. Dr. David mercifully said no. She came daily. John enjoyed the garden where she often took him outside to sit. They talked, reminisced, and tried desperately to hold fast to the moment.

Then came the yellow sputum again. The well-balanced triangle was now without one of its points, so the two remaining decided to forego the hospital and parenteral antibiotics and a ventilator in favor of oral antibiotics and continued close attention to respiratory therapy. Without speaking it, they knew what this would mean. She telephoned her office to cancel outpatients and lectures for the next several days. Fortunately, she was not on service; her partners had already accommodated her father's illness many times, and she was glad she would not have to ask yet another time. The students had just turned in their final exams from the introductory ethics course, and she carried those to his bedside as she sat and they talked and waited together.

As the hours passed, John talked less and she thought more. The questions she graded took on a haunting significance: define and give an example of microallocation and macroallocation of health care; should health care for the elderly be limited—why or why not; develop two arguments for or against physician-assisted suicide; is physician participation in active euthanasia compatible with the practice of medicine in today's world and justify your answer; contrast three differences between the traditional Hippocratic oath and any one of the modern versions studied in class. She thought of Quinlan and Brophy and Cruzan, of Debbie and her ovarian cancer, and especially of Diane and Dr. Quill and the covenants that bind parent to child or physician to patient.

Seventy-two hours was a very long time. In the papers she held, innocent young students argued the pros and cons of assisted suicide and euthanasia. Before her eyes, John struggled and fought for every breath. In her mind, she saw tulips and heard the echoes of his wish for a trip to Holland. In her heart, she cried and wished for the courage to act.

Would it be so wrong to use the skills he had encouraged her to gain? The battling forces she faced were not good and evil, but rather the little girl who loved her daddy and wanted to stop his suffering, and the trained physician who wondered if medicine has the right to assert absolute control over every process of life. The decision to withhold John's care was a definable act with both an intent and a soon-to-be-seen effect. A syringe of stolen morphine, easily obtained and used compassionately, would also have intent and effect. Could she truly say that between these two acts there existed a moral difference of such magnitude that the scene before her was justified? In the end, she was powerless against the person he taught her to be. When the time came, she quietly held him in her arms and kissed him goodbye. Then she rang for the nurse: "My father just died. The time was 3:49 a.m."

— *Maryella Desak Sirmon*
Clinical Associate Professor of Medicine,
University of South Alabama College of Medicine
Private practice, Nephrology Associates of Mobile (Mobile, Alabama)

John Albert Desak died June 1, 1991.

The Friendship of Women

Recently, I was asked to make a comment at a dinner meeting that brought together women physicians of many different ages in celebration of Women in Medicine month. I had been impressed with the many conversations around me on which I had been eavesdropping and also with the spirit of camaraderie that prevailed in the room. Women seemed relaxed and at ease with each other. As I thought for a few minutes about what I would like to say, it came to me that my many different friendships with women had been the richest part of my life. After I made this comment a young medical student sitting nearby asked me if I had known I would be asked to comment. I assume she was questioning whether this was a spontaneous response or an expected prepared remark.

It was indeed a spontaneous response, and I have often thought since then about the why and the truth of the answer. I think back to my childhood as an only child, growing up in a friendly neighborhood in a small town in Kansas. Early friendships were with the women in my extended family, my mother with whom I had more of a friendship than a mother-daughter relationship, aunts, cousins, women friends of our family, and of course, also with girl friends. I was lucky to have a girlfriend next door and my best friend close by. Annette and I walked to and from school together for 12 years. Much was shared as we took our circuitous route up driveways and alleys together. We read the same books, played duets, participated in neighborhood theatricals, and had funerals for dead birds. One summer we tree-sat and wept together as we read *Little Women* aloud. Even our china pattern was the same, a beautiful blue and white Spode Geisha ornamented with prunus blossoms, the Japanese symbol of love and joy. Annette died of Alzheimer's disease a few years ago. Although we lived in different states, we had stayed in close touch over the years, and I was able to become acquainted with her daughter, who returned to Kansas for college.

High school brought a wealth of friendships with women. I still occasionally have lunch with a friend who was in our Sub-Deb Club. A debate partner, who went on to become lawyer, was an important role model and friend. My memory of male friends is much scantier, although there were some important ones. Perhaps I felt less comfortable with men because I had no brothers, and my relationship with my father, while satisfactory, was not one of sharing ideas, cares, and concerns.

I still correspond with a friend in Chicago whom I first met at age 11 while visiting relatives. We stayed in touch through letters in which we shared intimate feelings of joy and sorrow. Although we have arranged visits at concerts, operas, and art exhibits, the letters remain at the heart of the friendship.

Living in a dormitory and a sorority house in college gave me an even broader chance to develop new friendships. In my experience, sororities provide special bonds that strengthen friendships and give them lasting qualities. My closest college friend recently died of Alzheimer's disease. It was such a sadness to watch Pete move away into her own lonely world.

My friendships with women medical colleagues have been less satisfying. I have often thought about this and have come to the conclusion that careers, particularly demanding and challenging ones, sap energy and fill so much space in our lives that there is little room left for the attention that real friendships require. Even now I am losing touch with one of my few contemporary women physician friends, another victim of Alzheimer's—another great sadness.

Secretaries and assistants have been good friends to me and have contributed greatly to my comfort and well-being at work. I remain in contact with one special secretary and joke about how she used to watch me "vanish into the cavern of the hospital."

I am thankful for newer friendships with a younger generation of women, including my one daughter, but in these I find for myself a different role. Old memories and shared experiences are not readily available, and the generation gap invades. My friendships with young women physicians give me a special kind of satisfaction as I watch them find their own way both in their professional and personal lives. Even more challenging is finding ways to develop friendships with five delightful granddaughters.

So much richness has been added to my life by women friends, each of whom has brought her unique personality, individual needs, and special way of sharing herself with me. And I have found a similar richness in returning such things in kind. This combination of receiving and giving is the lifeblood of true friendships, the real treasures in our lives.

— *Marjorie Spurrier Sirridge*
Professor of Medicine, Director of the Office of Medical Humanities and former Dean, University of Missouri–Kansas City School of Medicine

A Doctor in the Family[4]

My father walked barefoot to
the municipal school
with no money for lunch
and torn, fourth-hand books.
And every day his feet stung
from giant spider bites.
His friend had a mother
who squatted on street corners
and fried snacks in hot oil
so her son could have slippers
My father was motherless.

As a child, I heard him
mutter at beggars, those
who swarmed at the entrances
to temples and stores.
His eyes gave him away.
"Go on," he'd say, slipping
coins in a trickle into each of their hands.

Once, near a bookshop
where he bought me
my first Thomas Hardy,
I saw him reach down
to stroke this old cow
that blocked the pavement.
People stared at him while
he talked to the animal.
I looked away, pretended
I didn't know this mad man.
I was fourteen. He only smiled.

In his growing-up days, long
before I, his only daughter, was born,
my father's notion of a feast
was a handful of rice, an onion slice
and one chili, searing hot, green.
I never knew how it felt
to go hungry for days and
simply accept.

My father made a bookcase,
repaired clocks, planted flowers, among other
things. His fine surgeon's hands
painted oil pictures and watercolor words,
made kites that I flew with my brothers.
He brought in a dog, a mongrel, one day,
that had one fiery eye, seemed half dead.

My father named him first. Cyclops.
Lucky stray. Then nurtured him to health.

When I graduated, my father said—
his face almost expressionless—
"You are the first doctor, ever,
on my side of the family."
His eyes gave him away. He
saw in me the dreams of that
boy, too poor to practice the art
of medicine. My father was wrong.
I simply followed in his footsteps
where I'll always belong.

— *Bhuvana Chandra*
Pediatric psychiatrist and writer

The Two-Casserole Test[5]

The other day I saw a friend from house-staff days whom I hadn't seen
for a year. I asked him, "What is the best part of your life?" He said, "Just
like yours . . ." In the moment before he finished his sentence, my mind
whirled through the list of what he might think was best in my life. To
my surprise and relief, he continued, "My family and friends, of course."
Why was I surprised? Because physicians don't always rank family and
friends so high. Why was I relieved? Because it is always pleasant to
discover kindred spirits.

Physicians may have difficulty maintaining personal relationships.
Being a physician is one of the few socially acceptable reasons to
abandon a family. Some physicians perhaps never should have had a
family in the first place, but custom forced marriage and escape from
home life becomes attractive. Surely the demands of our profession can
absorb time and energy that could be used to build close ties. As we
insulate ourselves from patients' suffering, we may also insulate
ourselves from family and community. Spiro and Mandell (1998) point
out, "Professional detachment spreads from office to home, turning into a

kind of alexithymia so that many physicians no longer recognize when or if they have any emotion at all." Finally, sometimes, interests diverge, love withers, and duty alone may not be enough to keep a family together.

Why are relationships useful beyond our own and others' needs? For one thing, sharing love and affection forms the basis of trust and self-esteem that children need to grow into effective adults; effective adults need encouragement and support when challenges arise. Family and friends are part of the *glue* that keeps society together. People who pull together within families, friendly groups, and neighborhoods set the tone for the way a society works as a whole. Glue is under-appreciated; invisible things often are. Certain kinds of forces—or glue—little-valued but persistent—keep molecules, mayonnaise, individuals, families, and communities together. The goodness generated by healthy relationships adds love to the world at large. The world can stand a good deal more love.

Family and friends can also be leavening agents—sources of pleasure, wisdom, and good memories. All ages can supply strength and inspiration. When our daughter, Sarah, was in high school, we were asked to be part of a panel involving families in which both parents worked. We called our part of the program, "A Three-Career Family," figuring that Sarah's work was as important as ours and that being a student was her career at the time. As we prepared for our session, we tried to think of themes that kept our family not only glued together but profoundly enjoyable. We settled on "Negotiate, Accommodate, and Recreate." We recognized that the need to negotiate, and the ability to accommodate arose from our busy lives and the respect each of us had for the others' tasks; we realized that the planning, experiences, and recollections that came from our travels and adventures together provided us with deep pleasure.

Certainly, patients, colleagues, and the work that we do can be satisfying and uplifting. Take a moment, however, to take the "two-casserole test." Who in your life will bring you more than one casserole when life gets difficult: when your mother dies, your father dies, your professional life sours, your life's love gets cancer? Neighbors may bring one; the office may send one. But your family and friends will remember six weeks and six months later that you need another casserole, bouquet, note, or hug. How many people in your life will bring two casseroles? Patients are unlikely to send casseroles, and they are unlikely to be there at the end. They send best wishes if you yourself are out of commission because they are concerned, but it may just be that they want you back at work to care for them. It will be people who care for you because of who you are, not just what you do, who have the staying power.

It should be noted that colleagues aren't necessarily the same as friends. Friends aren't competitive. You can share the deepest feelings with friends. A woman who survived the Holocaust once defined the word friend as "someone who will take you in in the middle of the night when you are running away." Not many colleagues would do that.

E. B. White wrote a paean to friendship in *Charlotte's Web,* the story of a spider who saves a pig's life by weaving messages above his pen, making him a hero instead of a ham. At the end of the book, Wilbur, the pig, asks Charlotte, the spider, whose short life is ebbing away, "Why did you do all this for me? I don't deserve it. I've never done anything for you."

"You have been my friend," replied Charlotte. "That in itself is a tremendous thing. I wove my webs for you because I liked you. After all, what's a life anyway? We are born, we live a little, we die. A spider's life can't help being something of a mess, with all this trapping and eating flies. By helping you, perhaps I was trying to lift up my life a trifle. Heaven knows anyone's life can stand a little of that" (p. 164).

If your edges, or your core, are chipped or broken and in need of glue, it is time to open up, reach out, and build and rebuild personal and community relationships. Add some people to your "two-casserole list." One good way to start is to volunteer. Another is to take William Osler's advice to physicians: do the kind thing and do it first. As we lift up family and friends, so they lift us. We carry on together.

— Linda Hawes Clever

Chief of Occupational Health at California Pacific Medical Center
Clinical Professor of Medicine, University of California San Francisco

References

Spiro, F. M., & Mandell, H. N. (1998). When doctors get sick. *Annals of Internal Medicine, 128*, 152.

White, E. B. (1952). *Charlotte's web*. New York: Harper Collins.

The Cafeteria

It's been 24 years since Ann and I began our rotations as medical students—she, a dark-skinned Italian from New York City, and I, a fair-skinned Southern girl from rural Florida. At the end of the day, we'd meet in the cafeteria and discuss the day's events over coffee and cigarettes. We had ended up by chance in the same place—first in Kansas City for medical school and later, Akron, Ohio for postgraduate training. Over the years, we've had many experiences together, including husbands, children, divorce, teenagers, illness, and very busy practices that we own.

I did emergency surgery on her, and she held my hand through my mastectomies. We were like salt and pepper, night and day, but with time, our many differences have dissolved. We've looked to each other for strength and support both in good times and in tough times, always trying to maintain a sense of humor.

As young medical students in an environment where less than 10% of the class was female, we had some interesting experiences. People often mistook us for the TV ladies coming to collect money or employees at the hospital snack bar. Fortunately, we were blessed with a sense of humor and attempted to enlighten the public. Even 20 some years later, as the chair of a hospital department and director of a residency program, I encountered a very pleasant looking, well-dressed lady in the hospital cafeteria who commented on what good muffins I make. I simply smiled and thanked her.

I still meet Ann in the cafeteria to share these experiences, both of us now over 50. No more cigarettes and the coffee now decaffeinated, but the friendship remains unchanged.

Life is full of curve balls; they will make you stronger only if you let them. The answers are simply family and good friends. Relax, let life take you where it may, and remember to live, laugh, and love.

— *Lou Elizabeth Mac Manus*
Surgery, obstetrics and gynecology
Cuyahoga Valley Women's Healthcare, Inc., Akron, Ohio

Memories of Our Mother

With blue eyes and strawberry blonde hair
Your lilting voice serenaded us with music
Big Band and patriotic songs
God Bless America and *You Are My Sunshine*
Twirling through rooms and filling our home.
We'd laugh, dry dishes, sing harmony.

Your voice, the first I heard each morning
Telling my sleepy head to rise and shine
Oatmeal with raisin faces, Cream of Wheat, or sunny side eggs
Packing us off to school.
Every Saturday, a drive to see
Grandma and Grandpa
We'd sit on the porch swing and talk,
Eat apple kuchen and drink tea
Until fireflies came out twinkling in the dark.

You were a homemaker.
Monday was wash day
Sheets flapping in the breeze
Fresh with sunshine, delicious to crawl into
Tuesday was ironing day
I still hear the iron hiss on Daddy's shirts
We all were scrubbed and neatly dressed
An All-American Family of the 1950's.

You were a saver.
You saved cards, letters and pictures I drew as a little girl
You made scrapbooks and picture albums.
So I was surprised when you gave me your favorite things.
You said you wanted the pleasure of giving me
great grandma's crystal pitcher,
and your mother's garnet ring.
Not wanting me to wait until you were gone.

At first I didn't notice the hesitation in your step
Searching for names of common things
The newspaper unopened
No more bookmarks
Sleeping all day
Rummaging through the desk drawers at night
Looking for stamps
Not wanting to leave your house or Daddy's side.

The answer was found in the microscopic tangles
that were weaving around in your brain.
Blocking out the sunlight, the songs,
the crickets and fireflies,
until all was soft, gray and silent.

Diane Merritt's mother died from Alzheimer's Disease on Father's Day
June 20, 1999.

— *Diane F. Merritt*
Professor of Obstetrics and Gynecology,
Washington University School of Medicine
Director, Division of Pediatric and Adolescent Gynecology

Notes

1. Excerpted from Lindbergh, A. M. (1975). *Gift from the sea* (p. 28). New York: Pantheon. Reprinted with permission.
2. From Johnson, M. F. (1999). The doctor in the family. *Annals of Internal Medicine, 130,* 859–860. Reprinted by permission of the American College of Physicians-American Society of Internal Medicine.
3. From Sirmon, M. D. (1993). Tobacco, tulips, and terminal care. *Annals of Internal Medicine, 119,* 1043–1044. Abridged and reprinted by permission of the American College of Physicians-American Society of Internal Medicine.
4. From Chandra, B. (2000). A doctor in the family *Annals of Internal Medicine, 132*(10), 838–839. Reprinted by permission of the American College of Physicians-American Society of Internal Medicine.
5. From Clever, L. H. (1998). The two-casserole test. *Western Journal of Medicine, 168,* 288. This article was first published in the *Western Journal of Medicine* and is reproduced by permission of *Western Journal of Medicine.*

10

BALANCING

The term balance is often misconstrued to mean
a static state of affairs, a final "perfect" solution in
our role-juggling act. In truth, balance is a dynamic
process, akin to the way we repeatedly adjust our course
as we walk across a stream on slippery rocks. The real
goals of balance are to support each other through
periods of imbalance in work, marital, family, or
individual concerns, and to take responsibility for
remembering to regularly adjust course in order to
attend to some heretofore neglected areas of life.

— Wayne M. Sotile
— Mary O. Sotile[1]

August 1994: Letter to My Student[2]

August 1994

> *We forget all too soon the things we*
> *thought we could never forget.*
>
> — *Joan Didion*[*]

"Is it possible to have it all?" you asked in our conversation earlier this week. I've thought about that some more. This certainly is an issue I have struggled with much of my career, particularly the tension between the responsibilities of parenthood and one's professional role.

Some of the things you bring to the profession because of your gender, and socialization as a woman, will make your work life both harder and easier. Again I go back to the writing of Harriet Lerner, who first pointed out for me in a way that I understood, how often women take care of others at the expense of themselves. Sometimes you will be up all night with a woman in labor, instead of snoozing in the call room down the hall; or you will go the extra mile and do a home visit on an elderly patient both to make it easier for her, and to see the home where the family lives in order to understand the caregiving situation better. You will do this with ease, because of your socialization.

On the other hand, occasionally you will work in the extra patient once too often, miss your child's soccer game because you said "yes" to a patient, cover for a colleague instead of going to the art fair. Then, your inbreeding as a woman will cause you difficulty. Your patients will love you for it. Your male colleagues will occasionally be suspicious and resentful of your popularity. The stacks of presents from grateful patients may be a barometer of how big this struggle is for you. Ultimately you must find your own set of rules, your own boundaries between responsibility and self-care, your own understanding of how you fit into this role you have accepted. The Zen diagram of your many roles (friend, mother, partner, physician, self) changes from day to day and year to year. Only you can determine where, for you, the lines overlap and where they cannot. You must pay attention to where one circle is getting too big, overshadowing others. Be thoughtful about it. Find mentors and trusted friends with whom you can discuss these issues on an ongoing basis. Your patients, also, will be good teachers if you listen to what they tell you. Write in your journal. Keep a log of your time. Keep a journal of your stories. They are the vitamins which will help you grow as a person and as a professional. These stories are also a roadmap of where you have been and where you are going. They are the accounting of how much of the "all" you have, and how much you really want.

I wish you peace.

— Beth Alexander
Professor, Department of Family Practice,
College of Human Medicine, and
University Physician, Michigan State University

---

*Excerpt from "On Keeping a Notebook" from *Slouching Towards Bethlehem* by Joan Didion. Copyright © 1966, 1968, renewed 1996 by Joan Didion. Reprinted by permission of Farrar, Straus and Giroux, LLC.

Balancing, Juggling, and Other Feats

Finding a way to manage home and work simultaneously allows you to see the best in both arenas. When things get hectic at work, you can think about the joys of home, and when your family is overwhelming, remember that you will have the respite of adult interaction soon. Whatever path you choose, remember to cordon off time to do things you enjoy, such as hobbies, exercise, or simple quiet time. This is a time to rejuvenate and revisit the reasons you are attempting to accomplish so much. Above all, having a full life will improve your outlook as physician, partner, and parent and allow you to grow as a person.

— Donna L. Parker
Associate Dean for Student and Faculty Development,
University of Maryland School of Medicine

Juggling the Personal and Professional Life[3]

The most important single factor in the career of a woman doctor is the man she marries—who, I might add, is like anyone else, capable of change."

— *Marcia Angell*
Senior Lecturer at Harvard Medical School
Former Editor-in-Chief, New England Journal of Medicine

Workday Mornings—Three Weeks

My baby spit up her cereal
My two-year-old threw a tantrum
I wiped the rice cereal off my dress
We watched the garbage truck operate on our block
The baby had diarrhea as we were walking out the door

My son went pee pee in the potty
My son is learning how to dress himself
The baby is teething
I forgot to bring show-n-tell
My child showed me his project at daycare

The baby cried inconsolably
I read a book to my child
I breastfed my infant
My son is a sidewalk dawdler
My baby likes to be held

Sorry, I was late to Morning Report.

— *Stephanie Nagy-Agren*
Assistant Professor of Internal Medicine, University of Virginia
Chief, Infectious Diseases Section,
Veterans Affairs Medical Center, Salem, Virginia

Where Is the Self?

Self is what gets lost in our battle to balance home and medicine. We feel that we can handle more than average women; after all, we survived internship. We therefore take on more than we should: "Sure, I'll be on that committee," "I'll help the nursing staff understand the new protocol," "I'll be happy to lead the third-grade field trip." But in reality we are only one person with many roles: doctor, mother, wife, partner, daughter, friend, community leader, teacher, hospital politician, role model, and more.

Where is the *self?* There are pieces of me everywhere. There are only rare times when I pull it all together to be myself: a complete woman. Sometimes that happens when I say no to more demands on my time. Often it happens when I'm alone, a quiet late evening when the paperwork is done, the laundry is done, my family is asleep, and I'm relaxed enough to look forward to doing it all again tomorrow.

— Gayle Shore Moyer
Clinical Faculty, University of Michigan
Private practice, obstetrics and gynecology

The Multitude of Little Things[4]

There is a vast difference between being a doctor and a husband and being a doctor and a wife. There are many things a wife does for a husband—and I do not mean mechanical chores such as vacuuming and cleaning that can be done by someone else. I mean truly wifely chores such as arranging the social life, buying gifts, sending Christmas cards—all the dozens and dozens of things that make life run smoothly for a married couple. It takes some degree of executive ability to arrange life so that the multitude of little things that must be done get done. I am sure that every working woman, whether she be doctor or in an other profession, has at times wished she had a wife.

— Dorothy V. Whipple
Pediatrician, private practice, Washington, D.C.

Is It Worth It?[5]

We are proud of using our intellect and skills in leadership roles that were rarely open to our mothers' generation. We delight in coming in from the outside to sit in the halls of power and speak in our own voices. We love our connections with family and feel that nurturing the next generation, by mothering and mentoring, is at the core of life's meaning. We rarely feel bored or empty because the *New England Journal of Medicine* and *Gourmet* equally stimulate our creativity.

. . . Filling a complex array of roles, we feel that we have never reached our full potential in any area. No matter how shared the domestic tasks, we still track the family agenda in our heads while inside the boardroom and cringe when our kids ask why we don't serve hot dogs at the school like the other mothers. We have chosen partners who are stimulating and supportive, but we are often so tired by evening that our interaction is cursory. We feel blocked on our career path by not knowing the rules of play or, worse yet, discover that the payoff in power and prestige that goes to the winner is not as intoxicating as we had dreamed.

Potentially, we are *all* of these women and that is the dilemma.

— Nancy B. Kaltreider
Professor of Psychiatry Emerita, University of California San Francisco
Editor of Dilemmas of a Double Life *(1997)*

Can It Be Done?

Now that I have reached the ripe old age of 40 and my kids are 12, 10, and seven, it seems that every few days I am asked, "Can it really be done?" It might be a medical student at the beginning of that long road, an intern or resident in the heat of her childbearing years, or a junior faculty member trying to keep up with mounting responsibilities as she tries to hoist herself over the tenure and promotion hurdle. "Can it really be done?" "Can you have both a career and children?"

In my mind I scream out, "Yes. Definitely, yes. Don't pass up the opportunity. You deserve the chance to have your own bundle of joy."

But I hold myself back, wondering, *What is it that makes you even consider not having kids?*

Is it that you haven't found a spouse because you have spent all of your waking moments at work to the point where you are the one covering all of the holidays so those with a family can take off?

Is it because if you had kids, you would want to be a mom just like your mom, but she didn't work and was always at home ready to greet you at the door?

Is it because you are a perfectionist in everything you do, and you can't imagine how you would ever meet your expectations for yourself as doctor, wife, and mother?

Is it because you have worked so hard to become a surgeon or researcher or academician, yet there's more that you want to do? You want tenure, promotions, partnership. You want to reap the rewards for all your hard work.

Is it because the culture you so desperately want to be a full-fledged member of doesn't have any other women with children? And even if they are there, they aren't the role models you were hoping for?

Is it that you strongly suspect that your boss, Chairman, Dean, colleagues, and coworkers would not be happy if you turned up pregnant and asked for a maternity leave?

Is it that you worry that the bulk of the responsibilities for this baby will fall on your shoulders when you are already struggling just to work and take care of yourself?

This is all running through my brain as I try gently to explore where the question is coming from.

"Can it be done?" she asks again. Usually the concerns get blurted out pretty quickly. It can be one or all of the above considerations or some other worry that I haven't even imagined. "What if I had a baby with major problems?" "I'm not going to get married—is there any way that I can even have a baby?"

I gently explain, "Even though I love my work, if somehow I was told, *You must choose work or family, you can no longer have both,* I would race for the door and never look back. There is no comparison between work and family. There is no question of where my (and most parents') priorities are. Family is tops."

But the fact of the matter is, there is room for both work and family under most circumstances. There can be a balance between personal and professional goals. Women and men can find great personal satisfaction in being effective and happy in both spheres of their lives. Luckily in the last century, women forged inroads in every facet of medicine. The brave souls who got into the "boys' clubs" took the heat, gained competence, and survived are heroes to those women who are coming up behind them. In some domains, such as neurosurgery and transplant, they have just gotten a toehold; in other areas such as pediatrics and OB/GYN, they are a major part of the workforce. Nowhere are they clear leaders across the field, although there are rare Deans and department Chairs with no Y chromosomes.

As I explain all this to my interviewer, she begins to relax her shoulders and looks me straight in the eye. She now knows that I support her secret dream to have kids and pursue a demanding career. Her questions come much more quickly and urgently now. She wants to know the recipe for success. "When is the best time to have a baby?"

My mind becomes crowded with many friends and colleagues. I can picture Rita with four kids in medical school, transcribing the co-op notes for pharmacology and setting the curve. Janice coming to her internship pregnant because she thought she was infertile and, lo and behold, she wasn't. It was a miracle. Who cared if it was unacceptable at that prestigious residency (pediatrics nonetheless) to start her family the first year there? I see myself and my friend Lori as third-year residents, scheming to cover for each other during our brief maternity leaves so no colleagues could say that they had to work even one day for us. There's Karen who had three babies after she took her junior faculty position, cut back to 80% time, got a tenure rollback of one year, and still managed to scrape over the promotion and tenure hurdle. And finally, Roberta, who wanted so badly to be a famous academic neurosurgeon that she completed all her training and seven years as a faculty member, including tenure and promotion, before she even tried to get pregnant. She did it, although with life-threatening complications. I can see many more friends and colleagues walking around with round bellies at various stages of their education and careers. I share some of these vignettes with my interviewer so that she will see that it has been done at all phases and that it can be done no matter what the specialty or what the timing. The right time is the time that she (and her partner) determines it is.

She shares her fear that she might get into some trouble at work if she gets pregnant.

I agree with her that those around her might not be thrilled with her timing. I encourage her to try to obtain the written maternity and paternity leave policies at her institution. I also encourage her to avoid starting a new phase visibly pregnant so that people have a chance to get to know her and her work before they have to plan for a leave of absence. I recommend that she think through what she wants for maternity leave and any alternative arrangements that she might seek after the baby is born (part-time, one day at home, flextime). I encourage her (when the time is right) to make suggestions about how her work will be covered. I tell her to look at other women in her practice or department who are juggling work and kids and ask them the same questions she asks me. I encourage her to tell her boss, colleagues, or supervisors as early in the pregnancy as she is comfortable so that the necessary planning can be accomplished. As I see the guilt cross her brow, I remind her that many people, even men, have to take off for skiing accidents (you can't operate with a cast on your arm), heart attacks, and cancer, and none of these come with the four- to six-month warning that she will give her boss. She relaxes again, a little.

The final, most eagerly asked question is coming now. I can see it, and I brace myself for it.

"So how do you do it? Tell me your secret."

Again my head is full of friends and colleagues . . . Lori and Rebecca who practice pediatrics two and a half days a week, sing in the church choir, go to Gym 'n' Swim with their tots. Becca and six girlfriends who created their own private OB/GYN practice where everybody works four days a week, everybody has had at least one or two kids, and everybody shares in the profits. My friend Wendy, who works full-time with me in academic medicine. She's a medical oncologist and I'm a pediatric oncologist. Both of us care deeply for our families and our patients and have managed to scramble over the tenure hurdle. We now carry the title of tenured Associate Professors as we simultaneously revel in our school-age kids' accomplishments and antics. And Roberta. Ah, Roberta. She who is truly carving a path through stone. She is practicing neurosurgery three and half days a week and baking cakes with her kids, organizing play groups, and running a lab.

"There isn't a magic recipe for a perfect work/family soufflé," I tell my mentee. I describe a few key elements that have helped me. I pursued an area of medicine that I absolutely love. I live close to work. I go to my kids' school often and have dedicated, in-home child care that I love (in my case, a new au pair every year). My husband has learned how to split a lot of the work and responsibilities for our family with me, and he reaps the joy as well. We take regularly scheduled vacations every year no matter what, and I rarely work at home except for taking call. Most important, I savor and soak up the sheer joy that both my family and my work bring to me.

She looks a little worried now. "But how will I ever be able to do everything?"

I try to reassure her. "You will. Somehow, some way. The most important thing is that you believe that you can do this and you go for it. Have confidence that it will be great. I have never met a physician-mother who expressed regrets about opening her life and her heart to her child. You can do it. It can be done."

— *Mary Lou Schmidt*
Associate Professor of Pediatrics
University of Illinois College of Medicine

A Few Thoughts on Part-time Faculty: The Push for the Summit and the Long Climb Down[6]

I sat down for my daily "personal time" one night last week. It was 10:00 p.m. I had finally completed the complex assortment of managerial and brute force tasks that make up the day of any busy physician/parent/ whatever. My 15 minutes of restorative contact with the external world often consists of picking up the day's *The New York Times* and scanning for major world events. For example, I knew *in advance* that a former professional wrestler was running for governor of Minnesota. My full-time working spouse was in awe of my grasp of the American political scene.

On this particular evening of personal interface with "life as we know it" my eye was drawn immediately to the front page article entitled "Part-Time Work for Some Adds Up to Full-Time Job" by Reed Ableson (November 2, 1998).[1] This is news, I wondered, or just common knowledge and common sense? I have been trying with some intermittent success to work at my medical career at 75% time. My modified schedule allows me to meet the school bus, as it were, three days out of five. Some days it works out, other days it can't. I hardly consider this a major home presence in the lives of my children, but I know I have more flexibility than many other working docs/parents. Just this morning I said to my middle-schooler, "I'll be home when you get here after school," and I did see that little smile that creeps across his face when he is genuinely pleased. "Gosh," I thought, "he really does need me." What my beamish boy and my exuberant first grader don't know is that I will quite literally be running out of my office, a flat-out blur and praying for no traffic, so that our moment of tranquil reunion can occur as if quite naturally and without concern.

The article describes the current state of the U.S. corporate work force. In particular, the number of women in professional and managerial positions has grown right along with the number of dual-career couples, according to corporate analysts. More women in these professions are now deciding to work part-time or to work at home, willing to accept the option of reduced hours and reduced pay for more scheduling leeway. Face-time is less, but the job essentially remains the same. The corporate situation, which is identical to our own in some respects, got me thinking about the fundamental reality of what it means to be "part-time."

I see two groups on this mountain, those who are pushing for the summit and those who are climbing down. Our jobs are not counted by the hour and vary according to the academic season, the need to staff clinics or wards, attend and chair committee meetings, develop research, and take our share of call. We balance this with the need to attend parent-teacher conferences, our own medical appointments, or school band concerts, and to apply our healing skills to small scraped knees and aging loved ones. Our face time may not be as concentrated, but *we* are. I guess the business world is catching up with us.

Why are we willing to climb the professional Everest so very slowly, ". . . to stop and draw three or four lungfuls of air after each ponderous step"?[2] I can only speak for those who have gone before me. "Because it is there." My colleague and friend, Dr. Rebecca Wang-Cheng, summarized her experience in this way: ". . . Of course much of the work I did was on my 'own time,' but being part-time actually gave me more autonomy and control over my time. I could choose whether to spend my afternoon going to the library story hour with my son or writing a manuscript."[3] Senior faculty, in reflection, are on the long climb back from the summit, maintaining an active face in research and teaching, having achieved the pinnacle. There is plenty of company in this cohort.

Yes, I have worked 80-hour-plus weeks this year, just like my full-time colleagues. I have been staffing my ward team at awful hours and finishing up committee meetings or consults late in the day. Other days, I have the flexibility to help cook the sixth-grade luau. For the most part, however, I am trying to manage nearly the same workload as a full-time colleague by working more via the "electronic umbilical cord"[4] and by working more efficiently. Like the corporate women quoted in the newspaper article, I am willing to accept lower salary in exchange for flexibility and freedom. Does it bother me that I am in a sense being penalized for my efficiency? It does not.

Those faster climbers who pass me are using oxygen.

— Charlotte Heidenreich

Medical Director, Fortis Health

Former Associate Professor of Medicine, Medical College of Wisconsin

Notes

1. Abelson, R (1998, November 2). Part-time work for some adds up to full-time job. *New York Times*, p. A1.
2. Krakauer, J. (1997). *Into thin air* (p. 236). New York: Doubleday.
3. Wang-Cheng, R. (1996). The echo of my mother's footsteps. In D. Wear (Ed.), *Women in medical education: An anthology of experience*. Albany: State University of New York Press.
4. McGowan, J. J. (1994). A vertical curriculum in applied medical informatics in support of rural primary-care education. *Academic Medicine, 69,* 430–431.

Centered in the Deep Connections[7]

I am a person whose values from the 1960s have not waned; rather, they have deepened. My commitment to the social change has taken the form of a long-term dedication to the teaching and practicing of family medicine in an inner-city health center, where awareness of our society's inequalities is ever-present. I like to think that I practice in an egalitarian fashion; I attempt to put patients in charge of interactions as much as possible. By this I don't mean that I hold them responsible for their health (or sickness); rather, that I try to let the time be their time with me, to use the way they think necessary. This means I am committed to understanding and working through patient agendas, not just doctor-based agendas.

Feminism is a strong current in my orientation. In my practice, feminism means struggling to enable women to discover their strengths and to recover from the innumerable restrictions, hurts, and violations that have curtailed their freedom to grow and choose for themselves and their children. Physical and sexual abuse are frequent realities in the current and past lives of my patients. I believe that helping them heal from these assaults is one of the most rewarding tasks of feminist practice.

Nonetheless to say, this is not short work. I have made my *practice* and not my career the centerpiece of my work. This means that I have chosen to remain in one setting for the past fifteen years, the same site where I completed my family practice residency. A doctor used to be a person who came and stayed. Staying means staying in labor, staying in the practice, and staying in the community. I believe that the real work of family practice cannot be done in a few years, that the magic in the work lies in all the shared history.

Rare is the woman who has the good fortune to find a life partner who shares equally in her values and her commitment to her work. When Richard Schmitt, a committed socialist and feminist philosopher, joined me in Worcester in 1983, I knew that I was such a woman. Our daily joint engagement in both intellectual and family work makes my life rich and full. The depth of our relationship has enabled each of us to confront painful past histories and turn our understandings into growth in our work.

I am employed part-time. What this means is that I am in the health center a little more than two and a half days; I take one night per week of call and eight weekends a year. I do obstetrics and attempt to deliver my own patients when I am not on call. For this I am paid at 67% of a full-time salary, which is ample to live on. The two days I am at home, I spend reading and writing. This arrangement enables me to pursue my ideas as freely as possible with only occasional clinical interruptions, which are, after all, what I read and write about anyway.

We have two children, Addie, 6, in first grade, and Eli, 16 months, at family day care; three acres on a pond; a large garden; and a sister city project with a town in Nicaragua. How is it possible to do it all? First, for many years even before I met him, Richard had also chosen to work for pay on a half-time basis. His career was well established, and his position secure. In practice, he teaches first semester and has nine months to read and write. Secondly, we share all the responsibilities around the children equally, including transportation and doctors' appointments. Third, I spend no time commuting; our home is ten minutes from the health center and the hospitals. Fourth, we have forty hours a week of child care; Addie joins Eli at Debra Keating's family day care home after school for snacks and play until five o'clock. The days we are home are really available to us. Lastly, we watch no television and do not have a VCR. Our children's time with us, and ours with them, is intense, busy, engaged.

For me, my various roles—doctor, teacher, writer, mother, lover—are compatible, not conflicting. In many ways, each role is essential to the well-being of the others. Take away any, and all would suffer.

A sharing life partner, part-time employment, truly open time for creative work, excellent day care—these things are the essential ingredients in my recipe. And these are exactly what any person with children needs in stretching to reach his or her full potential. That's why I will keep working towards a society based on equal relationships, meaningful work for adequate pay, and respect for the enormity of human possibility. In the meantime, I will continue to struggle against oppressive and hierarchical relationships in families, between races, and between countries. I am centered in the deep connections which link my politics, my personal life, and my practice.

A Postscript

Twelve years later, I have now been 27 years at the same community health center. I work three days a week, take full call, and still deliver my own patients when I can. Last week, I went in to deliver the baby of a young woman whom I had brought into the world 15 years ago. Afterward, the teen father's mother came in and said, "You're Dr. Candib."

"That's right," I said.

"You delivered Jonathan! [the teen father]"

I think that was a first, to have delivered both parents.

In the meantime, Richard and I continue reading and writing together, and our lives only get more enriched, although the tragedy of widening inequality and lack of health care in our nation remains deplorable.

— *Lucy M. Candib*
Professor of Family Medicine and Community Health,
University of Massachusetts Medical School
Staff physician, Family Health Center of Worcester

An Independent Scientist[8]

One Friday afternoon in late April of last year, so tired I could hardly reach the telephone, I received a call from an editor of a Major Medical Journal. After the briefest of introductions, the editor explained that she wanted my long-time research partner, Melinda, and me to write an editorial to accompany a special article. Still perceiving myself to be a novice in academia, I was flabbergasted and struggled to maintain my poise. She explained a few details, then said something to the effect of, "Here's the bad news: we need the final version on May 12." Eighteen days. I experienced an anginal-like sensation, felt the opportunity start to slip away, paused, then tightened my grip. I blurted, "There is something I feel obligated to tell you. I am pregnant and my due date is in eight days, but I don't think it will be a problem." The silence that followed was painful; then she said in measured cadence, "Well, that's what coauthors are for."

I immediately phoned Melinda. Ideas for the piece started tumbling out. We acknowledged my pending delivery as only a minor potential obstacle. There could not, however, be mistakes or bad luck. I called my husband, Ron, with some trepidation. I had broken a sacred rule of our marriage by accepting a project without consulting with him to review its potential effect on our family. He was congratulatory, downright gleeful, even though he was keenly aware of the implications for us. After discussing the practical aspects of the project, we agreed that my parents would need to be drawn into the plans. My mother, true to form, was supportive but mystified that I had not chosen an easier life. Three hours by car, my parents arrived that night, after canceling their plans for golf

and bridge and commitments to my sister and her four children. The next
morning they spirited Dana, my 4-year-old, back to their home for a long
weekend.

The word of my good fortune spread. Two secretaries and a
co-worker of my husband offered to help care for Dana, should I need
time to write after the birth. A plate of baked goods arrived from the
neighbors. Our friend Larry brought us a massive pot of matzo ball
soup. Other friends and colleagues just asked how they could help. At
my next prenatal appointment, Phyllis, my obstetrician, sympathized
with my physical discomfort and assumed that I was anxious to deliver,
only to find out that I was hoping to stave off labor for as long as
possible. The need to finish the editorial became part of a boutique birth
plan.

So close to delivery, I had respite from my clinical duties. Ron and
I went out for dinner each of the next three nights and discussed ideas.
Soon I had a first draft and Melinda attacked it. I reported my aches and
pains to her several times a day. She and her husband bore the brunt of
running the manuscript back and forth.

A week after I accepted the assignment, in the evening, my
membranes broke. I called Phyllis. She asked about contractions,
the fluid's color, the presence of blood, and the status of the editorial.
I quickly packed an overnight bag. Larry, who had brought supper,
agreed to stay with Dana. My parents headed back to Portland, and
Ron and I headed for the hospital. Checking into labor and delivery,
Ron carried my overnight bag. I carried a briefcase. At midnight I was
still not in labor, and the nurse teasingly asked me if I wanted to work or
to take a sleeping pill. I chose the latter. Twenty hours later, Alexandra
appeared. Her sweet, good-natured disposition was quickly apparent:
even she was going to be a good sport about this.

The next day at the hospital my husband and I traded Alex and the
editorial back and forth. I was in my office typing a revision the following
day. As Alex slept, my secretary played the heavy and limited viewing of
the baby to two minutes. Two days later my colleague Melinda and I
shared caring for Alex as we completed a draft that was then FedExed to
associates across the country for review. Six days later, when the friendly

reviews returned, Melinda came to my home. She and I sat at the head of a king-sized bed, Alex sleeping between us, Dana snuggled on my other side, reviews and manuscript pages spread about. We hammered out final wording as Ron, my parents, and Larry cleared supper dishes and visited in the kitchen. Over the next week the journal's editors talked with me by phone in hushed voices, as though they were afraid to wake the baby. When the editorial[1] was published seven weeks later, I was thoroughly settled into maternity leave. I completed a telephone interview for *All Things Considered* while nursing.

During that summer I tried to reconcile the convergence of Alex's birth and writing the editorial with an important value in academia, that of the "independent scientist." A week before my delivery, I completed my first year on my school of medicine's promotion and tenure committee. Finding an applicant to be an independent researcher was often crucial for promotion. Everyone on the committee seemed more knowledgeable about independence than I, but I began to pick it up from context. Publishing with the same group over many years was problematic. Principal investigator status from the National Institutes of Health was more independent than the same position on a grant from a private foundation, even if the amount of money was the same. Single-authored publications were definitively independent. Particularly illuminating, last-place "senior" authorship was really independent apparently because it no longer mattered where one was in the lineup. (I wondered if this argument would fly with Dana's preschool class queuing up to go for a walk.) Though I could not put my finger on why, I found this emphasis on the paramount importance of independence disturbing.

The year since Alex's birth has been rigorous. I have pragmatically passed up opportunities for "professional advancement." I rarely travel, but when I do my entourage includes Ron, both children, and my parents. I share time-management tips with other "mom-docs"—wasted minutes at work ultimately come out of time with my family. Freedom is five minutes alone in the car singing loudly with a rock-and-roll radio station. But my passion for research remains and frequently gets me up at 4 a.m. for quiet time to think, read, and write.

When women friends talk about striving for balance, I experience humiliating memories of the gymnastic beam in high school. My goal is not to find balance, but to harmonize the worlds of work and family, without letting thoughts of one world unduly dominate the other. I am only variably successful. Even now as I jot these ideas, Alex tips over the Razzle Dazzle Rice Krispies and Dana dances in them, laughing wildly as she grinds them into the carpet.

A few weeks ago a fellow psychiatrist gently asked me how I might have professionally assessed a woman who checked into labor and delivery with a briefcase. I felt at a loss in explaining to him that those three weeks were exhilarating. Freed from a variety of everyday cares, surrounded by love and support, I knew that the barriers that compartmentalize my life were gone and I immersed myself in my two great passions.

Yet for me to claim to be an "independent scientist" seems a sham. As I reviewed successful applicants for promotion this year, I often wondered who made it possible for them to complete such prodigious amounts of work. I bemusedly imagined an alternate universe in which editors allow acknowledgment of child providers and spouses on manuscripts, department heads frown on failure to include a junior colleague on a publication, promotion and tenure committees view publishing with the same group over time like society views a good marriage, and both interdependence and generativity are rewarded.

— Linda Ganzini

Director of Geriatric Psychiatry, Portland Veterans Affairs Medical Center
Professor of Psychiatry, Oregon Health Sciences University

Note

1. Ganzini, L. (1997). Psychiatry and assisted suicide in the United States. *New England Journal of Medicine, 336,* 1824–1826.

How to Do It All at Once

I have been told there are two kinds of people in this world.
List makers, and those who don't make lists.
I don't really believe that.

I believe there are *six* kinds of people in this world.
Those who have a heart of gold, and those who don't.
Those who lie, and those who don't.
Those who get things done, and those who don't.
I always wondered how my busiest friends managed. Then people started asking *me* how I managed.
I thought I would tell you a little secret.
People that seem to manage do it *all at once*.
For example,
If there is a good program on television I want to watch, that's the day I do the laundry. This is called multi-tasking. The laundry is coded so even the 5-year-old can separate it to its rightful owner. The other trick, of course, is to own 30 pairs of underwear.
If I must drive to Seattle, I have a CME tape in my car.
Grocery shopping turns into a forum for discussing sex, vitamins, and cultural diversity. It's a great time to teach negotiating strategy (no, you can only have one Lunchable, not three), to reminisce (when I was your age all we got was yucky oatmeal, powdered milk, and moldy bread), and to talk about birth control. It also teaches addition, subtraction and division, and finally, the true meaning of buying on credit.
While eating dinner, we plan the next day's schedule and menu, and hear all the happenings at school.
While I sew, I call a friend on the speaker phone.
Cleaning the bathroom is easy when done while waiting for the bathtub to fill.
When cleaning the bedrooms, I use the lowest drawer approach. Anything on the floor gets shoved into the lowest drawer. If they don't ask for it for a month, it disappears as a donation to the poor.

Combining food groups can be challenging. The perfect food would probably be popcorn (fiber) covered with chocolate (endorphins) and spinach (folate to decrease dementia).

When the kids were little, they slept in their clothes so I could shovel them from bed to car to sitter's door without arousing them. Now, although they don't have to wear uniforms, they do: jeans and Abercrombie.

To exercise, I chase the children around the house and tickle them.

I recommend vigorous exercise like sit ups (just two) and jumping jacks *before* sex. It increases the heart rate and keeps the bed warm.

Laugh. It uses up more muscles and calories.

Finding time to keep in touch with my sisters in all corners of the U.S. means having to have both a routine and a time limit. (We like to gab.)

So, for my sister in Boston, it's e-mail in the morning while I drink my coffee, cut short by the necessity to dress the baby for kindergarten.

For my sister in San Jose, it's a lunch phone call between patients, her only free time that coincides with mine.

For my sister in Miami, it's a phone call from the cell phone while I drive home, the time she has just finished tucking in her four boys.

The danger comes when a hyperorganized person gets behind on her agenda, and must do four things at once. That can be a little overwhelming.

I have been known after a bad call night, to do some of the following:

Back out of the garage with the garage door *down*.

Back right into a car. In our own driveway. Our own car. State Farm was *not* happy.

Take my husband's beeper instead of mine by mistake. Now, mine has a neon pink coil of telephone cord permanently attached. Not easy to mistake his for hers ever again.

Lock myself out of the car and forget the combination. (I *know* it has to be someone's birthday.)

Lose my bifocals at the YMCA, thus making it *impossible* to open my locker combination.

Put the laundry in with all the hangers still attached to the shirts.

Boil the hard boiled eggs (twice).

Freeze the milk accidentally or put the ice cream in the refrigerator, only to wake up to the mess in the morning.

Get dressed in the dark and leave for work with my clothes on inside out or backwards. Now that may seem odd to those of you who are slender, but believe me, it happens.

The secret to my success, thus, are these comforting rituals that developed over a lifetime of sleep deprivation and the need to survive 5 children and a husband who can be called away at a moment's notice to crack a chest and save a life.

So if you see me zipping by in my red minivan, I am not ignoring you. am probably trying to make it on time to my daughter's Girl Scout meeting (late again).

And yes, I composed this article in my head first. While doing the dishes.

P.S. No, I do not balance the checkbook. Every New Years we open a new one and close the old one.

— *Teresa Clabots*
Assistant Clinical Professor of Pediatrics,
University of Washington School of Medicine

Late Lunch

The late lunch line at 2:00 or 3:00,
a scattering of doctors among the off-hour others;
a colleague's nod, a brief exchange,
acknowledging the rarity of this,
　　a sheltered peace-place;
protected by what others recognize as needs,
　　yet only when conditions are just right
　　will we allow ourselves—
rare respite, only briefly restful,
the press of things undone still live and warm.

Incessant insistent demands of the day
   fill time between the scheduled and the crises
   the way a river flows behind the paddle;
clamor of competing claims on finite time:
Rounds and the charts; the OR, the clinic, the charts;
   the office, the calls and the charts,
and the committees, the undone chapter, the grants—
the need to research, teach, and write, *and* be at home
   where spouses also working
   and children always growing
   wait—but not for long.

The old tradition, revered within red brick and columns:
portraits on the paneled walls look down,
starched white coats march by,
stethoscopes as medals hanging—
Commitment is a privilege and a duty,
to be thorough, to be there, to be prepared,
   to do it all and do it well—
from our first admission to the School,
to be In Medicine is to accept.

And in the quiet afternoon cafeteria
twice in one week my sighed remarks meet with others',
our common pressures find expression,
   speaking aloud this situation
   and our powerlessness in it.

And surprise—
   they feel it too, the
   macho model medical men
   who match the portraits.

— *Mary Williams Clark*
Chief of Pediatric Orthopedics, Sparrow Regional Children's Center
Clinical Professor of Orthopedics, Michigan State University

Balancing Family and Career:
Advice From the Trenches[9]

Ideally, the art of balancing family and career is equally important to men and women, but as long as women are the traditional caregivers, this balance is more of an issue for them. This is particularly the case in academic medicine; because the academic clock and biological clock tick in synchrony, efforts to build a family and a career typically converge for a woman in her twenties and thirties.

To start, set personal and professional goals and plot a course toward achieving those goals. Look in the mirror and ask yourself, "Who am I, and what do I want to be? Do I want to be a department chairman? Do I want to have a national reputation? Do I want to be a parent? Do I want to work full- or part-time? Do I want to do research? Do I want to live in a rural or urban area?" and so on. There is no right or wrong answer to any of these questions; they are personal decisions. I periodically ask myself, "If something catastrophic happened to me today, would I have any overwhelming regrets about the way I have lived my life?" If you ask yourself this question and the answer is "yes," I encourage you to change something soon.

Once you have established your goals, be sure to choose a partner who shares these goals. Although I did not realize it at the time, this was the single most important decision enabling me to achieve both personal and professional success. Thus, I would caution a woman to be wary of choosing a life partner who was raised to think that the worst form of humiliation was to be "beaten by a girl." I also advise women to avoid selecting partners who think that housework falls under the purview of the female sex. If a woman's goal is to be a tenured professor and her spouse's goal is to marry a domestic goddess, the relationship is doomed to fail. In my case, hiring someone to help with housework and laundry was the best thing for my marriage and my mood. For all the men reading this, I am here to tell you that dirty socks, underwear, and dishes are no more appealing to the X chromosome than to the Y chromosome. The time you save is time you can spend with the kids, your spouse, or getting extra work done.

Strive for geographic proximity—that is, have all your activities close together. This is something I did not actively seek to do, but it turned out to be crucial in balancing everything, especially when the kids were small. I live close to work and can park right outside the building in which my laboratory, my office, and most of my clinical work are located. In addition, I have chosen to live in a moderately sized city where such things as day care, schools, grocery stores, and the pediatrician are readily accessible. Keeping all your activities spinning successfully is simpler when the distance between them is not too great.

You must establish priorities in your life. My husband and I make every attempt to attend our children's school performances or sports events and to ensure that we have some family time every weekend and almost every weeknight. I have never heard one of my terminally ill patients say they wished they had attended that meeting, served on that committee, or made that grant deadline. I have, however, heard many of them express regrets about the amount of time they spent with their children and family. After all, very few of us will be remembered for our professional accomplishments. It is far more likely that we will be remembered as someone's daughter, son, mother, spouse, or brother.

Get up 1 to 2 hours earlier than you have to each morning. My mother gave me this advice. She worked full-time, went to school, and ran the household. That extra time in the morning, when the house is quiet and your mind is fresh, allows you to complete tasks and arrive at work feeling like you have already accomplished something. Don't fritter this time away on routine items; use it to attack some significant project. In addition, use technology as much as possible to blend work and home life; have a computer at home so you can work while the kids are sleeping and a cellular phone so you can take calls in the car or grocery store.

One of the best aspects of "having it all" is having two potential spheres of support. Sometimes, at home, the kids or my husband are grouchy and whiny, and no one listens to anything I say. At these moments, it is heartening to go to work, where I get a little respect, I have some control over things, and I write orders and someone follows them. Sometimes things don't go well at work. Perhaps I get a nasty manuscript review, one of my patients is not doing well, or a colleague is driving me crazy. At these times, it is gratifying to go home and cuddle with the kids, bake cookies, read together, and be a mom. There are also those special times when it all comes together; things are going great at work and at home. These are peak moments to be savored.

As with anything, there is a down side to "having it all." Balancing a full-time career in academic medicine and a family means that you serve many "bosses." The clinicians want you to see more patients, the educators want you to do more teaching and curriculum development, the researchers want you to write more grants and papers, and, of course, your children want you to be at their beck and call 24 hours a day. To prevent yourself from burning out by trying to please everyone, you need to set personal and professional limits. Decide what you want to do and what you are willing to do. Compromises and negotiations can be made, but try to emerge with your self-respect intact.

Another down side is meal preparation. When both parents work full-time, it is impossible to provide a home-cooked dinner every night. If this is something valued by you or your spouse, my advice is to hire a cook. Our solution has been to have home-cooked meals on the weekends and, with good planning, as many as 3 nights per week. Thursdays are pizza, and Fridays are fast food. We all take a Flintstone vitamin daily. It works for us.

As women climb the academic ladder, there are fewer and fewer female colleagues or role models. I view myself as being just at the bottom side of the glass ceiling looking through and, frankly, there are few persons on the other side whom I aspire to be like. This makes it a little lonely at times, and I get tired of sports discussions. Nevertheless, I am pleased to be guiding other female faculty members up the ladder and look forward to the day when one or two male colleagues will have to listen politely to an enthusiastic discussion of a sale at Marshall Field's.

— *Molly Carnes*

Professor of Medicine and Director,
Center for Women's Health, University of Wisconsin
Jean Manchester Biddick Professor of Women's Health Research

One Page at a Time

Eight o'clock and my husband Steve is going to tell the kids a Fred-and-the Finger-Monster story. Fred, a small green swivel clip, stars in many adventures spun from Steve's imagination. Just opening a door can be a huge ordeal for these little buddies, but they manage to hide in backpacks, get themselves mailed, and even drive trucks. For me, an F & the FM story means I might not be required for any bedtime duties; I may even have some time for myself.

I lay back on the sofa (I seem to have to read lying down, perhaps due to poor brain circulation), crack open a can of soda, and start to read. I'm whisked away, but within a minute, the phone rings. It's a school friend with homework questions for our nine-year-old. Up the stairs I trudge to tell Thomas to pick up the extension. In the midst of the next paragraph, the phone rings again. It's Cathy. Can our dog play with her dog, just wanted to phone first to see if it's okay (*They only play together everyday*, I mutter to myself). *Sure, sure, okay.*

I am rereading the same sentence when the doorbell rings, but I am determined to finish the sentence. By the time I open the door, our new neighbor is backing off the porch holding a warehouse-size can of lighter fluid and fumbling with the red cap. I'm hoping that she hasn't gone off the deep end or freaked out about cultural differences, but she's saying, "Okay, I opened it."

"You're sure?" I ask.

"Yes, yes, but do you know how much you use?"

"Just a *little* bit," I warn and gesture repeatedly with my thumb and forefinger squeezed tight. I'm thinking, should I go with her? Or wait for the explosion? But she's already backed off the front yard, and I return to the sofa.

Ahhh, yes, reading, I'm actually reading.

The doorbell again. Cathy has arrived with her dog to pick up Roxy. *Thank you, thank you.* I turn from the door, and there is Becca. When Fred became hungry in the story, she suddenly remembered that she needs to bring in five of "something to eat" for her kindergarten math class. We find a box that has five unbroken crackers in it, I label it, put it on the foyer table, and she skips up the stairs. What is it about bedtime that gives kids that energy boost?

A sip of soda and back to the book. The phone again. It's actually a call for me, not a kid or dog. My resident for the next day needs to review patients' histories with me to determine anesthetic plans. One patient has numerous complicated medical problems, so we spend time on that, and I begin to worry about the next day.

Okay, back on the sofa. Instantly: Ding, dong. It's Cathy back with Roxy, who refuses to release the plastic ball for Cathy, but one look from me and she's dropped it. I hand the slimy thing back to Cathy, thanking her profusely. I check—our neighbor's house is not on fire.

Okay, back on the sofa. By this point, Naddie the pup is so frustrated that she didn't get to go out, she insists on playing fetch with me, dropping her saliva-soaked ball on my chest, neck, and stomach, jumping on me if I refuse to throw it. But I refuse even more to get up again to push her into the backyard. I finally maneuver my body into a position between the sofa and the coffee table where she can't approach my face and book.

9:15. Thomas appears at the doorway. "My throat hurts." Getting the flashlight from the earthquake supply, I make a mental note to tell the sitter in the morning that he may not be able to go to school. She'll arrive at 6:30, and even with school-age kids, we need a plan for child care everyday. I beam the light in: not bad, just slightly red for now.

We head upstairs, I give him Tylenol, coax Roxy up on the bed, and tell Thomas the story of my trying to read one page. He laughs as I rub his back. He asks me to check that Fred is comfortable in his special little wooden shoe bed. Eventually, he murmurs and falls asleep. And as any parent knows while trying to get a kid to sleep, more sleep-inducing neurotransmitters are released in the parent's brain compared with the child's. I step, heavy lidded and yawning, from his bedroom.

— *Audrey Shafer*

Associate Professor of Anesthesia, Stanford University School of Medicine
Author of Sleep Talker: Poems by a Doctor/Mother *(2001)*

To Rachel

You taught me
life couldn't be planned.
I had your arrival scheduled
between manuscripts and grants,
mapped out on a pregnancy wheel
But you decided differently.
At 24 weeks — contractions
Intestinal cramps, I thought,
during my research presentation
— I had no idea.
Those scary first weeks
bed rest and terbutaline
still six contractions an hour
then gestational diabetes.
But you survived
past 28, 32, then 36 weeks
while I slowed down
the frantic pace of academic life.
You arrived five days late
on your own time,
our little 6 lb. wonder.

— Joan C. Lo
Assistant Professor of Medicine, University of California San Francisco

Pregnancy and the Professional Woman[10]

Although managing the practical difficulties of balancing career and children is undeniably challenging, a woman's unconscious fantasies about how she decides to do this will still come into play. Since there is no prescribed "right" balance, her fantasies about the impact of her working on her children, and about the effect of day care on children, will be reflected in how she prioritizes her time and how conflicted she feels about this. She can deal with her uncertainty by trying to be a "supermom" (Applegarth, 1986), feeling that she must meet all challenges of home and work life in order to relieve guilt about pursuing her own goals, which she may feel are selfish. Even if she acknowledges that she cannot be omnipotent in this way and is able to delineate a balance for herself between raising children and pursuing career goals, she will still have to cope with feeling sad, frustrated, or even depressed at the loss of the full scope of her work, much as men traditionally struggle with these reactions at the time of retirement. There is both a gain and a loss.

— Amy A. Tyson
Clinical Faculty, University of California San Francisco
Private practice psychiatry, psychoanalysis

Reference

Applegarth, A. (1986). Woman and work. In T. Bernay & W. E. Cantor (Eds.), *The psychology of today's woman: New psychoanalytic visions* (pp. 211–330). Hillsdale, NJ: Lawrence Erlbaum.

The Changing Role of Physicians as Working Mothers

When my mother wanted to become a doctor 80 years ago, she wrote to her uncle, Dr. Gerrit Van Zwaluwenburg, Chief of Radiology at the University of Michigan, for advice. I still have his letter to her strongly recommending that she should forget medicine and place her first priority on marriage and family. She persisted with medicine and attended the Women's Medical College in Philadelphia, married after graduation, and successfully raised four children.

My parents were missionaries in South India where I was born. As I was growing up, the only other doctors I knew were women. At that time, my mother's training as a doctor was considered secondary to her position as a missionary's wife. So she set up her office in one side room of our home. Every morning, the front porch was crowded with women and children waiting to be seen in her small examining room. But despite her work, she was always available for us, never complaining if we interrupted her between patients.

Many times we were awakened at night by a bullock cart bringing in a patient from some distant village. Too often, they had first tried the village herbalist or Hindu priest and arrived too late for modern medical help. Not having electricity, we used kerosene lamps or lanterns. I remember one night when Dad drove the car around to shine the headlight onto the operating table so that Mom could see more clearly. Eventually, he supervised the building of a small hospital with a battery-operated generator that provided electricity for the hospital as well as our home.

Thirty years after my mother first sought admission, I also applied to the University of Michigan Medical School. I was given the same excuses for excluding women: "Our experience is that most women who become doctors leave the profession as soon as they get married and have children." I assured the interviewer of my plans to continue practicing even after marriage and family and was later accepted as one of six women in a class of 90 students.

I had hoped for a residency in pediatrics but decided the demanding call schedule would be disastrous to our family life. By chance, I learned of a new psychiatric residency program for physician mothers at the New York Medical College. Recognizing the special needs of mothers, this program had established a 40-hour workweek for residents with only one overnight call per month and up to three months vacation leave per year. Time taken off was then added to extend the period of residency.

Our youngest daughter was two and a half when I started my residency in child psychiatry, a program that ultimately lasted five years because of extended leaves each summer. I could never have finished without the continued support and encouragement of my husband, who has always been actively involved in raising the children, from changing diapers to shuttling them back and forth to music lessons.

Those years working full-time during my residency were the most difficult for our family. My youngest daughter has daytime memories of the baby-sitter in our home but remembers me only coming home from work for supper and then reading stories and singing to her at bedtime. Still, these were precious times for us both. The older children had to take on more responsibilities after school and help prepare supper. It meant chore lists on the refrigerator and taking turns with dishes and housework. At one time, friction between our two oldest who shared a room was so severe that I even considered postponing the last two years of my residency. Our teenager, however, suggested having family meetings where everyone was given an equal opportunity to air grievances. This practice became a regular part of our Sunday routine. Not only were minor problems settled, but we also could plan different activities to suit the varied interests of each child.

After residency, I found a position that required only 30 hours per week, allowing me to be home soon after the children returned from school. In later years when they left for college, I returned to full-time private practice. I realized I was envious of my daughter, who worked school hours as a guidance counselor and later as a teacher, having summers off to be with her children. So again I chose to work part-time and take summers off to accompany my husband on his assignments to Africa, the island of Anguilla, India, or Nepal. In my preretirement years, this has also allowed me freedom to spend more time with 10 active, curious, and delightful grandchildren.

These major life decisions have limited my income as a physician and restricted advancement in my career. But they have added to the fullness and enrichment of my life in the multiple roles I love—wife, mother, grandmother, and child psychiatrist.

— *Marian Korteling Levai*
Psychiatrist formerly in private practice, now part-time locum tenens

Reflections on Balance

I graduated from medical school in 1967 and, after my internship year, applied for residencies in obstetrics and gynecology. When I interviewed at Columbia University Presbyterian Hospital, I was told that they had once taken a woman resident, but since it had not worked out, they were unwilling to take a chance on another woman. Fortunately, the chairman at Cornell was from Europe, where many residents were women. He recruited me to his program where I was one of two women. In the subsequent 30 years, it is interesting to reflect on how the tables have turned, as now more than 50% of ob-gyn residents are women.

As a physician and mother, here's some advice that I would give to women today.

Have your children young and hire as much household help as you can afford. There is never a convenient time to have children when building a career, but it is much easier biologically when you are young. Until my children were in school, I always had live-in child care, an arrangement that allowed me considerable flexibility when I worked late in the evenings. The meals were always served on time, regardless of when I got home.

My husband once said to me, "Just because you don't have time or don't want to do something doesn't mean I want to do it." Our solution was to hire ample household help, so my time at home could be spent actively involved with the children.

When my children were young, I increased my research time because it offered more flexibility. As my career advanced, they became old enough to enjoy trips when I traveled to meetings. By the time I became a department head at the age of 45, my youngest child was in college, and I had the freedom to move.

With a little creative scheduling, I could still participate in my children's activities despite working full-time. I once joined a carpool with four other neighbors, arranging my schedule so I could be absent every Friday afternoon from 3:00 to 4:00. Even though this meant returning later to work, scheduling that "regular meeting" allowed me to pick up five first-graders from school and deliver them to their respective homes, along the way of course, hearing firsthand about their day's activities. My son then stayed with our nanny until I returned home later that evening. Likewise, with school activities or sports, it again required only advance planning for me to leave the hospital.

Guilt can be a major deterrent for any working mother, but having had a wonderful nanny in my own childhood, I never experienced the same level of guilt when leaving the children with their nanny. Clearly, in an extended family model, many relatives take care of the children, not just the mother. It can be potentially beneficial for children to be exposed to other caregivers as well.

Having a family may slow down your career but need not end it. There are many innovative options for combining work and family for those who seek to be active participants in both arenas.

— Jennifer R. Niebyl
Professor and Head, Department of Obstetrics and Gynecology,
University of Iowa College of Medicine
Co-editor of Obstetrics: Normal and Problem Pregnancies

Notes from a Personal Journey[11]

I had a successful role model. My mother, a smart and beautiful woman, became a dentist at a time when women seldom ventured in the career of health sciences. She married my father, a physician, also from a household where women received an education but chose not to work except for economic need. My mother chose to work full-time all her life because she liked her career. She had an academic and a private practice career and was the mother of three children.

Still, it was a traditional household. My mother, as smart if not smarter than my father, consistently in the home deferred to him for any "pearls of wisdom" in the domain of cultural subjects or current events. She never budged though in reference to the "girls"; they were going to be given the same opportunity as my brother. What she learned and taught me was to be flexible with goals and to be ready to change in midstream; to not only prioritize, including herself in the priority list, but to learn to evaluate the crisis; to trust her judgment and to live with the consequences. She told me to learn to live with the loss that results from not being with the children as much but also to enjoy the reason that would be taking me away from them. She taught me to delegate as much as I could if delegating meant that I would have more time for my family. Where she could not go against her times was in the way she compromised with my father, playing a more traditional role within the relationship than the one she believed in.

I was blessed with a role model that I seldom see in my friends or patients. This role model has given me tools to pursue my struggle; it did not free me from my struggle. Choosing to work and knowing that I could be a professional in a committed relationship with children I did not doubt. Learning to trust that my mate was going to accept me at my best and not resent me (my mother's conflict with my father) was more uncertain. Having learned to trust my mate's acceptance of my choices has made me that much aware of similar struggles with my patients, women and men.

Here, we have succeeded in having full careers. What has suffered is the time we could spend with each other, as we chose one of us to be with the children, sacrificing the time we would have had together. This put a strain in the relationship, creating difficult moments along our life together. Still, as a woman, the choice we made gave me the possibility of pursuing another source of gratification, more often available to men than to women—namely, my own career.

— *Silvia Wybert Olarte*
Clinical Professor of Psychiatry, New York Medical College
President, Association of Women Psychiatrists

Notes

1. Excerpted from Sotile, W. M., & Sotile, M. O. (2000). *The medical marriage: Sustaining healthy relationships for physicians and their families* (p. 11). Chicago: American Medical Association. Reprinted by permission of the American Medical Association, *The Medical Marriage*, © 2000.

2. Excerpted from Alexander, B. (1996). Moments of becoming. In D. Wear (Ed.), *Women in medical education: An anthology of experience* (p. 158). Albany: State University of New York Press. Reprinted with permission of State University of New York Press.

3. Excerpted from Angell, M. (1982). Juggling the personal and professional life. *Journal of the American Medical Women's Association, 37*(3), 68. Copyright © 1982 American Medical Women's Association, Inc. All rights reserved. Reprinted with permission for education use only.

4. From Whipple, D. V. (1968). *Practice and family life.* Speech given at the Conference on Meeting Medical Manpower Needs: The Fuller Utilization of the Woman Physician.

5. Excerpted from Kaltreider, N. B. (1997). Is it worth it? In N. B. Kaltreider (Ed.), *Dilemmas of a double life: Women balancing careers and relationships* (p. 30). Northvale, NJ: Jason Aronson. Reprinted with permission.

6. From Heidenreich, C. (1998). A few thoughts on part-time faculty: The push for the summit and the long climb down. *Society of General Internal Medicine Forum, 21*(12), 9–10. Reprinted and abridged with permission.

7. From Candib, L. M. (1985). In M. A. Bowman & D. I. Allen (Eds.), *Stress and women physicians.* New York: Springer-Verlag. Reprinted by permission of Springer-Verlag, New York.

8. From Ganzini, L. (1998). An independent scientist. *Journal of the American Medical Association, 280*(11), 950. Copyrighted © 1998, American Medical Association. Reprinted with permission.

9. From Carnes, M. (1996). Balancing family and career: Advice from the trenches. *Annals of Internal Medicine, 125*, 618–620. Abridged and reprinted by permission of the American College of Physicians–American Society of Internal Medicine.

10. Excerpted from Tyson, A. A. (1997). Pregnancy and the professional woman: The psychological transition. In N. B. Kaltreider (Ed.), *Dilemmas of a double life: Women balancing careers and relationships* (p. 69). Northvale, NJ: Jason Aronson. Reprinted with permission.

11. Excerpted from Olarte, S. W. (2000). The female professional: Parenting, career, choices, and compromises. *American Journal of Psychoanalysis, 60*(3), 293–306. Reprinted by permission of Kluwer Academic/Plenum Publishers.

11

OUR FAMILIES' PERSPECTIVES

*But a household requires sustained attention to
many different needs, a very different kind of attention.
Time, space, and tools need to be used for multiple
purposes, leftovers must be varied and combined.
Integration becomes more important than specialization.
Leftover fabric from a dress will reappear in patchwork
five years later; one task may be put aside when the baby
wakes up for a different task that allows interaction. Some
tasks are undone within minutes, like a cup of tea that is
drunk as soon as it is made. Others endure for decades.*

— *Mary Catherine Bateson*[1]

Jelly[2]

Our daughter, age about 7 at the time, was passing cookies at a party
when some idiot of a woman commiserated with her because her mother
worked. Ann pulled herself up to all of her 4 feet and said: "In our house,
daddy makes the bread and butter and mommy makes the jelly."

— *Dr. W.*

From *Balm in Gilead: Journey of a Healer*³

Even as a young child, I knew both the passion and the reverence my mother brought to her work. At the dinner table, while protecting the privacy and anonymity of her patients, she would reenact the dramas of the clinic, providing enough details for us to get caught up in the story. I would hear tightness and anger in her voice when children and their families got hopelessly wrapped up in bureaucratic red tape, or when a colleague, out of fear or ignorance, acted unprofessionally. Sometimes I would feel waves of jealousy and abandonment when my mother would go off to help a child in trouble, leaving her three "real" children behind. A Saturday family adventure would be shattered, a cooking project stopped in the middle, the pansies half-planted. I always screamed loudly as she walked out the door, her cape streaming, her gait purposeful. When she returned to us, leaving the clinical emergencies safely out of her view, we would confront her with "how we felt" about her leaving, and she would carefully and candidly explain her devotion to her work *and* her mother-love for us. Didn't we know that the latter was deeper, that it would last "forever"?

From time to time, I remember my mother saying, without sentimentality, "I love my work," a statement I puzzled over as a child. It made me imagine a day at the office full of pleasure and sunshine. Since the home scene, with all its love and laughter, had its inevitable crises and struggles, I occasionally worried whether my mother liked going to work more than staying at home. Many years later, I understood everything she meant by that brief affirmation. Her work—with its frustrations and imperfections—offered her endless challenges and a few victories, offered her the chance to use her wisdom and skills, and offered her the "privilege" of healing others. Now that I am middle-aged, and "loving my work" as well, I know even more clearly how much my mother gained fulfillment from balancing work and family. And I also understand some of the high costs of this balance, and of her struggle with many unyielding institutions to live out these deep, dual commitments.

— *Sara Lawrence Lightfoot*
Professor of Education, Harvard University
Daughter of Margaret Lawrence
Author of Balm in Gilead: Journey of a Healer *(1988)*

Our Medical Marriage[4]

for Susanne

We kneeled on the bookstore floor
two students scanning the bodies
of new books, checking out
each other's *Principles*
of Internal Medicine.
Scores of textbooks later
we're a pair of pagers and missed dinners,
companions in sleep-deprived nights.
We suffered the long delay
before our only child while we ran
to slashed wrists and ODs,
sprinted from half-read journal
to school play to board meeting.
In conversation long as summer light
we talked patients and drugs,
recited the crushed prayers of the dying,
learned how we both took medicine
as a life-long lover.

One hushed June evening in mid-life
scented rose and thick with fireflies,
the phone steals her.
I sit with my unfilled glass
and a life we knew we were choosing,
our marriage a joining of two strains
of mint, planted close, cross-pollinated
to form a single type, the small, unfailing
flowers arrayed in purple spikes
I can see most clearly
when I'm down on my knees.

— *Richard M. Berlin*
Associate Professor of Psychiatry,
University of Massachusetts Medical School
Husband of Susanne King

From *Her Infinite Variety*[5]

I didn't meet Rosalie until I was twenty-eight, and had been running around a lot, all through law school and after. I'd known plenty of girls, some nice and some not so nice, and had even been more or less engaged a couple of times, but I always had the feeling they were trying to *land* me, one way or another, and I wriggled off the hook each time in a cold sweat. Then I went off to Fire Island one summer weekend and saw this tall good-looking blonde on the beach, studying Anderson's textbook of pathology, of all things. It amused the hell out of me. She was pretty cool at first, but I was persistent in a nice sort of way. She told me, finally, that she was a medical student, and it didn't take me long to realize that she wasn't just playing at it either. Her Dad was a fine orthopedist, and she was really bent on becoming one also. She was the first girl I'd ever met who had some goal in mind besides finding a guy. What struck me about her wasn't just that she and I had so very much to talk about—we did, of course—but that she was such a good-looking girl outside and so much of a *person* inside. It just bowled me over. I had never felt that way about the girls I had known, or been so proud when they liked me.

Anyway, it didn't take us very long to know that we were right for each other. We got married that winter. My practice was growing fast and I could have afforded a nice place, but in order to save her travel time I moved in with her into her little dormitory room. For a year and a half, I'd come back to that little place after a long day in court, take her out for a quick dinner, and then help her study until late at night, or help her relax sometimes by telling her stories about my cases, or hobnobbing with the other med students. I got to be the best midnight scrambled-egg cook on an illegal electric burner that you ever heard of. It was a grind, but I really loved the whole atmosphere—it was almost like being on some kind of wartime mission.

Then she graduated and became an intern, and we set up a nice apartment near the hospital where she could come in her off-duty time. After a year of internship and several of residency she went into practice, and four years later we had our first boy, and three years later our younger one. I guess it's *always* been somewhat like a wartime mission—a busy, urgent kind of life, with servants coming and going, kids getting sick and then well again, me having an important evening conference just when she has an emergency operation during the maid's night off, and all that. There have been periods when for days at a time we met each other only in bed. There were times during her residency when I thought that if her phone rang once more at night at just the wrong moment, I'd rip the goddamned thing off the wall and throw it out the window. And nowadays she often worries because she can't spend more time with the kids, but they're turning out to be wonderful boys and I don't think they could possibly love her any more, even if she did.

There *are* times when I think how much simpler it all was for my father—he would just come home and take his ease, and let everybody fuss over him. He was the one who counted, and everything was arranged to suit him. Sometimes I wish it were that way with me. But then Rosalie and I go out to dinner and I see people our own age sitting opposite each other but staring around sideways or looking at their food, and not having anything at all to say to each other. *We're* still like each other's dates—after eighteen years. We always find each other interesting, and its amazing to see how she really looks especially pretty and full of bounce after she's just pulled off a tricky operation and is still all excited and pleased by it, even though she's really dead-tired. I can't be sure how all this would have worked out if I weren't pretty successful in my own field, but I am. She has great respect for what I do, and she has even come to court a few times to hear me. She's very much a woman with me, but once in a while, if she tries to take over a little too much, I call her "Doctor" very respectfully, and she gets nettled for a minute, and then laughs and turns it off.

— *A lawyer*

What's a Mother For?[6]

It was the start of one of those *off* days. Everything went wrong. The alarm clock failed to go off at 6:15, and the whole family overslept.

Marian was rousing the kids and me. All the while we were getting breakfast, pulling the previous night's load of clothes out of the dryer, making sandwiches for the children, and posting notes for the baby sitter, Nancy, our 9-year-old, kept hunting for her unmatched sock. "Gollie," she grumbled, "What's a mother for?"

The comment made Marian, who works as a physician, ponder as she finished making one of the six beds. Along with 16 million other American working women, she tries to care for the needs of five overcharged children, ages 14 to 4, and, incidentally, a working husband.

Sometimes every working mother has to ask herself some basic questions regarding the overall effect this double life has on her family: *What is my influence as a mother? Are the children deprived of a certain emotional and spiritual stability? Is there a sense of general well-being and family unity?*

Because no husband is fully convinced he wants his wife to work—especially when he has to pitch in washing dishes and baby sitting after a rugged day—it pays to come up with some frank answers.

Mothers work outside the home for various reasons, none of them pat. The most obvious reason is financial. Some mothers work because it provides an escape from the frustrating boredom of household chores and all the tedious tensions that go along with taking care of children. Still others feel trapped because the talents they have are not being used creatively. In *The Feminine Mystique*, Betty Friedan stresses this problem of conflicting ambitions. Motherhood and the home may not present the modern, well-educated wife with adequate challenges. Consequently, four of every ten mothers with school-age children work outside the home.

What really matters in this never-ending debate is how her temperament affects the rest of the members of the home. How well does she manage her other job as wife and mother after returning home each evening? There are many at-home wives who feel empty and exhausted. A mother's attitude is fundamental in making for a happy home, whether she works or not. Children have sensitive antennae; they detect with amazing accuracy whether the mother performs her duties with love and satisfaction or because she feels duty-bound.

Kathy, our eighth-grader, recently forced Marian and me to take an honest look at ourselves. She brought an essay home from school: "There's a kind of behavioral chain reaction in our family. Somehow it starts when Daddy brings work from the office. And when he loses his temper—then Mommie takes it out on us, and we feel like orphans. But we know that they don't mean it—not really."

The essay helped us see that, as parents, we neglect to find out the views of our children. How do they feel about their mother and father working outside the home?

Nancy, our fourth-grader summed it up this way: "So, I get mad when my clothes are still in the dryer. But gee, down deep, I'm proud of the work Mommie is doing. And her being away from home makes me appreciate her all the more when she's at home."

Here, it seems to me, is the answer. Frankly, what is immediately important is learning how to appreciate each other as individuals and using wisely the time we have together as a family. Maybe it's not the easiest way to live. There are inconveniences. And clashes are bound to be expected.

What's a mother for? She cooks, shops, washes dishes, does laundry, folds clothes, mends, chauffeurs, helps with homework, and puts the children to bed. Countless times she bends down to tie shoelaces, but she also points up to the stars, directing inquiring minds to spiritual values that stand eternal. And in these unshakable standards of God's word she replenishes her own strength and faith.

A mother's love makes home the one place on earth where all members of the family still feels they belong. It is where they find shelter from the stress of a competitive world that is often hard and unfair, but in which they can live courageously and in which they have a part.

— *Blaise Levai*
Pastoral counselor and family therapist
Husband of Marian Levai

Life With Mother, the M.D.

My parents were in the class of '32 at Columbia University, College of Physicians & Surgeons (P&S). My father had a lifelong love affair with medicine, practicing as a general surgeon until he was 80 years old. He was beloved by his patients, colleagues, and staff. My mother once commented that being married to a doctor was "a voice on the phone, and a draft in the hall."

My mother did not share that same "call" to medicine and rather seemed to have stumbled into it. Her family had always placed a great emphasis on education—her father was a professor of economics at Columbia University; her Aunt, a Ph.D. before the turn of the century; and her grandmother, Olympia Brown, the first ordained female minister in the United States. It is unclear just whose idea it was that brought her to P&S where she was one of four women in the class.

Life as the daughter of two physicians was interesting. While many families talk about sports or politics at the dinner table, my parents often discussed interesting medical cases. I learned more about medicine than I shall ever wish to know.

My mother actually allowed my father to be the doctor that he was. She understood his work, provided the necessary support, and gave him the peace of mind his job required. I adored my father but was relieved that my mother did not share his passion for medicine. Had she been as busy as he, we would have been very lonely children indeed. No doubt we would have survived, but selfishly, I am grateful for my mother's companionship. Working part-time at a woman's clinic allowed her the freedom to become actively involved in my life and to be at home when I needed her. A staunch supporter, she ultimately became one of my best friends. Realizing now how difficult it must have been to combine career and family in the 1940s, I appreciate all the more her choices and attendant sacrifices.

— *Cynthia Magowan*
Community volunteer and homemaker
Daughter of Katharine W. Hooton

What We Have Fashioned Together[7]

Fools write papers that are autobiographical; wiser men confine their confessions to their analysts.[1] If further proof of folly be needed, note our temerity as men in daring to opine about the conditions of women's lives. Our hubris fairly invites criticism from colleagues, from readers, worse yet, from our wives. Clearly, we are not easily deterred. In our role as participant-observers in that most intense of relationships with successful women—being married to them—we insist on our right to try to say something on the matter.

We have had—and continue to have—a quite extraordinary experience in marriage, not one we were perceptive enough to seek when we fell in love or even one we welcomed fully when its depth first became manifest but one with unique meaning for our growth: the experience of living with a complete woman. We had been socialized to expect less and to settle for the creature comforts that came with that acceptance. Along the way, we may have shown some lack of grace in surrendering the customary conveniences; yet in return we have been granted a love the richer and fuller for having its roots in mutual respect and growing maturity. That, we acknowledge, we owe to our wives. Had it not been for their capacity to insist on respect for their integrity, it is doubtful we would have achieved what we now enjoy. Of course it was not unilateral; we claim our due for what we have fashioned together; but we know it would not have happened without what they brought us.

We consider ourselves the most fortunate of men.

— *Theodore Nadelson*
Former Chief of Psychiatric Services, Boston VA Medical Center
Husband of Carol Nadelson

— *Leon Eisenberg*
Maude and Lillian Presley Professor of Social Medicine
and Professor of Psychiatry, Emeritus, Harvard Medical School
Husband of Carola Eisenberg

Note

1. Freud, personal correspondence.

I Remember as a Child[8]

Our mother was, I suppose, a pioneer for her time, especially so because of her natural domesticity and interest in her home as a place to reflect personal tastes and interests. There was, undeniably, a struggle to make both ends meet: not only the financial end but the time problem. My father's salary as a minister was at once a source of difficulty (making it hard to have as much help in the house as a professional woman really needs) and a source of stimulation. Without Mother's earnings (modest though they were because it was the work rather than the income that gratified her), Dave and I would have had a far harder time getting our education and enjoying the occasional trips and indulgences children really expect from their parents. . . .

I remember as a child sitting on the hard benches of the old Boston Dispensary on Saturday noons waiting for the endless line of patients to be finished. At one time Mother had 3 offices in operation; in Boston on Commonwealth Avenue for a brief period; in Wakefield where she had built up a substantial practice; and in Peabody when Father was transferred there. When we would go to Provincetown in the summers for my father's parish there, mother always saw patients as much as conditions allowed. She had Portuguese patients and summer visitors who always waited for this seasonal practice.

I used to worry about her when she drove back and forth, not always in the best of automobiles. On dark, snowy nights that was a nightmare. But chiefly I was proud of her work. For better or for worse, she gave me a sense of having to accomplish something in my own life from which I shall never escape. So perhaps I had to exchange indulgence and ease and reassurance for something more urgent and compelling and certainly a thousand times more rewarding in my own growing up. Isn't it true that a woman who works out of necessity (financial or just because she feels she has something to offer) would be a problem mother if she had to stay home all day?

— *Mary Cogan Bromage*
Professor, University of Michigan School of Business Administration
Daughter of Sarah Edith Ives Cogan

Renuka Gera

My mother is a special person with much to offer you
She works and works and never stops for she has much to do
She's a doctor, a maid, a mom, and a wife
To help someone out she halts her own life

From the house to the hospital my mother does dash
To treat patients with anything from cancer to rash
It's a hard job but must be done
Not everything in life is meant to be fun

My mom sees a patient then fills out the chart
Checks how many are left before she can part
Though her job seems easy, it really is not
Giving bad news is hard and happens a lot

After each long day of helping children survive
Making sure the next day they're not dead but alive
She makes her way home with stops here and there
The grocery, the mall, and a quick cut of hair

Well this of course, is not the end of her day
This you probably assumed, I didn't even have to say
She'll come home to a house that's desperate for a clean
It's the messiest thing that I've ever seen

She'll sit there and scrub, rinse, mop, and wipe
I'm sure there is no one else of her type
And by the end of the night it looks spotless and nice
You'll find nothing around, not one grain of rice

At night my mom watches the evening news
By eleven o'clock she'll have started to snooze
As the night hours pass by she rests peacefully
Now tired, worn out, she asks that we let her be.

— Lori Gera, age 12
Daughter of Renuka Gera

Notes

1. Bateson, M. C. (1990). *Composing a life* (p. 181). New York: Penguin Putnam.
2. From Eisenberg, L. (1981). The distaff of Aesculapius—The married woman as physician. *Journal of the American Medical Women's Association, 36*(2), 87. Copyright © American Medical Women's Association, Inc. All rights reserved. Reprinted with permission for education use only.
3. Excerpted from Lightfoot, S. L. (1988). *Balm in Gilead: Journey of a healer* (pp. 6–7). Reading, MA: Addison-Wesley. Copyright © 1988 S. L. Lightfoot. Reprinted by permission of Pearson Education, Inc.
4. From Berlin, R. (1998). Our medical marriage. *Annals of Internal Medicine, 131*(9), 711. Reprinted by permission of the American College of Physician-American Society of Internal Medicine.
5. Excerpt from Hunt, M. M. (1962). *Her infinite variety: The American woman as lover, mate and rival* (pp. 280–282). New York: Harper & Row. Copyright © 1962 by Morton M. Hunt. Reprinted by permission of HarperCollins Publishers, Inc.
6. Levai, B. (1967). What's a mother for? Reprinted with minor editorial changes by permission of The Associated Press.
7. From Nadelson, T., & Eisenberg, L. (1977). The successful professional woman: On being married to one. *American Journal of Psychiatry, 134*(10), 1071–1076. Reprinted and abridged by permission of the American Psychiatric Association.
8. Excerpt from Offenbach, B. (1966). Four of us: Sketches of the four women ophthalmologists of the Massachusetts Eye and Ear Infirmary. *Journal of the American Medical Women's Association, 21*(7), 594–598. Copyright © 1966 American Medical Women's Association, Inc. All rights reserved. Reprinted and abridged with permission for education use only.

12

REFLECTIONS

Sharing our stories is the beginning of wisdom and
the first step in understanding our strength as women.
— *Elizabeth Forsythe Hailey*[1]

The Feminization of Medicine[2]

Recently I told my four-year-old son that he was due for a check-up with his pediatrician. He looked distinctly nervous (rumors about shots had obviously been making their way around the day care center) and asked me anxiously, "Is she a nice doctor?" I thought about the doctors my son knows—me, my close friends, mostly female. I picked my words carefully; it was clearly one of those critical moments when all of a mother's wisdom and tact is required. "Benjamin," I said, "I have to tell you something. Boys can be doctors too, if they want to. If they go to school and learn how, boys can be very good doctors, really."

— *Perri Klass*
Assistant Professor of Pediatrics, Boston University School of Medicine
Medical Director, Reach Out and Read National Center
Author of Love and Modern Medicine *(2001)*

Double Helix[3]

Now a housewife, once a surgeon
a template for the DNA chain
like the double helix of her being
she's reduced to wearing latex gloves
only while housecleaning every week
meticulously she dons cap, mask, apron

on a trolley arranged with surgical precision
lie her gloves, brushes, dusters, solutions
she drapes furniture with sheets of cotton
then pulls on her gloves tightens them
her size a neat seven

she prepares the area to be cleaned
with a weak Savlon solution
swabs it as she would an abdomen
in precise deft strokes
from above below left to right
never using an extra movement

and just as she had once done in the OR
she keeps soft music on—Strauss, Vivaldi
she wonders if now her DNA double helix
carries two genes
one for housewife one for surgeon

squeeze-drying the mop each time
she scrubs the floor surgically clean
removes the trolley
absently counting her instruments
removes gloves, cap, mask, apron
the overshoes

washes off the excess powder
from her hands and creams them
looking at them critically thrombosed
blue-veined yet soft supple
she warms them with her mug of coffee
and then takes up her pen
to write a poem.

— *Angelee Deodhar*
Opthalmologist, writer, and homemaker

Identity Crisis

It's not so easy to change your name
as if changing it will make it better,
your maiden name a phantom limb
hurting when you least expect it,
an old world name that is too much
for the mouths and forms of the new world:
too painful to hear pronounced
or see amputated in an application.
Many names are called, but few are chosen,
Should we add, combine, or hyphenate
as if our names were a word salad,
mélange, medley, potpourri,
fancy names for casserole.
I am tired of all these names,
Let me take a number
So that I don't have to spell out who I am.

— *Anne Lipton*
Assistant Professor of Neurology and Psychiatry,
University of Texas–Southwestern Medical Center

A Personal Journey

Growing up in a middle-class family in Lima, Perú, during the 1950s (my father an engineer, my mother a housewife), it never occurred to me there might be limits on my future choices. I thought that I could have everything—a fulfilling career and a satisfying family life. Yet there were few role models for the professional wife and mother.

Achieving that delicate balance between a successful professional and personal life has not been easy. This road can be difficult, nearly impossible, if one attempts it alone.

Fortunately, I have never been alone on this journey. My husband Renato, also an academic physician, has supported me from the beginning. There have been many times when I felt I could not be a mother, wife, and physician without sacrificing one for the other, times when I even considered quitting. Certainly I would have, had it not been for Renato reminding me of my plans, my passions, and my dreams. In speaking with other successful academic women, I realize that most have had this same kind of support on the home front. Women who do not often flounder, lower their expectations and, in the end, resent the choices that were forced on them.

A crucial element in my professional development has been the support and mentorship of a number of *maestros*. Among these, two individuals stand out: one, a professor who mentored me in the early years, and the other, my division chief who helped shape my career after my return to the United States. In fact, when I came to the University of Alabama at Birmingham as a fellow, I could have been regarded (and almost certainly was by some) as an outsider carrying several liabilities: I was a foreigner, a woman, a wife, and the mother of three children— one still very young. Instead, my division chief viewed these attributes as a source of strength and motivation. Looking back at the evolution of my career from a Visiting Research Fellow in 1980 to an Endowed Chair in the late 1990s, I truly believe that he was right.

I know these are different times, and women of a younger generation are entering academics with different expectations. Greater in number than the women physicians of my generation, they are also more assertive and less willing to tolerate overt or covert gender-based discrimination. They move at ease within the academic medical center, generally well liked by their colleagues and patients. They are less likely to be called "nurse" or to hear praises preceded by statements such as, "considering you are a woman, you have done quite well." Fortunately, the path to higher academic ranks is less cumbersome now than it was even a decade ago. In fact, most academic institutions, professional practices, and organizations have established policies toward maternity leave and other child-rearing activities. Beyond institutional or group practice policies, however, strong family support and academic mentorship remain as important and as decisive for these women as they have been for me.

I have been a physician, wife and mother for over 30 years. While it has been a challenge, my experience has been infinitely more rewarding because of it. As women, the world has always been placed on our shoulders; our burden has always been great. This is simply one more balancing act. I can only encourage young women in medicine today to pursue their goals with vigor and conviction.

— Graciela S. Alarcón

Jane Knight Lowe Chair of Medicine in Rheumatology,
University of Alabama at Birmingham

My Experience as a Woman in Medicine

The key to my admission to medical school was my parents' impeccable timing. They conceived me at just the right moment so that I graduated from high school in the upswell of the women's lib movement. By 1970, medical schools had increased their enrollment of female students from 1% in the 1960s to 15% in my class at the University of Chicago.

Once in medical school, I steered clear of the more radical women who clamored for equality and objected to sexist remarks in lectures. As a Chinese-American, the issue for me was not gender but ethnicity. Having been taught that minorities cannot compete on an equal basis with the majority, I concentrated on being better than anyone else in my work.

I completed medical school at another fortunate time. The end of the Vietnam War had drastically reduced the numbers of men applying for research training positions at the National Institutes of Health, an appointment that had exempted men from the military draft. This created such a vacuum that the institute resorted to recruiting at medical schools. I applied and was accepted as the first female clinical associate at the National Heart, Lung, and Blood Institute. Being a woman and a minority posed no problems for me there. In fact, I gained many skills later useful in my academic career.

My love for research stems from childhood. My parents, both researchers in virology, introduced me to the fun of science. I spent many a Saturday in my father's lab at Johns Hopkins University, dissecting chick embryos or talking with the graduate students. My mother bought books on creative science experiments that could be performed at home with rudimentary instruments. Their encouragement helped me ignore the stigma of getting good grades in calculus and being the only girl to take physics, at a time when girls were considered intellectually inferior to boys. Fortunately, I had my mother as a role model. Seeing that she had successfully established a career in science, there was no question that I could also. In college, I let boys know by the third date of my intentions to pursue a career. A lot disappeared, but at least I found out before getting emotionally attached.

My career development I owe to my mentor, a senior faculty member who gave me incredible resources, financial backing, and intellectual freedom. His support of my career, at a time when I had yet to establish my own name, was critical because it allowed me to devote my energies creatively in independent investigation. Thus, I avoided wasting time struggling for grants or managing heavy clinical loads to earn my salary. He also guided me back from my occasional foray into avenues that his experience predicted would prove unrewarding, an exercise that ultimately sharpened my critical thinking.

Research and teaching are the goals of my career. I chose gradually to withdraw from patient care, a decision not made lightly considering the long hours of training and the clinical skills that I had worked so hard to acquire. But given a choice, I always ran to the lab, not to the clinic. Eventually, patient care became a distraction to my research goals. In retrospect, my decision to accept a research position was the right one. Managed health care has so eroded the financial base of our division that the faculty have taken severe salary cuts while being burdened with ever increasing clinical loads. As a research professor, my work was unaffected.

A word about the woman's role: I have two children, and although I felt some guilt for not staying home with them, I learned early on that being a stay-at-home mom just wasn't my forte. My husband also found that my temper was much worse when I stayed home than when I worked. The key to our family was the decision to hire a nanny, a wonderful woman who lived with us for most of 19 years. She provided the daily continuity that buffered my fractured schedule. Having a nanny at home meant never worrying about getting sleepy children to day care in the morning, rushing home to pick them up in the evening, or staying home unexpectedly when a child became ill. Having a nanny at home meant that there were three adults loving my children instead of two. Having a nanny at home was like having a wife for me, so I understand exactly why a man might want a stay-at-home wife.

When my children were young, they sometimes wished for a "mommy like the other mommies." This opinion changed, however, as they grew older. By college, both assured me that they were very proud of their mother.

My husband has been fully supportive, not just verbally but in sharing housework and meeting the needs of our children. More than once, I returned from a spring meeting, relieved to find that the Easter bunny had not forgotten to visit our children. I think verbal support is the minimum that a woman should look for in a prospective spouse, that at least he won't complain if dinner is late. Lending a hand is even better. But most important is the emotional support. When I feel defeated by division politics or overwhelmed by grant proposal deadlines, my husband feeds me a good dinner and sees that I get a good night's rest before pushing me out early the next morning with a pep talk. It would have been much more difficult for me to achieve my current position without this active support on the home front.

The greatest drawback to having a career has been the loss of personal time. Work became my personal time, with every other moment devoted to family. It was hard for me to read a book, much less exercise, and pursuing a hobby on my own was simply out of the question. I was so torn between my responsibilities that I felt guilty leaving the children to go out on a "date" with my husband. What a revelation to discover that I could enjoy myself after our children left home. Now at the age of 50, my husband and I have taken up mountain climbing. We take classes on snowshoeing, map and compass navigation, and avalanche safety. This is our second life as we continue to enjoy both our careers and our time together.

— *Florence H. Sheehan*
Research Professor of Medicine, University of Washington

Scopes, Hopes, and Learning the Ropes[4]

When I was visiting professor at St. Raphael's Hospital in New Haven last spring, several older clinicians expressed their concern about the multiple demands on their junior colleagues. As someone who had a successful career and a family, what advice did I have for their younger colleagues (male and female) raising families. À la David Letterman, here is my top-10 list—what I know now but wish I had known then.

10. Do whatever decreases your guilt the most.
9. Lower your expectations.
8. Choose your battles.
7. Cherish your 2-casserole friends.
6. Find novel ways to be with your family.
5. Don't always say no.
4. If it's important, just do it.
3. Learn the culture and the rules.
2. Follow your heart.
1. My golden rule: "People will forget what you say. They will sometimes remember what you show them to do. They will never forget how you make them feel."

Let me expand. *First the guilt*: guilt seems to be an integral part of motherhood—fortunately not fatherhood, or at least not as much. When our children were very young, all my women friends felt guilty—those who worked outside the home felt guilty for working and the others felt guilty for not working. No single solution works for all. Remember, one oft quoted aphorism for working mothers and fathers: You can do it all, just not all at the same time.

Lower your expectations. After decades of laundry duty, we sort clean clothes, five laundry baskets for each person—located in the basement next to the dryer—we don't fold or iron. The clean clothes of my 3 teenage sons never even make it to their rooms. The uncluttered kitchen countertops I admire will be a reality to me only in magazine photos. We now consider pizza a weekly staple (and I don't mean homemade).

Work can be consuming—try not to let it be. For my father's generation, work was valued above all. Sometimes it was an escape or even a refuge, but one that implied service and sacrifice to humanity. But often the truly brave person is the one at home with the children during the arsenic hour (usually 5-7 p.m.) where chaos reigns. The controlled environment of office or hospital where no one throws tantrums (hopefully), your requests are obeyed, you are treated with respect and civility, and not called "stupidhead," and peanut butter is not smeared on your clothes—this is the coward's domain.

Choose your battles. As a mother of teens, this has been a huge lesson for me, but one I have incorporated into my work as well. I try to see the other's point of view, and I spend less time trying to change people's minds to my point of view.

Cherish your 2-casserole friends. Linda Clever, Editor of *Western Journal of Medicine,* uses this term. When you are sick, in the hospital, most people will find the time to drop off a casserole for the family at home. But who will go to the trouble of bringing a casserole a second time? For me, it is my book club friends, among others. They even provided biting but honest criticism of early drafts of this speech.

Find novel ways to spend time with your family. My friend Anabel was inspired that I shopped for a new car last year with my son Joe: Why not? He was far more interested than my husband. Of course doing this regularly can be expensive. Taking one child with you on a business trip makes an ideal way to mix business and pleasure and decreases the burden for the caretaker at home.

Don't always say no. My career in *Clostridium difficile* was a direct result of saying yes when colleagues in medicinal chemistry needed someone to do physical exams for their project on digoxin metabolism. I was asked surely because I was the most junior person in the Division at the time. I said yes because being colleagues at the University means helping one another. When that group began work on the hamster *C. difficile* model, I was the natural person they turned to, a happy, collaboration that has lasted 15 years.

If it's important, "just do it." If a need exists, consider developing a plan to get the job done; even if it is not your immediate concern, if you think it's important go for it. Others may never see the need, but the results will be satisfying to you. Some examples—I started a women's group at my hospital after seeing how important it was while visiting another institution, and as a new parent to an elementary school, I put together a parent guide to answer all the questions I had had when my children started in that school.

Learn the culture and the rules. Understand communication styles and differences. The Deborah Tannen book, *You Just Don't Understand,* was an eye-opener for me; learning about gender differences in communication enabled me to understand my sons, my husband, and the men at work better. We can't change behavior, but it sure helps to understand it. It works both ways—when Larry Brandt was President [of the American College of Gastroenterology], he stopped by the Women's Committee which I chaired, saw everyone was talking at once, and later asked me if I was in control or needed help. The horizontal meeting style looked like chaos to him, but was typical for an efficient meeting of that all-female group.

Follow your heart. When a project is too boring, it may be OK to move on—a lesson which I had learned earlier in my 3 and ¾ years of fellowship and a fruitless horseradish peroxidase study.

Finally, my *golden rule*—I found it posted in our ICU several years ago—"People will forget what you say, they may remember what you show them to do, but they will never forget how you make them feel." Think about it—it's true, isn't it?

— Christina M. Surawicz

Professor of Medicine, University of Washington School of Medicine
Section Chief, Gastroenterology at Harborview Medical Center
President, American College of Gastroenterology

Defining Ourselves

Defining myself, as opposed to being defined by others,
is one of the most difficult challenges I face.

— *Carol Moseley Braun*[1]

I do not define myself solely by my gender or ethnicity but, rather, by the strength and support of my family and African American ancestors who have steered the course to my career in medicine. I no longer question my choice to become a physician, and I continue to embrace all the challenges and privileges this profession poses.

The most important advice I can offer in pursuing any dream or career goal is not to limit your scope. There will be countless naysayers who will doubt your potential and limit your efforts, but never be discouraged.

— *Carol Merchant*
Assistant Professor of Neurology, Columbia University
College of Physicians & Surgeons
Director, Memory Center, Columbia University

Note
1. Quoted in an interview in *The New Republic*, November 15, 1993.

Looking Good

When I was first starting practice, an exhausted patient of mine, a single mother, discouraged at how much of her small income went to looking fashionable for her job told me, "You're so lucky, you're a doctor: You don't have to look good." That about says it all. Otherwise being a woman physician has been like being a woman and being a physician.

— *Martha Stitelman*
Rural family practice

What It's Been Like[5]

I was a girl medical student, a lady intern, a woman resident, a member of the fair sex, chief resident; but finally, just a surgeon.

— *Kathryn D. Anderson*
Surgeon-in-Chief, Children's Hospital Los Angeles
Professor of Surgery, University of Southern California
Vice President, American College of Surgeons

Reminiscences of My Medical Career

On the first day of medical school, we were introduced with the usual flurry of welcomes and instructions, including a parting admonition (in Latin) from the pipe-smoking Dean of Admissions at Cornell: "Don't let the bastards get you down."

As I left the amphitheater, I wondered who "the bastards" were meant to be. The teachers? The other students? Even the patients, perhaps? In any case, there fortunately turned out to be very few of them in any category. I was one of six women in the class, and we were well treated overall, despite the occasional prank. For example, once while fishing for my keys at night, I found a mouse that had been slipped into my lab coat pocket.

I do remember, however, being very dismayed that no ladies' rooms were built in the new science building, forcing me to go to another floor and borrow a key to the secretaries' private bathroom. Another irritating experience was the lack of scrubs in small sizes. I also remember being told that anatomy was a good field for women because "it did not change much and thus was easy to keep up with."

When I started on my first clinical rotation, I was so proud to stand on the East River Drive in a white coat and thumb a ride with the other medical students to Bellevue Hospital. My father sometimes drove by and gave us a ride, exclaiming, "No one would ever pick up a lawyer!" I worked with several attendings whose excellent clinical skills and wonderful sense of humor provided role models for many students; they treated each of us with respect and kindness, regardless of gender.

A series of internships in the last year of medical school kept me very busy. During my surgery rotation, we had one night in four off and were on call every weekend. I spent most of two months with another classmate who went home one day and called his new wife by my name. I can also remember falling asleep in the elevator.

The chief surgical resident on that service kept rotating my schedule because one of the attendings did not want a woman assistant in the operating room. Later, that same attending specifically asked to have me transferred to his service when his intern came down with hepatitis. I felt pleased that, despite the palpable reluctance to accept women in surgery, my hard work had been appreciated.

I finally decided to pursue internal medicine and was accepted as an intern at Bellevue Hospital in the Cornell division. After picking up a white uniform with a newly embroidered patch showing unequivocally that I was a doctor (I had been told to sit with the nurses at our combined RN-MD graduation at Cornell, a common mistake in those days), I waited at an elevator surrounded by a group of very sick looking prospective patients. When the elevator arrived to reveal space for only a few more passengers, the operator barred the way and said, "Let the doctor on." He meant me. I was stunned. I checked to make sure I was really the doctor he was talking about and then, rather flustered, took my place in the elevator.

Thirty-five years have elapsed since that day. That incident reflected the high regard in which physicians were held at that time. Attitudes toward the profession have since shifted because of many issues revolving around commercialization of medicine, access to care, and poor press, particularly in the 1980s when doctor bashing was at its height. Now a doctor is a "health care provider" and women have become mainstream in the profession.

While at Bellevue, I continued to learn about critical illness and the drama that accompanied it. The experience fostered close bonding with the other house staff. We could have never survived the long hours and difficult work without the camaraderie of working as a team. It was not unusual to start laughing and joking in the early morning hours. Once, a patient's family brought me a birthday cake that I did not have the

THIS SIDE OF DOCTORING

chance to eat. It was gone the next day with a card in its place reading "Happy Birthday, Michelle." During my time at Bellevue, New York City had its first blackout, and I roamed the corridors with an otoscope for light. President Kennedy was assassinated while I rotated in neurology. The event was announced to me by a patient who was demented. It was several hours before I realized he was right. I learned all about homelessness in the TB wards and human drama in the emergency room corridors that were always crowded with weeping families.

I left Bellevue feeling I could handle anything and pursued a fellowship in endocrinology, an evolving specialty that had been revolutionized by the recent discovery of a method to measure small amounts of hormones in the blood: the radioimmunoassay. I became fascinated by the effects of starvation on women's hormones and found my niche as an expert in amenorrhea at a time when this disease was just becoming prevalent, particularly among dancers and athletes. New York became an interesting area of opportunity. I started my own practice, which grew rapidly.

I had married during my second year of residency, and while my husband pursued his training in orthopedic surgery, I raised two sons. These were extremely happy years, but I was not prepared for the physical and emotional fatigue of full-time work while caring for two small children—despite the help of both my family and my in-laws. One particularly difficult time was studying for my specialty boards, which I could do only when the children were asleep. When I finally completed my exams, all my patients asked, "Did you pass, Dr. Warren?" Thank goodness, I did.

Finally, the full-time help of a French woman seemed to tip the precarious balance, and I was able to manage with her help for nine years. Despite that, I felt guilty and worried all the time, particularly when the children were sick. I still regret not having taken more time off.

Looking back over my experiences, I feel privileged to have trained at a time when every year a new treatment or drug changed the face of a disease. Yet these same technologic advances have effectively distanced doctors from their patients and made the practice of medicine increasingly difficult and expensive. But overall, the science and human dialogue that drew me into medicine so many years ago have continued to provide a fascinating and rewarding area of work. Now, issues of women's health have been spotlighted by the increasing longevity of women, but many more challenges remain.

— *Michelle Palmieri Warren*
Professor of Medicine and Obstetrics & Gynecology,
Wyeth Ayerst Professor of Women's Health, Columbia University,
Director, Center for Menopause, Hormonal Disorders, & Women's Health

Enjoying the Moment

When I first heard of the "Women in Medicine Anthology" from a colleague in the medical community, it struck a strong chord within me. For a month, I mulled over the issues, wondering all the while what I should write. I struggle to balance my career and family on a daily basis, a dilemma that constantly tears at me. At times, I feel no longer able to shoulder the burden of juggling medicine and motherhood, but at other times, I would not have it any other way.

Once I arrive at work and am busy, though, I am content. I know that I am appreciated, that I provide a needed service in the community. A solo practitioner in an affluent seaside community, I care for a young, healthy population, mostly female. I see patients three and a half days a week and share call with a colleague, an arrangement that allows me considerable time at home with our two young children. I can take the girls to gymnastics, head for the pool, or enjoy ice cream cones on a hot, sunny day. Because our nanny helps run the household, I am free to spend quality time with my family.

Certainly the rewards of practicing medicine are great. I experience immense satisfaction in my work and am proud of my profession. After a particularly grueling day at work, especially if I have seen a patient with cancer or another life-threatening illness, I enjoy my children all the more. My contentment with work allows me to relax and savor each moment with them. I have read that happier mothers, working or not, make better mothers.

Still, there remain those difficult days when each hour drags, times I feel like an outsider both at work and at home. Because I don't spend a lot of time at the hospital, many physicians do not know me. I usually refer to the same cadre of specialists time after time, never expanding my narrow group of professional acquaintances. Meanwhile, I live in a neighborhood where only a handful of women work. I am always out of the loop when it comes to school information, neighborhood gossip, and the ever-critical carpool scheduling. Luckily, some wonderful neighbors help keep me in the know.

Perhaps the most difficult concept to master has been the importance of self-care. I used to feel guilt-ridden if every free moment was not spent doing something constructive with the children, but eventually I realized trying to do that was too draining. I now make room for personal time, exercising three mornings a week and reading books on adventure traveling. My husband and I also have a weekly "date night." Our marriage is strong but requires continual efforts to keep it refreshed and enduring.

I trained a long time for a career in medicine but received no training for the role of motherhood—unquestionably the most life-altering experience I have ever known. My daughters are an ever-renewing source of inspiration, joy, and laughter. I can hardly remember my life before children ("B.C.," as we jokingly refer to that time). Some days when my husband and I arrive home at the same time, we toss our briefcases aside and lie down on the floor in exhaustion. As our girls dance around our heads, ecstatic that we are home, we wink knowingly to one another. Life is good, let's enjoy the moment.

— *Catherine Chang*
Private practice, internal medicine

Navigating the Maze of Academic Medicine

My path in medicine has been self-styled and somewhat unconventional. After several detours from my original trajectory to become an academic endocrinologist, I have finally found a semblance of balance in my life. Despite the long hours and times of uncertainty, I truly believe that the rewards have outweighed the sacrifices. Now, at age 46 as a tenured professor, division chief, practicing endocrinologist, and mother of two, I am often asked how I survived and avoided terminal burnout. How was I able to juggle clinical practice, research, teaching, and family responsibilities while (arguably) maintaining my sanity? The question is probably best answered by sharing a few of the lessons I've learned over the years.

Find something that you have a passion for, something that truly interests and excites you. Because you will be working long hours and many years to reach your goals, it will be much easier to stay the course if the work is of inherent interest to you. Choose an area to which you are committed, even if it entails more challenges than others. I was fortunate to find two such areas: endocrinology and women's health. Although the journey was long and the hours often late, the excitement of the work sustained me through the times of personal sacrifice.

Have the courage to take risks. Be willing to challenge conventional assumptions, ask the difficult questions, and pursue avenues that don't necessarily guarantee success. Most new ideas and innovations in medicine and science involve taking risks and thinking outside of the box. My additional years of training in epidemiology turned out to be a risk worth taking; I've been better equipped to pursue my goals because of this detour and the attendant sacrifices.

Know your priorities and never compromise them. For me, family ranks the highest. Certain times of the week are absolutely sacrosanct in terms of being with my family. Of course, it's important to choose your husband or partner well: someone who shares your values, who will support you in reaching your goals, and who will be an involved parent. I've been very fortunate to have a wonderful and supportive husband who adores our children. There's no accomplishment I'm more proud of than our children and the strength of our 20-year marriage.

Support your colleagues. Medicine and science are not zero sum games but, rather, collaborations. Take pride in mentoring junior faculty members and provide opportunities for them to reach their potential. A common mistake is for investigators to feel that their stature is in some way diminished by the successes of their colleagues. Helping to nurture the careers of junior faculty members is one of the greatest rewards of entering the ranks of senior faculty.

— JoAnn Elisabeth Manson
Chief, Division of Preventive Medicine, Brigham and Women's Hospital
Professor of Medicine, Harvard Medical School
Editor-in-Chief of Prevention of Myocardial Infarction *(1996)*

From Teacher to Psychiatrist With Family

I don't know why, but I recall wanting to become a psychiatrist since the age of eight. Only as an adult did I discover two male psychiatrist and male psychologist cousins. Raised in a happy nuclear and extended family, I also hoped to marry and have a family.

As a 17-year-old first-year Brooklyn College student, I was told by a noted psychologist and first year adviser that I had no scientific ability. So I became an elementary school teacher and, instead, supported my husband through his medical training. Then we agreed it was my turn, and I completed the prerequisites as we joyfully welcomed our first child. After a series of applications, I enrolled at the University of Louisville School of Medicine, an institution with a family-friendly curriculum suitable for my unique situation.

In medical school, I was one of six women; two of us were mothers. During the academic year, Stuart was cared for by a wonderful baby-sitter and later at a day care center. I studied early and late, reserving most Saturdays for leisurely excursions to the park. I also took summers off to be a full-time mother, well aware that my classmates were meanwhile gaining useful research experience. My priorities were clear. My goal was to rank in the middle of the class, and I avoided leadership opportunities in order to spend more time at home. I accepted my position as a nontraditional student despite the lack of role models.

My family grew during my internship and residency years, and by the time I joined the University of Louisville psychiatry department as a faculty member, I was the mother of three. During those early years, much of my time and energy were focused on the children. Although I did not neglect my professional responsibilities, my full-time academic career did not begin until much later. In the meantime, I developed educational programs in response to the clinical needs I observed in students, one program being the University Student Mental Health Service. As my children grew, I involved them in my work. All three young men are into their own careers now, the younger two completing residency training in pediatrics and adult and child psychiatry, yet they still remain close-knit as brothers and close to us.

Of paramount importance, we as women physicians must first know ourselves honestly. We must recognize life's different stages and that goals may and should change with time. Don't make life choices that will result in life regrets. Respect yourself, your values and decisions. Don't hide from yourself. Being a wife, mother, and physician have all been extraordinary experiences. I would *not* have wanted to miss any.

— Leah J. Dickstein

Associate Dean for Faculty and Student Advocacy
Professor and Associate Chair for Academic Affairs
Department of Psychiatry, University of Louisville School of Medicine

Generation to Generation: Mother-Daughter Physicians

Out of a wish to do research together and curiosity about the relationships between mothers and daughters who are both physicians, we embarked on a long-term research project called Generation to Generation: Mother-Daughter Physicians. What makes a daughter follow her mother into a career in medicine? How does the mother's experience as a physician influence her daughter's experience? We wondered how relationships between other mother-daughter pairs differed from, or were similar to, our own experiences.

Our background review of the literature taught us that, compared with male physicians, female physicians are less likely to have mentors or role models, less likely to hold positions of leadership in medicine, more likely to experience gender discrimination and sexual harassment, and more likely to have their careers adversely affected by family responsibilities. Women physicians whose mothers were also physicians might have an advantage in dealing with these issues. Perhaps something could be learned that might help other women. And we were very interested in the varying experiences of women in medicine from different generations and in their individual life stories.

Diane, Mother

I grew up in a typical working-class community of the 1950s when most women married early and stayed home to raise their children. If women had careers rather than jobs, they were teachers, nurses, or social workers. No one in my family was a physician; my college didn't even have a premedical program. But I was good in science and had an uncle who was a medical researcher. For reasons not entirely clear to me, I decided to attend medical school after my junior year in college. Miraculously, my parents, who had neither a college education nor much money, supported my decision. Unlike most men in our generation, my future husband, Adam, was intrigued by the idea and encouraged my ambitions.

I began my medical education at Washington University in St. Louis, and after my first year there, I married Adam, who was a graduate student in chemical engineering at Yale. In those days, it was almost universal that the wife would be the one to transfer. Yale reluctantly accepted the transfer despite my breaking their 6% quota for women students.

In that prefeminist era, discrimination against women was overt and the norm. We were cautioned that no one would marry us if we were too smart or too capable. Women who pursued careers outside the home were told they would cause lasting, irrevocable damage to their children. A decade later, when the feminist revolution was in full swing, I was no longer viewed as a deviant but as an admired role model.

My husband and I were determined to have it all. How naïve we were to think that balancing careers and family would come easily or naturally. We eventually had four children, the first during my fourth year in medical school and the last while I was in private practice as a psychiatrist. I took a brief leave of absence during those years to spend some time at home, and after the birth of my last child, I worked part-time while also beginning psychoanalytic training.

I had always wanted an academic career, one that included research, teaching, and administration, but I felt obligated to put those ambitions on hold until my children were older. It wasn't until the age of 39 and eight years post-training that I took on a full-time academic position at the New Jersey Medical School in their new program for child and adolescent psychiatry. I spent 14 exciting years there, eventually becoming Director of Child and Adolescent Psychiatry and building a large inner-city program that often felt like a M.A.S.H. unit. I moved up the academic ranks to full professor on the nontenured track, while also becoming active in professional organizations. Juggling career and family was complicated, especially given the difficulties of finding and keeping competent child care. There were no role models or mentors, but for 10 years I co-taught a course to first-year medical students called Parenting and Professionalism: Combining Career and Family, which taught me a great deal about the different ways physicians and their families manage. What made it all possible was having a loving and supportive husband who was an equal partner in all ways at a time when that was rare.

Lydia, Daughter

One of my earliest memories dates back to the age of four, when I announced to my mother that I wanted to be a nurse. "Why not a doctor?" my mother asked, to which I responded authoritatively, "Women can't be doctors." My misperceptions were gently but firmly corrected, and from that time on, I eagerly sought out opportunities to expose myself to the medical field. As a child, I loved shadowing my mother when she rounded at the hospital. Several personal encounters with illness during my adolescent years taught me firsthand what it was like to be the patient. Realizing the important roles that doctors play in the lives of others helped reinforce my desire to study medicine. By the time I was in junior high school, it was no longer unusual for a girl to voice such aspirations.

Although most young women in my mother's generation planned on staying home to raise their children, I knew many women during my undergraduate years at Yale who aspired to careers in medicine. Nearly 40% of my entering class at Albany Medical College were women. I enjoyed excellent mentoring in both research and clinical medicine, but unlike most of my peers, I was fortunate to have my mother as a constant, steady role model. She gave me the confidence that I could succeed, not just in medicine but also in the challenging task of balancing that career with a fulfilling personal life. We were both deeply moved when she participated in the hooding ceremony at my graduation.

After a residency in pediatrics and a fellowship in adolescent medicine, I accepted a faculty position at Children's Hospital Boston. My Division Chief is a woman, as are the majority of my colleagues. I have had wonderful mentors, both male and female, who have helped guide my career in academic medicine. My opportunities stand in stark contrast to the overt discrimination that my mother faced at a time when female role models in medicine were rare. I have always felt supported in and respected for my career choice by family, friends, colleagues, and society at large.

But I have followed only half the model. There was no societal or family pressure on me to marry or to have children at an early age. Although I am in a serious relationship, I am not married nor have I started a family. My generation is blessed to have more choices—but having so many options can sometimes be more challenging.

One unfortunate similarity to my mother's experience has been my exposure to sexual harassment, ranging from sexually explicit remarks to quid pro quo situations, such as when a male superior asked me on a date while giving me his superlative recommendation. During my mother's career, such conduct was socially acceptable, at times even officially sanctioned. The challenge for my generation is the insidious form this harassment now takes. At times I have been told that the femininity and confidence I bring to the workplace actually provoke the sexually explicit comments. How ironic that the very social evolution allowing me to pursue medicine with ease has created an environment in which such behavior toward women still thrives.

Nonetheless, I have found medicine to be an incredibly rewarding profession, all the more so because I have had the opportunity to learn from my mother's experiences. In pursuing my own career, I have been able to use my mother as a mentor, discussing how to balance the multiple demands of the job, develop effective negotiating strategies, and advance up the academic ladder while preserving the patient care aspects that drew me to medicine in the first place. At the same time, I have begun to mentor my mother in research, as we work together on our study of mother-daughter physicians. And what fun it has been to refer cases to one another and to cite each other's work! Being the daughter of a woman physician has enriched the process of my medical career in so many wonderful ways.

— Diane K. Shrier
Clinical Professor of Psychiatry and Pediatrics,
George Washington University Medical Center
Senior Consultant, Walter Reed Army Medical Center

— Lydia A. Shrier
Assistant Professor of Pediatrics, Harvard Medical School
Attending, Adolescent Medicine, Children's Hospital Boston

Notes

1. From Giese J. (1998). *A woman's path.* New York: Golden Books.

2. Excerpted from Klass, P. (1992). *Baby doctor: A pediatrician's training* (p. 284). New York: Random House. Used with permission.

3. From Deodhar, A. (1999). Double helix. *Annals of Internal Medicine, 130,* 941. Reprinted by permission of the American College of Physicians–American Society of Internal Medicine.

4. Excerpted from the presidential address of the American College of Gastroenterology. Abridged and reprinted from Surawicz, C. M. (2000). Scopes, hopes and learning the ropes. *American Journal of Gastroenterology, 95*(2), 345–348. Copyright © 2000, with permission from Excerpta Medica, Inc.

5. Excerpted from Anderson, K. (1974). What it's been like. *Harvard Medical Alumni Bulletin, 48*(6), 22. Reprinted by permission of the author.

AFTERWORD

Compiling and editing this anthology was like gathering together a circle of women to share life experiences and stories. Within their narratives, I found strength, reassurance, and validation of my own struggles as a woman and physician. Together, these writings represent our collective heritage. Although the social and political milieu has evolved over the years, certain issues remain constant, and the universal dilemmas at the heart of mothering and doctoring will always persist. Some authors touched on a compelling theme of interconnectedness, the sense that one's work as a physician cannot easily be separated from the other lives that we lead—as wife, mother, daughter, friend. How these different roles become integrated varies tremendously from individual to individual and, for most, requires some degree of compromise, sacrifice, or even unlearning of traditions. The way chosen need not be conventional or well traveled but simply one that reconciles personal and professional goals.

Support in both the workplace and the home remains of paramount importance in allowing women to achieve the delicate balance required to maintain their very full lives. Fortunately, overt barriers of earlier centuries have largely been broken down, but subtle inequities still linger at varying levels within the medical profession and within our society at large. Only by confronting these traditional biases may we hope to create an environment in which all women may realize their full potential as physicians, as women, and as mothers.

Although we each must find our own path, the sharing of experiences, lessons, and frustrations may help illuminate the way or, at the very least, provide a network of encouragement and support. As those looking back have told us, the rewards of this struggle are well worth the effort. Women bring an intuition, sensitivity, and nurturing much needed in the practice of medicine; allowing them to realize their professional aspirations encourages a richer family life. These stories, essays, and poems attest to the amazing range of professional and domestic capacities that women physicians have achieved. Ultimately, the decisions made and the responsibilities borne by the present generation will better define the perceived roles and expectations of our daughters. Like our predecessors, hopefully, we will have made their burdens lighter.

For more than a century and a half, American women physicians have grappled with the dilemma of how to be a woman and a physician, how to be different from yet equal to their male colleagues. . . . The ideal of balance has been a virtue and a conscious goal throughout their history in the American medical profession, the hoped-for solution to the dilemma of difference.

. . . can women physicians "restore the balance" in their profession, in their own lives, and perhaps even in the lives of their patients? It seems clear that the answer is yes, but they can not, should not — and may no longer have to — do it alone.

— Ellen S. More[1]

Note

1. From More, E. S. (2001). *Restoring the balance* (pp. 2, 258). Cambridge, MA: Harvard University Press.

GLOSSARY

adenocarcinoma   a type of cancer arising from glandular tissue or structures

angina   a suffocating type of pain, generally used in reference to chest pain, a warning symptom of heart disease

aphasia   inability to speak or understand language

arthrodesis   fusion of a joint

ascites   an accumulation of fluid within the abdomen

astrocytoma   a type of tumor composed of astrocytes

asystole   the condition in which the heart has stopped beating

attending   staff or faculty physician

axilla   armpit

beta agonists   a drug that stimulates the beta-adrenergic receptors, often used in the treatment of asthma and obstructive lung disease

blighted ovum   a fertilized egg in which development has stopped

Braxton Hicks contractions   light, generally painless uterine contractions that normally occur in the third trimester

call	generally, "on call"—the term used when doctors must be available either in (as is the case for interns and residents) or out of the hospital for emergency calls
catheterization	the act of passing a tube through a hollow organ—for example, to access or visualize blood vessels, heart chambers, or the urinary bladder
cautery	a heated instrument used to destroy tissues or stop bleeding
CCU	coronary care unit—cardiac unit that provides close monitoring of patients with critical heart disease
cephalothorax	of or pertaining to the head and chest
chemotherapy	the use of chemical substances to treat disease, most typically cancer chemotherapy
colonoscope	a fiberoptic instrument that when inserted into the intestine allows visualization of the entire lining
colonoscopy	the procedure in which a colonoscope is passed into the intestine to look for abnormalities
commissurotomies	a surgical procedure to increase the size of an opening—for example, a mitral commissurotomy used to help open up the mitral valve of the heart
craniotomy	surgical removal of part of the skull to expose the underlying brain
cricothyrotomy	an emergency procedure to cut an opening in the neck (at the site of the cricothyroid membrane) to relieve airway obstruction
CT	cat scan—diagnostic radiology with the use of X-rays and computerized integration
D&C	dilatation and curretage—treatment in which the lining of the uterus is scraped away; used primarily to remove fetal tissue—for example, after a miscarriage
defibrillator	a machine used to deliver electric shocks to the heart to restore its rhythm to normal

diabetes	most commonly refers to diabetes mellitus, a metabolic disease due to lack of or resistance to insulin, a hormone produced by the pancreas—the net result being the accumulation of sugar in the blood, which may lead to increased urination, electrolyte disturbances, kidney failure, heart disease, and visual problems
diabetic ketoacidosis	an acute metabolic complication that can occur in patients with diabetes mellitus as a result of insulin deficiency
dialysis	usually refers to hemodialysis, a technique used in patients with kidney failure to remove waste materials from the blood
digitalize	the process of administering the drug digitalis to a patient with heart failure in order to achieve optimum tissue levels
diplopia	double vision
diverticulitis	an inflammatory condition of the large intestine
DSHS	form of welfare in Washington State linked with health insurance on a capitated basis
dura	the outermost membrane covering the brain
dysarthria	a disorder of speech affecting pronunciation of words
dyspnea	shortness of breath
edema	accumulation of fluid within tissues
EEG	a recording of the electrical activity of the brain used to determine level of consciousness, detect structural disease, and diagnose seizures
EKG	a recording of the electrical activity of the heart, used in the diagnosis of heart disease
embolization	the process in which an embolus (material substance such as a blood clot, fat, air, or foreign body) is carried by the blood stream until it becomes lodged in a more distal blood vessel

epidural hematoma	bleeding in the extradural space (the space just on or over the dura, which is the outermost membrane covering the brain)
episiotomy	a surgical incision made during birth to enlarge the vaginal opening
esophagus	the tubular, muscular organ that channels solid and liquid food from the mouth to the stomach
fellowship	generally one to three years of subspecialty training following residency
fracture	a break in a bony structure
gallstones	the presence of stones in the gallbladder, which may cause pain or obstruction
gastroenterology	the study and treatment of diseases of the digestive tract
gastroesophageal reflux	the backflow of acidic stomach contents into the esophagus, usually causing symptoms of heartburn and indigestion
gastroscope	a fiberoptic scope used to visualize the interior of the stomach
geriatrics	the study and treatment of diseases in the elderly
GI	gastrointestinal—pertaining to the digestive tract
heart block	a condition in which conduction of the electrical impulse of the heart is delayed
hematoma	an accumulation of blood within tissues
hemoglobin	a substance within red blood cells that carries oxygen to the tissues
hemostasis	the process by which bleeding is stopped
hepatitis B	inflammation of the liver due to the virus Hepatitis B
hepatitis serologies	a blood test that determines whether or not an individual has been infected with the hepatitis viruses

herniation	the process in which tissue or organs protrude out of the body cavity in which they are located
Hippocratic oath	the oath taken by a doctor to observe a code of behavior and practice modeled by the Greek physician Hippocrates
house officer	an intern or resident
humerus	bone of the upper arm
hypertension	high blood pressure
hypothyroid	abnormally low activity of the thyroid gland
hypoxia	lack of oxygen
ICU	intensive care unit
internship	the first year of training after medical school, often the most rigorous in terms of amount of overnight call
intracranial	within the skull
intramedullary rodding	a metal rod placed through the shaft of a bone to stabilize a fracture
intrapulmonic	within the lungs
intubate	the process of placing a breathing tube through the mouth and into the trachea to bring air into the lungs
IV	intravenous—within a vein
juvenile rheumatoid arthritis	an autoimmune disease with arthritis and other manifestations occurring in children and teenagers
leukemia	a cancer of the white blood cells
lobectomy	the surgical removal of a lobe of an organ
lupus	an autoimmune disease affecting multiple organs, but commonly the skin, joints, heart, lungs, and brain
lymphadenopathy	disease of the lymph nodes
mastoiditis	inflammation of the mastoid process of the temporal bone, often a complication from ear infections

Medical Scientist Training Program (MSTP)	a program funded by the National Institutes of Health in which medical students will receive both an M.D. and Ph.D.
medical training	generally, four years of medical school followed by a year of internship, several years of residency in a particular specialty, and occasionally a subspecialty fellowship.
Medicare	a national, government-sponsored program that provides health care to persons over 65 years of age
metastasis	spread of cancer to distant organs
middle meningeal artery	a blood vessel in the head
mitral stenosis	narrowing of the mitral valve opening, one of the main valves in the heart
mitral valve prolapse	a structural anomaly of the mitral valve of the heart, allowing the valve leaflet to prolapse into the atria after the valve closes
morbidity and mortality	a regular conference to discuss complex cases and the cause of illness or death
morning report	a morning conference for residents in which interesting cases are presented and discussed
myocardial infarction	heart attack
nasogastric (NG) tube	a tube placed into the nose and threaded all the way to the stomach—generally for feeding or suctioning
necrotizing fasciitis	a rapidly progressive infection, often fatal, that spreads along the lining of the muscle
nephropathy	disease of the kidneys
neurofibromatosis	a congenital disease in which multiple benign tumors grow out from the fibrous coverings of nerves
oculoplastics	plastic surgery involving the eye

oligohydramnios	a condition during pregnancy characterized by abnormally small amounts of amniotic fluid (the fluid bathing the fetus)
oncology	the study and treatment of cancer
ophthalmology	study and treatment of diseases of the eye
orthopedics	study and treatment of diseases of the bone and joints
otitis media	inflammation of the middle ear, usually due to infection
otolaryngology	study and treatment of diseases of the ear, nose, and throat
ova	female reproductive eggs
ovary	the female reproductive organ that produces eggs
paracentesis	a technique for removing excess fluid from a body cavity, generally referring to the abdominal cavity
parenteral	administration of a drug into the body by routes other than the mouth—for example, by injection or by intravenous catheters
parotitis	inflammation of the parotid gland (in the cheek area), often caused by infection
PCP	phencyclidine—a street drug that causes confusion, agitation, delusions, and in severe cases, coma
pectoriloquy	an abnormal transmission of sounds made by the patient's voice that can be heard through a stethoscope
pelvic	pertaining to the bony structure formed by the hip bones and lower spine
pelvic diatheses	slight separation and loosening of the bones of the pelvis (the structure composed of the hip bones and lowermost spine) during pregnancy
pelvic inflammatory disease	an inflammation, usually due to infection, involving the female reproductive organs
penicillin	an antibiotic used in treating a variety of infections

placebo	a treatment that has no inherent healing powers but may work because of the patient's belief in it
pneumococcus	*Streptococcus pneumoniae*, the bacteria that causes pneumonia
polycystic kidney disease	an inherited disorder in which the kidneys have multiple large fluid-filled cavities or cysts
porphyria	a rare, inherited disease caused by abnormal breakdown of porphyrins (a component in the red blood pigment hemoglobin)
prednisone	a steroid drug used to treat inflammatory conditions such as rheumatic diseases, severe allergy, and asthma
proteinuria	the presence of protein in the urine
renal	pertaining to the kidney
residency	the years of training following internship in a particular specialty, generally still with long hours and overnight call
rongeur	an instrument for cutting tissue, particularly bone
rounds	the act of seeing patients, one by one, generally including chart review, interviews, examinations, and delineation of a treatment plan
scarlet fever	a contagious childhood disease characterized by fever, sore throat, and a scarlet-colored rash on the skin
schistosomiasis	a disease of the tropics caused by blood flukes
scut	the routine daily tasks that a house officer must carry out
semilunar hyperdensity	half moon shaped "density" that on a radiograph looks whiter than the surrounding area
SSI	Supplemental Security Income—a federal supplemental income program that provides money to aged, blind, and disabled people who have little or no income
strep throat	a bacterial disease that causes symptoms of fever, sore throat, and enlarged lymph nodes in the neck

subarachnoid bleeding	bleeding in the subarachnoid space surrounding the brain
subinternship	a rotation during the fourth year of medical school in which the student assumes added responsibilities in the care of patients—close to the role of an intern but with much more supervision
sulfadiazine	an antibiotic
syncope	fainting spell
tachycardia	abnormally fast heart rhythm
thoracostomy	surgical procedure to make an opening in the chest wall for drainage
thyroid	a gland in the neck that produces the hormones responsible for regulating the rate of metabolism
trimester	one of the three periods (each consisting of three months) that divide a pregnancy
triple arthrodesis	fusion of particular joints in the foot, a technically challenging operation
tuberculosis	a disease caused by the organism *Mycobacterium tuberculosis* that most commonly affects the lungs but can spread to other organs in the body. Before the development of antituberculosis drugs, patients were quarantined until no longer infectious
urinalysis	examination of the urine
urology	the study of diseases of the urinary tract
uterus	the womb in which the fetus grows and matures
vernix	the substance that coats the skin of a newborn baby

RESOURCES FOR WOMEN IN MEDICINE

Professional Organizations

General

Association of American Medical Colleges (AAMC), Women in Medicine Program (www.aamc.org/about/progemph/wommed)

American Medical Women's Association (www.amwa-doc.org)

American Medical Association, Women Physician's Congress (www.ama-assn.org/wps)

The Foundation for the History of Women in Medicine (www.fhwim.org)

Special Interests[1]

Committee on Women's Involvement in American Academy of Allergy, Asthma & Immunology

Women in Cancer Research

American Heart Association Women in Cardiology Committee

Committee on Women in Cardiology

Joint Committee for the Advancement of the Dermatologic Health of Women

American Association of Women Emergency Physicians

Women in Endocrinology, Endocrine Society

Subcommittee on Women in Family Medicine, American Academy of Family Physicians

Women in Gastroenterology Committee, American College of Gastroenterology

Gay and Lesbian Medical Association (www.glma.org)

Society of General Internal Medicine, Women's Caucus

Professional Women in Genetics, American Society of Human Genetics

Mommd, Connecting Women in Medicine (www.mommd.com)

Women in Nephrology

Women in Neurology Section, American Academy of Neurology

Women in Neurosurgery

Women in Ophthalmology

Ruth Jackson Orthopaedic Society

American Academy of Otolaryngology, Head and Neck Surgery, Women in Otolaryngology Task Force

American Society for Investigative Pathology, Committee on Career Development, Women and Minorities

American Academy of Pediatrics

Women Plastic Surgeons, American Society of Plastic Surgeons

Committee on Women and Caucus of Women Psychiatrists, American Psychiatric Association

Association of Women Psychiatrists

Women's Caucus of the Academy of Psychosomatic Medicine

American Association for Women Radiologists

Women in Rheumatology, American College of Rheumatology

Association for Women in Science

Association of Women Surgeons

Women in Thoracic Surgery

Women in Urology

Note

1. Most current contact information listed with the AAMC Women in Medicine office: www.aamc.org/about/progemph/wommed/wimspecialty1.htm

ABOUT THE EDITOR

Eliza Lo Chin, M.D., M.P.H., is a general internist with an interest in women's health. She received her M.D. from Harvard Medical School and an M.P.H. from Columbia University; she completed an internal medicine residency at Brigham and Women's Hospital in Boston. During her training she married her medical school classmate, Dr. Douglas Chin. Until recently, she was Assistant Clinical Professor of Medicine at Columbia University College of Physicians & Surgeons where she was actively involved in both the clinical and teaching programs. In August 2000, Dr. Chin moved to Los Angeles where her husband completed a fellowship in hand surgery. She devoted the year to her three children, Emily, Sarah, and Nathan, and the completion of this anthology. Currently residing in Northern California where her husband maintains a busy surgical practice, she is preparing to resume her medical career in a part-time capacity.

ABOUT THE CONTRIBUTORS

Dorina Rose Abdulah, M.D., M.P.H., is Clinical Instructor at Harvard Medical School's Division on Aging. Her research and clinical practice are based at the Beth Israel Deaconess Medical Center, a Dorchester community health center, and a senior center. She grew up in New York City and obtained her undergraduate degree in biochemistry from Harvard College. She went on to earn a master's in biology from New York University, a medical degree from Albert Einstein College of Medicine, and a master's in public health from Columbia University. She completed her internal medicine residency at Columbia–Presbyterian Medical Center and a geriatrics fellowship at Harvard.

Graciela S. Alarcón, M.D, M.P.H., is the *Jane Knight Lowe* Chair of Medicine in Rheumatology at the University of Alabama at Birmingham. A Peruvian native, she joined UAB as a Research Fellow in 1980 and as a faculty member in 1981. Her interests include adult and pediatric rheumatology and clinical outcomes, specifically in minority population groups. For her contributions to improve the quality of life of patients with arthritis, she was corecipient of the 1997 Arthritis Foundation Virginia Engalichteff Award for Impact on Quality of Life. She is the former editor of *Arthritis Care and Research* and serves on the editorial boards of numerous publications. She is married to Renato D. Alarcón, MD, MPH, Professor and Vice Chairman, Department of Psychiatry, Emory University. The Drs. Alarcón have three children: Patricia, Sylvia, and Daniel.

Beth Alexander, M.D., M.S., is Professor in the Department of Family Practice in the College of Human Medicine at Michigan State University. She came to MSU from the University of Kansas where she served on the faculty. In addition to her background in medicine, she also has a degree in counseling psychology. Her current administrative role is University Physician, Chief Health Officer for MSU, in addition to a part-time practice and teaching responsibilities. Her academic writing has primarily focused on adolescent health care, domestic violence, and human sexuality. Her avocational interests include competitive tennis, rose gardening, hiking, music, and rock carving.

Karen P. Alexander, M.D., is Assistant Professor of Medicine at Duke University where she works full-time as a cardiologist and outcomes researcher. Her research focuses on cardiovascular care and clinical outcomes of women and the elderly. She graduated from Duke University School of Medicine in 1992. She and her husband Dr. John Alexander married at the end of their internal medicine residencies at Brigham and Women's Hospital. She later completed a cardiology fellowship at Duke University in 1998. The Alexanders have a three-year-old daughter Emily and a newborn son Benjamin.

Elizabeth Garrett Anderson, M.D. (1836–1917) was Britain's first woman doctor. Initially unable to gain admission to medical schools, she trained as a nurse at Middlesex Hospital and attended medical lectures. In 1865, she passed the Apothecaries examination, thus obtaining the necessary certificate to practice medicine. Several years later, she received her formal medical degree from the University of Paris. In 1866, Dr. Garrett established a dispensary for women in London that later became a hospital (now called the Elizabeth Garrett Anderson Hospital). For over a decade, she served as Dean of the London Medical School for Women. A devoted feminist, she also helped advocate for women's suffrage in Britain. She was elected mayor of Aldeburgh 1908, becoming the first woman mayor in England.

Kathryn D. Anderson, M.D., is Surgeon-in-Chief and Vice President of Surgery at Childrens Hospital Los Angeles and Professor of Surgery at the University of Southern California. Born in Lancashire, England, she began her medical studies at Girton College, Cambridge. There, she met her husband Dr. French Anderson, married, and emigrated to the U.S. where she graduated from Harvard Medical School. After a year in pediatric medicine, she completed a surgical residency at Georgetown University Hospital. She was Secretary of the American College of Surgeons for nine years and is now the first Vice-President of the College. From 2000-2001, she was President of the American Pediatric Surgical Association. In 1999, Dr. Anderson was elected as a Fellow of the Royal College of Surgeons in England. She has published over 100 articles or book chapters.

Marcia Angell, M. D., is Senior Lecturer in the Department of Social Medicine at Harvard Medical School and former Editor-in-Chief of the *New England Journal of Medicine*. A graduate of Boston University School of Medicine, she trained in both internal medicine and anatomic pathology. Dr. Angell writes frequently on issues of medical ethics, health policy, the nature of medical evidence, the interface of medicine and the law, and end of life care. Her critically acclaimed book, *Science on Trial: The Clash of Medical Evidence and the Law in the Breast Implant Case*, was published in 1996. In addition, she is coauthor, with Dr. Stanley Robbins and, later, Dr. Vinay Kumar, of the first three editions of the textbook, *Basic Pathology*. In 1997, *Time* magazine named Marcia Angell one of the 25 most influential Americans.

Anne Armstrong-Coben, M.D., is Assistant Clinical Professor of Pediatrics at Columbia University. She is married to novelist Harlan Coben and is the mother of four children. She continues to strive for "the balance." Since writing her contribution, she has been at peace mostly being Mom but now has a flexible work situation doing curriculum development for Community Pediatrics at Columbia University and providing medical care for homeless youth as Medical Director of Covenant House in Newark, New Jersey.

Nassim Assefi, M.D., is a women's health specialist and clinician-teacher at Harborview, the county hospital at the University of Washington School of Medicine, where she cares for vulnerable populations, including immigrants, refugees, and the urban underserved. In her spare time, she is a salsa dancer and a fiction writer. Thanks to writing residencies at Hedgebrook writers' colony and the Whiteley Center, she has nearly completed her novel, *The Blood of Pomegranates*, a cross between epistolary and travelogue prose, which explores maternal bereavement across cultures.

S. Josephine Baker, M.D. (1873-1945), graduated from the Women's Medical College of the New York Infirmary in 1898. She was the former commissioner of health in New York City and later the director of the Bureau of Child Hygiene. Dr. Baker introduced many significant reforms, including preventive health care for children, child hygiene, midwifery standards, education for young mothers, and routine school inspections for infectious disease. In 1911, she organized and became President of the Babies Welfare Association, which later became the Children's Welfare Federation of New York. Her efforts resulted in a significant drop in New York City's infant mortality rate from 1918 to 1923. Much of her life is chronicled in her autobiography, *Fighting for Life* (1939).

Emily Dunning Barringer, M.D. (1877-1961), graduated from Cornell University Medical College in 1901. The first woman to train at Gouverneur Hospital in New York City, she endured substantial discrimination from her male colleagues. As New York's first woman ambulance surgeon, however, she won the support of the hospital staff and community. Her life story is told in her autobiography, *Bowery to Bellevue: The Story of New York's First Woman Ambulance Surgeon*. Dr. Barringer also served as president of the American Medical Women's Association and of the Women's Medical Association of New York. She was married to Dr. Benjamin

Barringer, former head of the Urological Department at New York's Memorial Hospital. They had two children, a son and a daughter.

Preetha Basaviah, M.D., is an Assistant Clinical Professor of Medicine and co-directs the Foundations of Patient Care Course at University of California, San Francisco. Prior to UCSF, she served as an Associate Firm Chief and as a Rabkin fellow in medical education at Beth Israel Hospital, Harvard Medical School. She received her M.D. from Brown University School of Medicine and completed her residency in medicine at Beth Israel, including time as a primary care chief resident at the West Roxbury VA. While at Harvard, she received the Lowell B. McGee Teaching Award as well as the Katherine Swan Ginsburg Award for Humanism in Medicine. While not pursuing her passion in medical education, Dr. Basaviah can be found either at dance studios or on the tennis courts. She currently resides in San Francisco with her husband.

Doris Rubin Bennett, M.D. (1924-1994), was one of 12 women at Harvard Medical School in 1945, the first year that women were admitted to that school. She married an upper classman and continued her training in pediatrics at the Massachusetts General Hospital. She began in private practice, later becoming director of child health of the Columbia Point Tufts Medical Center in Boston and Chief of Pediatrics at Harvard Community Health Plan (Kenmore Center). She was also a national consultant for the Head Start program. In 1976, Dr. Bennett was awarded the Radcliffe graduate medal for her work in child health. In later years, she became actively involved at Harvard Medical School, both in medical student teaching and as president of the Alumni Council.

Richard M. Berlin, M.D., is Associate Professor of Psychiatry at the University of Massachusetts Medical School. He is also a poet and physician with a private practice in Lenox, Massachusetts. His chapbook, *Code Blue*, was the winner of the 1999 Poetry Society of South Carolina's Chapbook Contest. His poetry is featured in his column "Poetry of the Times," which appears monthly in *Psychiatric Times*. His poetry has also appeared in numerous medical and literary journals where his work has received awards from the National Writer's Union, *Journal of General Internal Medicine, Slipstream, New Millennial Writing*, and finalist nominations for the Pearl Poetry Prize and the Kate Tufts Discovery Award. He lives with his wife Susanne King, M.D., a child and adolescent psychiatrist. Their daughter Rachel is a student at Williams College.

Anne E. Bernstein, M.D., is Clinical Professor of Psychiatry at Columbia University, College of Physicians & Surgeons and Attending Physician at New York-Presbyterian Hospital. She also maintains an active private practice. She received her M.D. from Albert Einstein College of Medicine in 1962 and completed her residency in psychiatry at Mt. Sinai Hospital where she was appointed Chief Resident. She has authored or coauthored three major textbooks, including *Psychodynamic Treatment of Women* (coauthored with Sharyn Lenhart, M.D., 1993) and over 30 articles in peer-reviewed journals. She is an active member of the American Medical Women's Association, having served for eight years as the Director for Members-in-Training. The mother of four, Dr. Bernstein now has three grandchildren with a fourth on the way.

Jennifer Best, M.D., is a second-year resident in internal medicine at the University of Washington. She completed her undergraduate work in science and the humanities at Seattle Pacific University, and in 2000, received her M.D. degree from Northwestern University Medical School in Chicago. Jennifer and her husband, Eric, enjoy time with family and friends, good food and wine, home improvement, and boating.

Janet Bickel, M.A., is Associate Vice President for Institutional Planning & Development and Director of Women's Programs at the Association of American Medical Colleges (AAMC). She has worked at the forefront of medical education for over 25 years, most recently concentrating on issues of women's professional development and faculty leadership development. Ms. Bickel has published on a broad spectrum of areas, including two books: *Women in Medicine: Getting in, Growing and Advancing* (Sage, 2000) and *Educating for Professionalism: Creating a Culture of Humanism in Medical Education* (2000), edited with Delese Wear. Under her direction, a series of AAMC professional development seminars for prospective women leaders in academic medicine has been offered since 1988.

Elizabeth Blackwell, M.D. (1821-1910), was the first female medical graduate in the United States. After graduation from Geneva Medical College in 1849, she pursued postgraduate studies in Europe, later returning to America where she worked and practiced for the next two decades. With her sister, Emily Blackwell, and Maria Zakrzewska, she cofounded the New York Infirmary for Women and Children in 1857 and its associated Women's Medical College in 1868. In 1869, she returned to England where she continued to fight for women's rights within the medical field. Her most notable works include her autobiography, *Pioneer Work in Opening the Medical Profession to Women* (1895), and *Medicine and Society in America: Essays in Medical Sociology* (1902).

Liza Sharpless Bonanno, M.D., is currently a board certified psychiatrist in part-time practice. She graduated from Brown University (Providence, RI), received her M.D. from the University of North Carolina at Chapel Hill, and completed residency training at Vanderbilt and Wake Forest University Hospitals. Dr. Bonanno developed an interest in writing because of the influence of her grandmother, Alice Gordon, author of several books published in the 1930s. She and her husband, Vinny, recently moved to Dayton, Ohio where he is studying aerospace medicine. They have three children, Vincent, Marianne, and Mitchell.

Deborah Young Bradshaw, M.D., is Clinical Associate Professor of Neurology and Instructor in Medical Humanities at State University of New York Upstate Medical University in Syracuse, New York. Her research interests include adult and pediatric electromyography, Guillain-Barre syndrome, and peripheral neuropathy. She was educated at Wellesley College, SUNY Upstate Medical University, Boston University and the Lahey Clinic Medical Center. She lives with her two daughters and enjoys reading classic fiction, Bible study, and outdoor activities.

Mary Cogan Bromage, M.D. (1906-1995), was former Associate Dean of Women, Professor of Written Communication at the Graduate School of Business Administration and Lecturer in the Department of English at the University of Michigan. She authored several monographs on Irish history and on the topic of written communication. She graduated *summa cum laude* from Radcliffe College in 1923 and was the daughter of Dr. Sarah Edith Ives Cogan, a graduate of the Women's Medical College of Pennsylvania in 1892 and one of the early women ophthalmologists at the Massachusetts Eye and Ear Infirmary.

Lucy M. Candib, M.D., is a family physician who has taught and practiced in an urban neighborhood health center in Worcester, Massachusetts, for the past 25 years. This health center is a residency training site of the University of Massachusetts where she is Professor of Family Medicine and Community Health. Within the context of long-term doctor-patient relationships, Dr. Candib has put feminist principles to work in a multicultural setting. She has lectured widely on sexual abuse and violence against women and has introduced a feminist critique of medical theory in numerous articles and in her book, *Medicine and the Family: A Feminist Perspective* (1995). In 1995, she received a Fulbright grant to teach family medicine in Ecuador. She lives with her life partner, Richard Schmitt, and their two children, Addie and Eli.

Molly Carnes, M.D., M.S., is Professor of Medicine at the University of Wisconsin Medical School and Program Director of the Women's Health Fellowship. She completed her undergraduate work at the University of Michigan, received her M.D. from the State University of New York at Buffalo, and earned a master's of science degree in population health from the University of Wisconsin where she trained in internal medicine and geriatrics. Dr. Carnes is the founding director of several programs with the dual focus of women's health research and developing women leaders in academic medicine. The National Institutes of Health has honored her with a Women's Health Academic Leadership Award. In 1999, she was appointed the first Jean Manchester Biddick Professor of Women's Health Research.

Kathryn A. Carolin, M.D., M.S., is Assistant Professor of Surgery at Wayne State University and Karmanos Cancer Institute. She completed her undergraduate degree in chemistry and cellular and molecular biology at the University of Michigan, Ann Arbor; her surgical residency at North Oakland Medical Centers in Pontiac, Michigan; and her breast surgery fellowship at the University of Michigan. Currently board certified, she primarily practices breast surgery at the Karmanos Cancer Institute and Harper Hospital. Dr. Carolin also works in the laboratory of Dr. Michael Tainsky where her research involves the molecular biology of breast cancer.

Bhuvana Chandra, M.D., was born and raised in India. Married to her college sweetheart, she took time off to raise their two children. She is the recipient of the first Outstanding Child and Adolescent Psychiatry Fellow Award as well as a Faculty Award for Outstanding Teaching, both from Cedars-Sinai Medical Center, Los Angeles. Her poems and essays have been published in various medical journals including the *Annals of Internal Medicine*, *JAMA*, and the *Lancet*. Her literary fiction was nominated in 1998 by the UCLA Writers' Program for the James Kirkwood Prize in Creative Writing. She is currently on sabbatical so she can finish her first book, a collection of short stories.

Catherine Chang, M.D., is a solo practitioner in Newport Beach, California. She was born in Rochester, New York, and raised in California. She completed her undergraduate education at the University of California, Berkeley, her medical education at the University of California, Los Angeles, School of Medicine, and her residency at Mt Zion Hospital of the University of California, San Francisco. Dr. Chang and her husband, Miles, reside in Irvine with their two daughters. Together, they enjoy biking, watching movies, reading adventure travel books, and family outings.

Rita Charon, M.D., Ph.D., is Professor of Clinical Medicine and Director of the Program in Narrative Medicine at the College of Physicians & Surgeons of Columbia University. She graduated from Harvard Medical School in 1978, undertook primary care internal medicine residency training at Montefiore Hospital, and completed a Ph.D. in English at Columbia University in 1999. She is in active general medicine practice and lectures and publishes widely on topics in narrative medicine.

Teresa Clabots (Garcia-Otero), M.D., is Assistant Clinical Professor of Pediatrics at the University of Washington, in Seattle; she practices pediatrics and pediatric endocrinology. Born in Cuba into a family of 10 children, her mentor was her father, a physician/inventor, who loved to tell stories. Writing became a way to pass on the family stories of their lives as immigrants. It also served as a way to share with others stories of her daily struggles as a woman physician, mother, patient advocate, and mentor to other female practitioners. She is working to complete a book and lives in Lakewood, Washington, with her husband and soulmate, Dr. Joseph Clabots, a cardiothoracic surgeon, and their five children, who range in age from eight to 22 years.

Mary Williams Clark, M.D., is a pediatric orthopedic surgeon at the Regional Children's Center, Sparrow Hospital System in Lansing, Michigan. She attended Swarthmore College and Yale University School of Medicine, completed her residency at the University of Pittsburgh, and remained on faculty there for the next five years before becoming Director of Rehabilitation at the Children's Hospital of New Orleans. There, her daughter was born, and four months later, her husband died suddenly. She is now happily remarried. Her career as an "academic migrant worker" has taken her to Charlottesville, Virginia; Hershey, Pennsylvania; Toledo, Ohio; and Lansing, Michigan. Her major interests include pediatric amputations, limb deficiencies, and the humanistic aspects of medicine, including poetry.

Linda Hawes Clever, M.D., is President of Renew!; Clinical Professor of Medicine at the University of California, San Francisco; founding Chair of the Department of Occupational Health at California Pacific Medical Center; and former editor of the *Western Journal of Medicine*. She is a graduate of Stanford University, where she also completed her training. Dr. Clever founded Renew!, an organization whose purpose is to return health to health professionals and others by helping them reaffirm values, replenish energy, and move ahead. She is active within the American College of Physicians and is a member of the National Academy of Sciences Institute of Medicine. She has written numerous papers and book chapters. Her husband is also an internist; their daughter is a Robert Wood Johnson Clinical Scholar.

Ruth Cohen, M.D., is in private practice in New York City and is Assistant Clinical Professor of Psychiatry at New York Hospital, Cornell University. She is grateful to New York University School of Medicine for educating her and giving her the opportunity to treat patients at Bellevue Hospital, where she saw people achieve their best under extreme circumstances. As one of 10 women in a class of 120 students during the 1970s, she was often overlooked as an oddity. Yet she made some wonderful friends and received remarkable support. At discouraging moments, she thinks back to what Dr. Saul Farber, Chairman of Medicine, told the students: "Pay close attention to your patients. They will win the Nobel Prize for you."

Sondra S. Crosby, M.D., is Assistant Professor of Medicine at Boston University School of Medicine. She practices internal medicine at Boston Medical Center where she has a special interest in refugee medicine. She received her M.D. from the University of Washington and completed her residency in internal medicine at the former Boston City Hospital (now Boston Medical Center). She lives in the Boston area with her husband and four children, from Sierra Leone, China, and Kazakhstan. They are "expecting" again, a 2 year old little boy from Kazakhstan.

Rosa E. Cuenca, M.D., is a Surgical Oncologist and Assistant Professor of Surgery at East Carolina University School of Medicine where she graduated from medical school in 1986. She continued her training at University of North Carolina at Chapel Hill and at Roswell Park Cancer Center in Buffalo. She specializes in breast cancer, melanoma, sarcoma, and endocrine diseases. Dr. Cuenca lives in Greenville, North Carolina, with her husband and two children.

Sayantani DasGupta, M.D., M.P.H., is Assistant Attending Pediatrician and Postdoctoral Research Fellow in urban community health at Columbia University and a faculty member for the Health Advocacy Program at Sarah Lawrence College. She is a graduate of Brown University, Johns Hopkins University School of Medicine, and a recent graduate of the residency program in social pediatrics at the Children's Hospital at Montefiore/Albert Einstein College of Medicine. Dr. DasGupta has published essays on issues of medical education, race, gender, sexuality, health, and the South Asian community. She is the coauthor of *The Demon Slayers and Other Stories: Bengali Folktales* (1995) and author of *Her Own Medicine: A Woman's Journey From Student to Doctor* (1998). She lives in New York City with her husband.

Janice E. Daugherty, M.D., is Director of Predoctoral Education, Department of Family Medicine, East Carolina University. She is an only child who grew up in Virginia, Tennessee, and North Carolina, moving often because of her father's work in retailing. Always being the "new kid" meant learning to adapt to many situations, which prepared her for the rapid changes in life and medicine today. A graduate of Wake Forest University School of Medicine, she is married to Dr. Richard Rawl, also a family physician. They are the proud parents of three children, who are also always changing and discovering, even into their teenage years and beyond. She enjoys teaching, especially in finding better ways to help students and physicians have the understanding needed to care well for their patients.

Angelee Deodhar, M.D., an Indian ophthalmologist, took to writing as a second career following a life-threatening, chronic, incapacitating pulmonary thromboembolism. For the last 11 years, she has been writing short stories, poems, and articles and feels that writing has significantly helped her heal. Her work has been published internationally. "Double Helix" is an autobiographical poem written during a hospitalization while she was on oxygen. She is a member of the Haiku Society of America and of the International Arts Medicine Association. Her main interest remains haiku and its related forms of poetry and art (haiga) and their use in healing. As a full-time writer/artist, Dr. Deodhar devotes her time to her home, her rheumatologist husband, Dr. S. D. Deodhar, her son, and their two dogs.

Gayatri Devi, M.D., is the Director of the New York Memory Services and an attending physician at Lenox Hill Hospital. She is board certified in neurology and psychiatry, with specialty training in behavioral neurology and memory disorders. She completed her training at State University of New York Downstate Medical Center and at Columbia–Presbyterian Medical Center. Prior to her current position, she was Assistant Professor of Neurology at Columbia University and Director of the Memory Disorders Center at Columbia–Presbyterian Eastside. She has authored many research papers as well as the book *Estrogen, Memory and Menopause* (2000) and has served as an expert consultant for *Psychology Today* and *Time*. She lives in New York City with her husband, her daughter, and their two dogs.

Leah J. Dickstein, M.A., M.D., was an inner-city Brooklyn sixth-grade public school teacher, with a master's in education, when she entered medical school. Her leadership roles include being President of the American Medical Women's Association and the American Association for Social Psychiatry, Vice President of the American Psychiatric Association, two-term President of the Association of Women Psychiatrists, National Chair of the AAMC Group on Student Affairs, and AAMC faculty member for their Women Faculty Development Seminars. Dr. Dickstein has published over 65 peer-reviewed papers and chapters, edited five books, and conducted research on gender and religious issues in Nazi camp survivors. In 1984, she created the Physicians and the Arts medical student elective to foster creativity in the arts.

Kathleen Dong, M.D., majored in English at Brown University (1982) where she also graduated from medical school (1985). She completed her internship and residency at the UCLA Neuropsychiatric Institute where she developed her interests in the unconscious, family dynamics, and psychoanalytically oriented psychotherapy. She has been in private practice, primarily as a psychotherapist from 1989 to 2001, during which time she served as clinical faculty at Stanford University and completed her analysis. Most recently, she moved to Tacoma, Washington, with her family to become a full-time mother to her delightful "two-nami" daughter. Her husband, a former academic and now private practitioner, is encouraging her to develop a career in writing.

Helen MacKnight Doyle, M.D. (1873–1957), also known as Dr. Nellie, began her life with happy days on a farm and moved to wretched days in a corset factory, to a Dakota homestead, to Bishop in eastern California to join her father, and then to medical school in San Francisco. Only a young woman of exceptional courage could have endured the insults and barriers she encountered while studying to become a doctor. But endure she did—with grace and humor—and returned to Bishop, barely 21 years old, to hang out her shingle. There, among the ranchers and miners of Owens Valley, she practiced for the next 22 years. In 1898, she married Dr. Guy Doyle; they had two children, Dorothy and Morris. In 1917, Dr. Nellie studied anesthesiology, a specialty she practiced for 10 years after moving to Berkeley in 1921.[1]

Amy L. Dryer is currently in her third year of medical school at the College of Physicians & Surgeons of Columbia University. She was born and raised in Maryland and received a B.A. in East Asian Studies from Smith College in 1992. She decided to pursue a career in medicine after teaching Japanese for three years in Massachusetts and earned a postbaccalaureate premedical certificate from Columbia University in 1999. She lives with her husband, Sean, in New York City.

Ambur L. Economou, M.D., graduated from Harvard Medical School in 1998 and now practices family medicine and obstetrics in a small town in Missouri. She has always enjoyed writing stories both to create art and for therapy and hopes someday to write a novel. She is married and has a nine-year-old daughter and a newborn son. "Jane" is her first nationally published story.

Leon Eisenberg, M.D., is the Maude and Lillian Presley Professor of Social Medicine and Professor of Psychiatry Emeritus at Harvard Medical School. His former positions include Chief of Child Psychiatry at Johns Hopkins Hospital, Chief of Psychiatry at the Massachusetts General Hospital, and Chair of the Department of Social Medicine and Health Policy at Harvard Medical School. Dr. Eisenberg has served as consultant to the World Health Organization in Geneva and has chaired international scientific groups in Bulgaria, Geneva, Mexico, Uraguay, and Italy. He is the recipient of numerous awards and honorary degrees and has published widely, most recently coediting *World Mental Health: Problems and Priorities in Low-Income Countries* (1995), and *Bridging Disciplines in the Brain, Behavioral and Clinical Sciences* (2000).

Grace H. Elta, M.D., is Professor of Medicine at the University of Michigan. She graduated from the University of Michigan Medical School and then pursued training in internal medicine and gastroenterology. She has been married for 28 years and has three children, ages 19, 17, and 15. Her oldest son recently completed his sophomore year at Indiana University. Over the past years, Dr. Elta's major interests have focused on the children, but now that they are older, she enjoys motorcycle riding, step aerobics, and reading romance and mystery novels. Her favorite music is country (which drives the GI fellows crazy when she plays it in the endoscopy rooms).

Melissa Fischer, M.D., M.A. Ed., is an Internist with a particular interest in graduate medical education. She received her medical degree from the New York University School of Medicine and was a resident and Chief Resident at Stanford before obtaining her master's in education, also from Stanford University. Her professional time is divided between patient care, resident and student education, and research on teaching, learning, and educational assessment. Dr. Fischer ultimately hopes to improve the methods and quality of medical education. She lives in the San Francisco Bay area where she is delighted by her husband, daughter, and three cats.

Kathleen Franco, M.D., is a psychiatrist at the Cleveland Clinic Foundation where she directs the consultation-liaison service, the medical student rotation in psychiatry, and the Center for the Study of Alternative Medicine. Her research interests have ranged from delirium to physician stress, maybe the latter leading to the former. Mentoring residents and students has been one of her greatest joys, one that keeps her from giving up at work when things get difficult. She is married to Dr. David Bronson, an internist. Together, they have six children ages 26 to 20- Rob, J.C., Carly, Jackie, Chad, and Jonathan. Her favorite pastimes include singing with the Federated Church Chancel Choir, gardening, and traveling. Other interests include spirituality and distant healing.

Beverly M. Gaines, M.D., is the President of Beverly M. Gaines, M.D. & Associates PSC, a general pediatric practice in downtown Louisville, Kentucky, which she established in 1984. Two full-time physicians, one part-time physician, and nine staff employees provide outpatient and inpatient care to a racially and ethnically diverse population. Dr. Gaines is an active member of the National Medical Association, having served as Chair and Vice Chair of Finance, Chair of the Mazique Symposium, Vice Chair of NMPAC, and Chair of the Pediatric Scientific Section. In August 2001, she was reelected to the office of Vice President. Within the Louisville community, she founded the annual African American Health Jamboree and has served on the Kentucky Health Policy Board, an independent agency appointed by the Governor.

Linda Ganzini, M.D., is Director of Geriatric Psychiatry at the Portland VAMC, Professor of Psychiatry and Director of the Geriatric Psychiatry Fellowship Program at Oregon Health Sciences University, and Senior Scholar at the OHSU Center on Ethics in Health Care. She is a 1978 graduate of Yale University and a 1983 graduate of OHSU. She completed her psychiatry residency in 1987 and a geriatric medicine fellowship in 1989. From 1989 to 1999, she served as Director of the Portland VAMC Consult-Liaison Psychiatry Service. Dr. Ganzini's major research interests are in end-of-life care and decision making. She is married and has two daughters Dana and Alexandra, ages eight and four.

Lori Gera is the daughter of two full time physicians and has a lot of respect for hardworking physician moms. She wrote the poem included in this volume when she was 12. It is her mother's most cherished Christmas gift. Lori is a freshman in high school. She is an honors student and is on the tennis team. She also enjoys playing basketball and volleyball, volunteering at a local hospital, and being with her friends.

Anju Goel, M.D., is a graduate of Stanford University School of Medicine (1999) and a third-year resident in primary care internal medicine at Montefiore Medical Center in the Bronx. She plans to pursue a master's of public health and, ultimately, a career in international health. She lives with her partner and two cats in Tuckahoe, New York.

Lori Gottlieb is a student at Stanford University School of Medicine. Previously, she was a film and television executive in Hollywood. She is the author of *Stick Figure: A Diary of My Former Self* (2000/2001), a compilation of her coming-of-age diaries, which has been cited by the American Library Association as one of the "Best Books for 2001." A national bestseller, *Stick Figure,* has been optioned for film by Martin Scorsese. For a list of media, reviews, and other information, please visit www.lorigottlieb.com. As a journalist, Ms. Gottlieb has written for the *New York Times, Time, People, Glamour, Mademoiselle, Redbook, Cosmo-Girl, Seventeen, Slate* (guest diarist), *Salon* (former monthly columnist), the *San Jose Mercury News,* the *San Francisco Chronicle, Daily Variety,* and the *Industry Standard,* among others.

Charlotte Heidenreich, M.D., is a general internist who completed the six-year B.A./M.D. combined degree program at Lehigh University and the Medical College of Pennsylvania. She met her future husband on the first day of residency at Northwestern University where they were both terrified interns. They now have two children, ages 14 and nine, who are an ongoing and joyful reality check. Her favorite hobby is singing with the Milwaukee Symphony Chorus, whose membership has no idea that her day job is medicine. Dr. Heidenreich spent 10 interesting years on the faculty at the Medical College of Wisconsin, combining teaching, clinical practice, and residency program administration while working part-time. Always ready for something new, she stepped away from academics in 2000 and is now Medical Director at Fortis Health in Milwaukee.

Marilyn Heins, M.D., graduated from Radcliffe College, received her M.D. from Columbia University College of Physicians & Surgeons, and completed a residency in pediatrics at Babies Hospital in New York. She was Associate Dean for Student Affairs at Wayne State University School of Medicine and Vice Dean and Professor of Pediatrics at the University of Arizona College of Medicine. Dr. Heins currently devotes her time to writing, consulting, lecturing, and conducting workshops for parents and those who work with children. She has written over 600 parenting columns for the *Arizona Daily Star,* and her second book, *ParenTips—for Effective, Enjoyable Parenting,* was published in 1999. Her web site, parentkidsright.com is a popular online resource. She and her husband, a veterinarian, have been married for 43 years and have two grown children.

Marion Hilliard, M.D. (1902–1958), graduated from the University of Toronto Faculty of Medicine in 1927. In 1928, she joined the staff of Women's College Hospital in Toronto, eventually becoming Chief of Obstetrics and Gynecology. She was one of the three physicians who pioneered the use of cervical scrapings for early cervical cancer detection. Her efforts helped establish a cancer detection clinic at the hospital and an affiliation with the University of Toronto as a teaching institution. A writer for *Chatelaine*, a woman's magazine, she authored two well-known books, *A Woman Doctor Looks at Love and Life* (1957) and *Women and Fatigue: A Woman Doctor's Answer* (1958, 1960). Dr. Hilliard was also a hockey star at the University of Toronto and named "Athlete of the Year" in 1925.

Grace Foege Holmes, M.D., entered medical school in the early 1950s as one of five women in a class of 75 students and there met her future husband, Fred Holmes. After internship at the University of Kansas Medical Center, they worked as missionary physicians in Malaya. In 1963, they returned to KUMC for postgraduate training, Grace in pediatrics and Fred in internal medicine, both later joining their respective faculties. Grace practiced general pediatrics and pursued research on the growth and development of children. From 1970 to 1972, they worked at the Kilimanjaro Christian Medical Centre in Moshi, Tanzania and then returned to medical academia in Kansas. Portions of Grace's life story are included in two autobiographical works, *Whither Thou Goest . . . I Will Go* (1992) and *On Safari: A Collection of Stories* (1998). The Holmes family includes six children (five adopted, three of Chinese origin).

Harriet Hunt, M.D. (1805–1875), was one of the most well-known early women physicians who learned the practice of medicine not by formal education but through apprenticeship. She was inspired to study medicine when her sister became afflicted with a severe illness that doctors were unable to cure. With Dr. Hunt's help, her sister eventually recovered, and together, they pursued medical apprenticeship. She was twice refused admission to Harvard Medical School but was later granted an honorary degree by the Female Medical College of Pennsylvania in 1853. She was an ardent feminist and spokesman for women's issues. Her autobiography, *Glances and Glimpses; or Fifty Years Social, Including Twenty Years Professional Life* was published in 1856.

Sheri Ann Hunt, M.D., is currently in private practice at the Northwest Psychoanalytic Building in Seattle, Washington, where she treats both adults and children. She graduated from the Medical College of Wisconsin in 1990 where she also completed her residency in general psychiatry. She practiced in Milwaukee for four years and then returned to her home state of Washington to complete a Child and

Adolescent Psychiatry Fellowship at the University of Washington. Dr. Hunt also began her Adult and Child Psychoanalytic Training at the Seattle Psychoanalytic Society and Institute. She is an affiliate member of the American Psychoanalytic Association and has published poetry and prose, as well as scientific articles in a variety of medical journals.

Jennifer Hyde, M.D., is a second-year resident in pediatrics in the Boston Combined Pediatrics Residency Program. She received her M.D. from Stanford University School of Medicine in 2000 and her B.S. in biology and women's studies from Duke University in 1994. Part of a foreign service family, she was born in Taipei, Taiwan, and then lived in Hong Kong and Tokyo, Japan, before settling in suburban Washington, D.C., at the age of eight. She studied marine mammals in Mexico as an undergraduate and participated in HIV research in Zimbabwe during medical school. Currently, she lives in Boston with her husband, Peter.

Mary Putnam Jacobi, M.D. (1842–1906), graduated from the Female (later Woman's) Medical College of Pennsylvania in 1864. One of the most brilliant women in her time, she was Professor of Material Medica and Therapeutics at the Woman's Medical College of the New York Infirmary and founding President of the Association for the Advancement of the Medical Education of Women (later Women's Medical Association of New York City). She authored more than 100 works, including several landmark essays and books and was the first female recipient of the esteemed 1876 Boylston Prize from Harvard. A selection of her writings has been compiled into a book, *Mary Putnam Jacobi, M.D.: A Pathfinder in Medicine* (1925). She was married to Dr. Abraham Jacobi, considered by many to be the founder of pediatrics in America.

Toby Jacobowitz, M.D., M.A., has a private practice in internal medicine and pediatrics. She is the Associate Medical Director for Hospice of Washtenaw and is a physician for Emergency Physicians Medical Group. Dr. Jacobowitz completed her master's degree in speech pathology at the University of Minnesota, Minneapolis and her M.D. at Wayne State University School of Medicine. Originally from Brooklyn, New York, she worked as a speech pathologist and as a teacher of the speech and hearing impaired prior to entering medicine. Her special areas of interest include international adoption, domestic violence, women's health, eating disorders, and physician well-being. She currently lives in Ann Arbor, Michigan, with her husband, Harry Haber, a biostatistician at Pfizer, and their two sons, David and Gabe.

Mildred Fay Jefferson, M.D., served as a general surgeon on the active staff of the former Boston University Medical Center and was formerly Assistant Clinical Professor of Surgery, Boston University School of Medicine. She was the first Negro woman graduate of Harvard Medical School, the first woman intern in surgery at the former Boston City Hospital, and the first female member of the Boston Surgical Society. A diplomate of the American Board of Surgery, she is the Chairman of the Citizens Select Committee on Public Health Oversight; a member of the House of Delegates, Massachusetts Medical Society (Suffolk District); a member of the American Medical Association; and the recipient of 28 honorary degrees from American colleges and universities. She is also a founder of the National Right to Life Movement.

Marie F. Johnson, M.D., is Assistant Professor of Geriatrics at the University of Colorado Health Sciences Center. She graduated from Johns Hopkins School of Medicine in 1992, followed by an internal medicine residency at the University of California, San Francisco. After working for several years as a general internist, she received additional training in geriatrics from the University of Colorado. Until 2001, Dr. Johnson was actively involved in health services research in the area of posthospital care for Medicare beneficiaries but has interrupted this work to raise her three children. She is currently on leave of absence from the University of Colorado, motivated in large part by the experience described in her essay included in this collection.

Nalini Juthani, M.D., is Professor of Clinical Psychiatry at the Albert Einstein College of Medicine and Director of Psychiatry Education and Assistant Dean for medical students at the Bronx Lebanon Hospital in New York. Raised in Bombay, India, she completed medical school at the Bombay University in 1970 and then immigrated to the United States with her husband, Dr. Virendra Juthani, where she specialized in psychiatry and raised three children. Their eldest daughter is a physician, their second daughter a law student, and their youngest, a son is a premedical student. As Dr. Juthani would say, if we observe and listen to our children they are our best teachers.

Nancy B. Kaltreider, M.D., is Professor of Psychiatry Emerita at the University of California, San Francisco, and is dividing her time among clinical work, community service, teaching in the women's program, and rowing a single scull on San Francisco Bay. She graduated from Harvard Medical School in 1964 and completed residency and fellowship training in adult psychiatry. She was appointed to a faculty position at UCSF, which lasted for the next 30 years. While at UCSF, she combined teaching activities with clinical practice and founded a program for women. She joined with colleagues to write and edit a book *Dilemmas of a Double Life: Women Balancing Careers and Relationships* (1997) and continues to be interested in the changing complexities of women's roles. She married a medical school classmate and has two adult children.

Cynthia J. Kapphahn, M.D., M.P.H., is Clinical Assistant Professor in the Division of Adolescent Medicine at Stanford University School of Medicine. She is also assistant editor for the *Journal of Adolescent Health*. She attended Yale University School of Medicine and completed a residency in pediatrics at Johns Hopkins Hospital. She received a master's degree in public health from Johns Hopkins University before completing her fellowship in adolescent medicine at the University of California, San Francisco. In addition to her clinical practice, Dr. Kapphahn has a research interest in health policy and adolescents' access to care. She lives in Menlo Park, California, with her husband, an architect, and their three-year-old son.

Kathy Kirkland, M.D., is Assistant Professor of Medicine at Dartmouth Medical School where she works in infectious diseases and hospital epidemiology. Her real passion is working with medical students to maintain humanity and connection during the process of becoming a physician. A graduate of Mount Holyoke College and Dartmouth Medical School, she completed a medical residency at Columbia-Presbyterian and married Marc Gautier, a medical school classmate and co-Chief Resident. Following an infectious disease fellowship at Duke University, she spent two years with the CDC's Epidemic Intelligence Service and then returned to Duke. After nine years in N. Carolina, she moved with her husband and three children to Vermont. Not a day goes by when she doesn't feel incredibly lucky to live where she wants to be living and doing what she wants to be doing.

Perri Klass, M.D., is Assistant Professor of Pediatrics at Boston University School of Medicine. She subspecializes in pediatric infectious diseases and has a primary care practice at Dorchester House, a neighborhood health center in Boston. At Boston Medical Center, she serves as Medical Director of the Reach Out and Read National Center, which makes literacy promotion part of pediatric primary care. Dr. Klass is the author of *Love and Modern Medicine* (2001), *Other Women's Children* (1990), *Baby Doctor: A Pediatrician's Train- ing* (1992), and *A Not Entirely Benign Procedure: Four Years as a Medical Student* (1987). Her short stories have won five O. Henry Awards and have been widely anthologized, and her essays have appeared in the *New York Times Magazine, Parenting, Discover, American Health, Esquire, Vogue, Knitters,* and many other publications.

Kathryn Ko, M.D., is the Chief of Neurosurgery at Brookdale University Hospital and Medical Center in Brooklyn. Of Korean, German, and Irish ancestry, she was born and educated in Honolulu, Hawaii, and graduated from the University of Hawaii School of Medicine in 1983. She completed a residency in neurosurgery at Mount Sinai Medical Center in New York City. She is a pioneer in medical holography and has authored several research papers on this topic. She is interested in the rendering of medical subject matter in true three dimensions and credits her art background for this awareness. Dr. Ko authored *The Survival Bible for Women in*

Medicine (1998) and is currently at work writing her second book, *A Brain Surgeon's Ambidextrous Affairs*.

Priya Krishna, M.D., is an otolaryngology resident at the Southern Illinois University School of Medicine in Springfield. She graduated from the University of Missouri–Kansas City School of Medicine six-year combined B.A./M.D. program in 1997 and then completed a one-year preliminary surgical internship at McGaw Medical Center of Northwestern University Medical School in Chicago in 1998. Newly appointed the national resident representative to the Society of University Otolaryngologists, Dr. Krishna also serves on a Graduate Medical Education Committee, a hospital ethics committee, and is involved with the school's Alpha Omega Alpha chapter. She is the proud owner of a 1923 restored Steinway and is an avid pianist.

Rebecca J. Kurth, M.D., is an Assistant Clinical Professor of Medicine at Columbia University College of Physicians and Surgeons who practices at Columbia Eastside PrimeCare. She received her A.B. in history and literature from Harvard College in 1983 and her M.D. from Columbia University College of Physicians & Surgeons in 1987. She completed her residency training in internal medicine at the Presbyterian Hospital in New York City in 1990. Dr. Kurth is actively involved in medical student education and directs the medical school's course in primary care. She is married to Dr. Randolph Marshall, an academic neurologist and kayaking enthusiast, and is the mother of three children: Trevor, Ginger, and Zoe.

Ann Klompus Lanzerotti, M.D., was born in 1940 and raised in central New Jersey. She received an A.B. from Radcliffe College in 1961 and an M.D. from Stanford University School of Medicine in 1968. Her internal medicine residency was completed in Dallas, Texas, and San Francisco, California, and her hematology-oncology fellowship in San Francisco. Since 1972, Dr. Lanzerotti has lived in San Francisco where she practiced at the U.S. Public Health Service Hospital (1975–1981) and Kaiser-Permanente, South San Francisco (1982–1998). Her current activities include daily tai chi, volunteer teaching at UCSF Medical Center, reading voraciously, and making sporadic forays into short story writing. She is married to Dr. Richard Lanzerotti and has two daughters.

Cynthia Gail Leichman, M.D., is Professor of Medicine at Albany Medical College and Director of the Multidisciplinary Gastrointestinal Oncology Program. Prior to her current position, she was Associate Professor of Medicine at Roswell Park Cancer Institute. Her area of interest is translational research in gastrointestinal malignancies, and she has conducted clinical trials on both national and institutional levels. Dr. Leichman grew up on a farm in western New York and was initially destined to be either a professor of history or a lawyer; her career in medicine came as something of an afterthought. She obtained her M.D. from Wayne State University

School of Medicine. Her husband, a partner at home and at work, is also an academic medical oncologist. They have three sons—ages 21 to 29—and two aging felines.

Blaise Levai, Ed.D., works as a pastoral counselor and family therapist with his wife, Dr. Marian Levai, in a family psychiatry practice in Jacksonville, Florida. He was trained at New Brunswick Theological Seminary and earned an M.A. from the University of Chicago and an Ed.D. from the University of Michigan. After teaching at Voorhees College, Vellore, India and Northwestern College in Orange City, Iowa, he worked for the Bible Society and Methodist Board in New York. He has pastored churches in India and Nepal as well as the U.S. He has published numerous articles, several books on overseas mission, and a novel, *Search For Freedom*, on India. He has been honored with a doctorate in humane letters from Hope College and a master's of divinity from New Brunswick Theological Seminary.

Marian Korteling Levai, M.D., spent her childhood in India where her mother, Dr. Anna Ruth Korteling, founded a rural hospital and clinic. She graduated from Hope College in Michigan and the University of Michigan School of Medicine in 1951. She worked with her husband Blaise Levai, Ed.D. at the internationally known Christian Medical Hospital in Vellore, India. On returning to the United States as the mother of five, she completed a residency in child psychiatry at the New York Medical College and later worked as the director of a child psychiatric unit in New Jersey and Florida. Both she and her husband received honorary doctorates in humanities from Hope College. Since moving to Florida, they have worked together in a family psychiatry practice. They have five children and 10 grandchildren.

Sara Lawrence Lightfoot, Ed.D., a MacArthur Prize Fellow, sociologist and daughter of Dr. Margaret Lawrence, is Professor of Education at Harvard University. She completed her undergraduate studies at Swarthmore College and her doctoral work in the sociology of education at Harvard. A prolific author, she has written seven books, including *Balm in Gilead: Journey of A Healer* (1988), a biography of her mother which received the 1988 Christopher Award. In 1993, the Sara Lawrence-Lightfoot Chair, an endowed professorship, was established at Swarthmore College. In 1998, she was the recipient of the Emily Hargroves Fisher Endowed Chair at Harvard University, which upon her retirement, will become the Sara Lawrence-Lightfoot Endowed Chair, the first endowed professorship at Harvard named in honor of an African American woman.

Anne M. (Peternel) Lipton, M.D., Ph.D., is Assistant Professor of Neurology and Psychiatry at the University of Texas–Southwestern Medical Center, specializing in neurobehavior and dementia. She graduated from a combined M.D.-Ph.D. program at Northwestern University Medical School in Chicago. She inherited her love of reading and writing from her mother, an English teacher. She has lived in 10 states and now enjoys living in Dallas and traveling with her husband.

Joan C. Lo, M.D., is Assistant Professor of Medicine at the University of California San Francisco (UCSF) and San Francisco General Hospital. She studied biochemistry at the University of California Los Angeles and received her medical degree from Harvard Medical School. She completed residency training in internal medicine at Brigham and Women's Hospital and a postdoctoral fellowship in diabetes, endocrinology and metabolism at UCSF. Dr. Lo is currently an endocrinologist at UCSF where her research has focused on the metabolic changes associated with HIV infection and therapy. She is married to her long-time friend and colleague, Dr. Alan Go, physician scientist at Kaiser Permanente Division of Research, and they are proud parents of Rachel Elizabeth Go born July 2001.

Lou Elizabeth Mac Manus, D.O., is a general surgeon, obstetrician, and gynecologist who presently resides in Akron, Ohio. Born in Tampa, Florida, she attended college at Emory University in Atlanta, Georgia, and then moved to Kansas City, Missouri, to complete medical school. Dr. Mac Manus has been in practice since 1982 and is the co-owner of Cuyahoga Valley Women's Healthcare, Inc. Her pleasures in life include training residents, playing golf, and enjoying her family and friends. At the age of 48, she was diagnosed with breast cancer. This has been an inspiration to her. Currently, she is well and busy in a full-time practice and still enjoys her chosen profession. She lives with her husband, Warren, who is a ceramic artist and her teenage daughters, Susan and Genelle.

Dugan Wiess Maddux, M.D., lives and works as a nephrologist in Danville, Virginia. She graduated from Vanderbilt University in 1980 and spent nine years in Chapel Hill, North Carolina, where she and her husband, Frank, completed medical school, internal medicine residency, and nephrology fellowship. Both are now nephrologists at the Danville Urologic Clinic. They have a daughter, Emma, and a son, Cabell. Her children and her chickens are the subject of a number of essays she has written.

Cynthia Magowan was born and raised in Montclair, New Jersey, where her parents (both graduates of Columbia University College of Physicians & Surgeons in 1932) made their home for nearly 60 years. Her father was a surgeon and chief of staff at Montclair Community Hospital. Her mother, Dr. Katharine W. Hooton, practiced medicine for some years, later becoming active in the Montclair Garden Club. Dr. Hooton is now retired and turned 96 in August 2001. Mrs. Magowan married Merrill L. Magowan in 1962. They have three sons and four grandchildren. She is active in her community with directorships and former directorships in Planned Parenthood, Children's Hospital Foundation, KQED, the San Francisco Symphony, the Cardiology Council for UCSF, and the Hillsborough Garden Club.

JoAnn Elisabeth Manson, M.D., Dr.P.H., is Chief of the Division of Preventive Medicine, Co-Director of Women's Health, and Director of Endocrinology in the Division of Preventive Medicine, Brigham and Women's Hospital. She is also Professor of Medicine at Harvard Medical School. She received an A.B. from Harvard University, an M.D. from Case Western Reserve University School of Medicine, and a doctorate in Public Health and Epidemiology from the Harvard School of Public Health. Dr. Manson is principal investigator of several NIH grants, including the Women's Health Initiative in Boston. A recipient of numerous awards, she has also published over 300 articles and seven books, including the textbook, *Prevention of Myocardial Infarction* (1996) and *The 30-Minute Fitness Solution: A Four-Step Plan for Women of All Ages* (2001).

Marcia Quereau McCrae, M.D., (1940-2001) graduated from Vassar College and Harvard Medical School. She completed an internship at the University of Pennsylvania Hospital, residencies at the Children's Hospital of Philadelphia and the Children's Hospital Medical Center in Boston, and a fellowship in developmental evaluation at the Children's Hospital of Boston. She practiced developmental pediatrics and published numerous articles within the field. In 1983, Dr. McCrae founded ProKids of Berks County, a nonprofit advocacy group that works to improve services and resources for Berks County children. Prokids has named its annual service award in her honor. She worked tirelessly to improve the lives of handicapped children and was a champion of all children. On top of this, she was a fabulous mother and is deeply missed.

Julia E. McMurray, M.D, is currently Associate Professor of Medicine at the University of Wisconsin, Madison. She has been in practice 20 years, working on a balance between a busy general internal medicine practice and family life with two children. One of four children of a dual-physician couple, her research interests have centered on the careers and work lives of women physicians.

Carol Merchant, M.D., M.P.H., is Assistant Professor of Neurology at Columbia University College of Physicians & Surgeons and director of the Memory Center, part of the Taub Institute of Research on Alzheimer's disease at Columbia University. A graduate of George Washington University College of Medicine and Health Sciences, Dr. Merchant completed her residency in neurology at Mount Sinai Medical Center in New York. She also earned her master's in public health at Columbia University Mailman School of Public Health. She has authored several publications on risk factors associated with Alzheimer's disease and preventive treatment. She is an active member of the National Medical Association and council delegate of the Council for the Concerns of Women Physicians.

Diane F. Merritt, M.D., is Professor of Obstetrics and Gynecology at Washington University Medical Center and Director of the Division of Pediatric and Adolescent

Gynecology. She graduated from Miami University and New York University School of Medicine, later completing her residency at Washington University Medical Center. Dr. Merritt is known internationally for her expertise in genital injuries, congenital reproductive tract anomalies, and hormonal disorders of puberty and menopause. For 20 years, she pioneered the program in pediatric and adolescent gynecology at Washington University Medical Center, now an established major referral center in the Midwest. A recipient of numerous awards, she has been consistently ranked among the Best Doctors in America. She and her husband (a cardiovascular biophysicist) have three children.

Daphne Miller, M.D., has a small neighborhood family practice in San Francisco while also teaching medical students and family practice residents at the University of California, San Francisco. She received her M.D. from Harvard Medical School and completed a family medicine residency and primary care research fellowship at UCSF. Her husband Ross Levy, an architect, designed her office. Her two children, Arlen and Emet, are frequently seen drawing pictures and doing homework in her waiting room.

Alison Moll, M.D., is a preceptor at York Hospital's Family Practice Residency Program in Pennsylvania. Following 13 years of clinical practice in family medicine, she turned to writing full-time. She has published a volume of poems, *Miracles Like Breathing* (1997) and her latest book about preventing childhood violence is due out from M. Evans & Co. in summer of 2002. Besides writing plays, fiction, nonfiction, and poetry, Dr. Moll speaks to schools and community groups about Colonial medicine, violence prevention, and poetry. She likes to hike, sing, canoe, and roller-skate with her two children. In recent years she has visited Peru, China, and the Dominican Republic on medical mission trips.

Michelle Monje is a student at the Stanford University School of Medicine, pursuing an M.D. and a Ph.D. in neuroscience. She grew up in the San Francisco Bay Area with her mother and maternal grandparents. She attended Vassar College in Poughkeepsie, New York, and graduated in 1998 with a bachelor's degree in biology. She plans to specialize in neurology and has a particular interest in cerebrovascular disease and critical care neurology.

Gayle Shore Moyer, M.D., has been in private practice for more than 10 years. A graduate of University of Michigan Medical School, she completed her residency in obstetrics and gynecology at the University of Illinois in Chicago. She and her husband, Bruce, moved back to Ann Arbor after residency to be closer to their families. Dr. Moyer and her husband try to stay active in the community while raising two sons, Alex, 13, and Justin, 11.

Gulli Lindh Muller, M.D. (1889-1972), paved the way for women at Columbia University, College of Physicians & Surgeons. Originally from Sweden, she graduated from Barnard College, and with the help of the Dean at Barnard, pleaded persistently with the Dean of the Medical School of Columbia University to be accepted into the class. She was accepted with the provision that they would raise $50,000 to help make the necessary renovations to accommodate women students. Graduating first in her class, she later served as a faculty member at Columbia University before moving to Massachusetts where she worked in research (clinical and anatomic pathology) at Boston City Hospital.

Theodore Nadelson, M.D., formerly Chief of the Psychiatric Service at the Boston VA Medical Center, has recently retired from clinical practice and is now writing a book. His interests have included consultation-liaison psychiatry and the issues surrounding dual-career marriages. He received his M.D. from the University of California in 1960, trained in psychiatry at the Sheppard Pratt Hospital in Towson, Maryland and the Beth Israel Hospital in Boston, and completed psychoanalytic training at the Boston Psychoanalytic Institute in 1968. In 1965, he married Dr. Carol Nadelson. They have two children, now adults.

Stephanie Nagy-Agren, M.D., is Assistant Professor of Medicine at the University of Virginia School of Medicine and Chief of the Infectious Diseases Section at the Veterans Affairs Medical Center in Salem, Virginia. She received a B.S. from the University of Illinois, an M.D. from the University of Chicago Pritzker School of Medicine, and completed a medicine residency at the Hospital of the University of Pennsylvania. Following two years of immunology research at Stockholm University in Sweden, she returned to the U.S. for an infectious diseases fellowship at Yale University School of Medicine. She began writing poems after the birth of her second child and believes the healing abilities gained through motherhood have enhanced her work as a physician. She has published poems in a small literary journal and an essay in *JAMA*.

Jennifer R. Niebyl, M.D., is Professor and Head of the Department of Obstetrics and Gynecology at the University of Iowa College of Medicine in Iowa City. She graduated from Yale University School of Medicine and did her residency training in obstetrics and gynecology at Cornell University–New York Hospital and the Johns Hopkins Hospital in Baltimore. She then completed a fellowship in maternal-fetal medicine at Johns Hopkins Hospital. Dr. Niebyl is Co-Editor-in-Chief of the *American Journal of Perinatology* and Associate Editor of the *Journal of the Society for Gynecologic Investigation*. She is co-editor of the textbook *Obstetrics: Normal and Problem Pregnancies,* and author of *Drug Use in Pregnancy,* as well as numerous articles and book chapters.

Danielle Ofri, M.D., Ph.D., is an attending physician at Bellevue Hospital and a faculty member of New York University School of Medicine. A recipient of the 2001 Missouri Review Editor's Prize in nonfiction, her stories have appeared in both medical and literary journals. She is Editor-in-Chief of the *Bellevue Literary Review* and has also edited a medical textbook, *The Bellevue Guide to Outpatient Medicine* (2001). She lives in New York City with her husband, daughter, and dog.

Silvia Wybert Olarte, M.D., was born in Mendoza, Argentina, where she completed her medical school education. Her postgraduate training at New York Medical College included a psychiatry residency, fellowship in group and family therapy, and psychoanalytic training. Her career has been devoted to both public psychiatry through her work with the Latino population in New York City and dynamic psychiatry through her private practice in the treatment of women and her role as a training psychoanalyst at the Psychiatric Institute of New York Medical College where she is a Clinical Professor of Psychiatry. Dr. Olarte met her husband in medical school, and both came to this country to train. He is Clinical Professor of Neurology at Columbia University College of Physicians and Surgeons. They are the proud parents of two sons and one daughter.

Bethenia A. Owens-Adair, M.D. (1840-1926), was the first woman with a medical degree in Oregon. She married at the age of 14, had a son, and then divorced to flee an abusive husband. Against the wishes of her family, she gave up her business as a milliner to pursue medicine. She received her first M.D. from the Eclectic School of Medicine in Philadelphia and years later a second M.D. from the University of Michigan. As the first woman doctor in Roseburg, Oregon, she was scorned by many. Eventually, she moved to Portland where she married Colonel Adair in 1884. She later practiced in Warrington, Oregon, often braving rugged travel while making house calls. She was also an activist in the movement to secure equal rights and suffrage for women.

Barbara Cammer Paris, M.D., is Clinical Associate Professor of Medicine and Geriatrics at Mount Sinai School of Medicine and Medical Director of Geriatric Inpatient Services, Mount Sinai Medical Center, in New York City. She was born and raised in New York City, and after completing her residency training in internal medicine, she married and moved to Boston where her husband attended graduate school. During the ensuing three years, she worked as an internist and had their first child. In 1983, the family moved back to New York City where Dr. Paris pursued a fellowship in geriatric medicine at Mount Sinai Medical Center, during which time her second child was born. She later joined the faculty at Mount Sinai where she continues to teach and see patients.

Melissa A. Parisi, M.D., Ph.D., is a clinical geneticist at Children's Hospital and Regional Medical Center, University of Washington, where she juggles patient care responsibilities and research into the basic genetic mechanisms of human development. She went to medical school in northern California where she learned to eat tofu and understand yeast genetics. She currently resides in Seattle, WA with her husband and two dogs. She remains inspired by the families she meets who daily cope with complex and rare genetic diseases.

Donna L. Parker, M.D., is Associate Dean for Student and Faculty Development at the University of Maryland School of Medicine (UMSoM). She graduated with a B.S. from McGill University and received her M.D. from the UMSoM. She completed her residency in internal medicine at Mercy Medical Center in Baltimore and later returned to the University of Maryland to become the Medical Director for the internal medicine clinic. Subsequently, she became the Associate Program Director for Ambulatory Education within the Department of Medicine and Assistant Dean of Admissions for the School of Medicine. She has achieved Fellowship in the American College of Physicians and was elected to Alpha Omega Alpha by the students at UMSoM. Dr. Parker enjoys family life with her husband, Nevins, and their two daughters, Audrey and Ava.

Barbara K. Pawley, M.D., is Assistant Professor of Radiology at the University of Louisville School of Medicine. Born in Louisville, Kentucky, she has lived there all her life. Her father was an electrician while her mother stayed home with their seven children. Barbara was a middle child, sandwiched between five brothers and a sister. She received a bachelor degree in engineering from the University of Louisville, but after three years of work as an engineer, she decided to pursue a medical career, a transition that involved night classes and a two-year detour teaching high school. She believes that her greatest commitment is in her 21-year marriage and her greatest wealth is in her five children who range in age from two to 16.

Veronica Piziak, M.D., Ph.D., is Professor of Medicine at Texas A&M University Health Science Center and Chief of Endocrinology at the Scott and White Clinic. She also holds appointments in the School of Nutrition and the School of Rural Public Health. Her research interests are in the areas of diabetes prevention and therapy and osteoporosis. She completed a Ph.D. in biochemistry from the University of Massachusetts, an M.D. from the University of Kentucky, and an Endocrinology Fellowship at the University of Cincinnati.

Cynthia Rasch, M.D., is in private practice in Shoreline, Washington, and is the former Medical Affairs Manager for Elixis.com. She graduated from the University of Washington School of Medicine in 1991 and completed internal medicine residency training at Kaiser Foundation Hospital, San Francisco. She remains active in the Alumni Association of the University of Washington School of Medicine and is a clinical tutor for second-year students.

Elsa Raskin, M.D., is presently in private practice in New York City. She practices general plastic surgery, both reconstructive and cosmetic with a special interest in oculoplastic surgery. Her hospital affiliations include the New York Hospital and the New York Eye and Ear Infirmary where she has teaching appointments in the plastic surgery clinics. Her daughters Vanessa and Alexis, now five and four years old, have grown into the most delightful, pleasant little girls.

Rachel Naomi Remen, M.D., is one of the pioneers of the mind-body health movement. She is an alumna of Cornell College of Medicine and Stanford Medical School. She is Clinical Professor of Family and Community Medicine at the University of California San Francisco School of Medicine, Co-founder and Medical Director of the Commonweal Cancer Help Program, and Founder and Director of the Institute for the Study of Health and Illness (ISHI). Dr. Remen has cared for many thousands of people with cancer in her 28 years of practice. Her bestselling books include *Kitchen Table Wisdom: Stories That Heal* (1996) and *My Grandfather's Blessings: Stories of Strength, Refuge and Belonging* (2000). She has a 48-year personal history of chronic illness, and her work represents a unique blend of the perspectives of patient and physician.

Joyce Rico, M.D., is Medical Director at Fujisawa Healthcare, Inc. She trained in dermatology and was a member of the faculty at Duke and New York University before moving recently to industry. She lives on Chicago's North Shore with her husband and two children and is an avid reader, traveler, and knitter.

Elizabeth A. Rider, M.S.W., M.D., is Codirector of the Academies of Medical Educators Collaborative and is also responsible for the Resident as Teacher Program for the Harvard pediatric residencies. A graduate of Harvard Medical School, she completed pediatric residency training at Boston's Children's Hospital and fellowship training in general academic pediatrics at Massachusetts General Hospital. She serves on the Board of Directors of the American Academy on Physician and Patient and is a National Pediatric Faculty Development Scholar. Dr. Rider teaches faculty and medical students and received the Harvard Medical School Morgan-Zinsser Teaching Award. She is a member of the Bayer-Fetzer Group on Physician-Patient Communication in Medical Education. Dr. Rider has a part-time private pediatric practice.

Mary Bennett Ritter, M.D. (1849-1939), was a graduate of Cooper Medical College, San Francisco (later Stanford University School of Medicine) in 1886. She practiced in Berkeley, California, where she became a regular medical examiner and counselor for women students at the University of California. Concerned about the poor facilities for student lodging, she led the efforts to establish "clubhouses" in which women students could live and eat together. One of the first dormitories was later named in her honor. In 1909, she moved to La Jolla, California, where her husband, Professor William Emerson Ritter founded the Marine Biological Station (now Scripps Institution of Oceanography). No longer in medical practice, Dr. Ritter devoted her time to the community.

Patricia A. Robertson, M.D., is Professor of Clinical Obstetrics and Gynecology at the University of California at San Francisco (UCSF) and a perinatologist, providing obstetrical care for high-risk pregnant women. She is Co-Director of the Center for Lesbian Health Research and Director of Medical Student Education for the Department of Obstetrics, Gynecology and Reproductive Sciences at UCSF. Her research interests center on obstetrical issues for lesbians. She is an Advisory Board member of the Lesbian Health Fund, which funds pilot research projects in lesbian health care; a cofounder of the Lyon-Martin Clinic, a full-service clinic for lesbians that began 20 years ago; and a cofounder of the Women in Medicine conference. Dr. Robertson lives in San Francisco with her partner and children.

Mary Canaga Rowland, M.D. (1873-1966), was born in Nebraska and received her medical degree from Kansas City Medical College in 1901. She practiced medicine on the frontier during the pioneer days, making house calls with horse and buggy. Her first husband, Dr. Walter Rowland, was murdered shortly after their child was born. She eventually moved to Oregon where she was the physician for Chemawa Federation Indian School from 1917 to 1927. After her resignation in 1927, she devoted her time to writing her memoirs, which have now been edited by her great great nephew into a book, *As Long as Life: The Memoirs of a Frontier Woman Doctor.*

Bonnie Salomon, M.D., is an emergency physician at Lake Forest Hospital in Illinois. Born and raised in Chicago, she graduated from Harvard College in 1983 and the University of Illinois at Chicago College of Medicine in 1987. After residency at Northwestern, she worked in academic and community hospitals. In 2000, she completed a fellowship in medical ethics at the University of Chicago. Her poems and essays have appeared in several journals, including *The Lancet, Annals of Internal Medicine*, and *The Pharos*. She lives with her husband, Michael, and son Jonathan, in Deerfield, Illinois.

Jessica Schorr Saxe, M.D., is a family practitioner at CMC-Biddle Point, a community health center in Charlotte, NC. A graduate of Tufts University School of Medicine, she completed her family practice residency at Duke. After over 20 years in the same practice, she now takes care of several four-generation families, including children whose mothers she delivered. Her husband Allen teaches anthropology, runs, bakes bread, and makes pickles. She has four children—Kafia, Eddie, Talia, and Jeremy—from whom she has learned invaluable lessons about negotiating life in public schools, how to throw a baseball, and what clothes are hopelessly out of style. Most of all they have taught her humility in answering questions about child rearing.

Mary Lou Schmidt, M.D., is Associate Professor at the University of Illinois College of Medicine where her primary clinical interest is children with cancer. She was born in Louisville, Kentucky, and received all her postgraduate training at Northwestern University's Children's Memorial Hospital. Board certified in pediatric hematology-oncology, her research interests include clinical trials and quality of life in neuroblastoma patients and clinical ethics. She is also actively involved in the teaching of medical students and residents. Dr. Schmidt resides in Chicago with Steve, her husband of 17 years, and her three children, Alexandra, Samantha, and Kevin.

Susan K. Schultz, M.D., is Associate Professor of Psychiatry at the University of Iowa College of Medicine, the institution where she completed psychiatry residency and a research fellowship. She is boarded in geriatric psychiatry and presently conducts research in the area of psychosis in dementia. Her research involves treatment trials using antipsychotic medication in late life as well as neuroimaging studies in dementia syndromes. She is active in the American Association for Geriatric Psychiatry and works as assistant to the Editor-in-Chief of the *American Journal of Psychiatry*.

Audrey Shafer, M.D., is Associate Professor of Anesthesia at Stanford University School of Medicine and staff anesthesiologist at the Veterans Affairs Palo Alto Health Care System. She teaches medical humanities courses for medical students and undergraduates and is the author of *Sleep Talker: Poems by a Doctor/Mother* (2001). She and her husband met in medical school and have two terrific children. They live a quiet suburban life, complete with swings hanging from the family room ceiling, drum set, and garage-cum- discothèque.

Florence H. Sheehan, M.D., is Research Professor of Medicine in the Division of Cardiology at the University of Washington where she is involved in three-dimensional echocardiography and image processing. She received her B.S. degree from the Massachusetts Institute of Technology and her M.D. from the University of Chicago. After her medicine residency at the Medical College of Virginia, she worked as a Clinical Associate at the National Heart, Lung, and Blood Institute for three years. Her research since 1980 has been oriented toward the development and validation of methods for quantitative analysis of cardiac images and the application of these methods to clinical and experimental research. In 1996, she founded a company to assist in translating her research into clinical practice.

Teena Shetty, M.D., M.Phil, completed degrees in English literature and comparative literature with honors at Brown University in 1995. She also studied English literature at Oxford University in England and won a Fulbright Scholarship to complete an M.Phil. degree in medicine at Gonville and Caius College, Cambridge University in 1998–1999. She is a graduate of the Brown University School of Medicine and presently in her first year of a neurology residency at New York–Presbyterian Hospital (Cornell University) and Memorial Sloan Kettering Cancer Center. Dr. Shetty is also the winner of the national Leah Dickstein Award for a female medical student distinguished in leadership and creativity.

Diane K. Shrier, M.D., is Clinical Professor of Psychiatry and Pediatrics at the George Washington University Medical Center, Senior Consultant in the Department of Psychiatry at Walter Reed Army Medical Center, and an Attending Physician in the Department of Psychiatry at Children's National Medical Center in Washington, D.C. She divides her work between part-time private practice, teaching, and research. She is currently principal investigator on a research project, Generation to Generation: Mother-Daughter Physicians. Dr. Shrier has published numerous articles and book chapters and has also edited a book. Her research interests include gender-related issues, sexual harassment, and balancing career and family. She married after her first year of medical school and has four children, one of whom is also a physician.

Lydia A. Shrier, M.D., M.P.H., joined the faculty at Children's Hospital Boston after completing a fellowship in adolescent medicine there in 1996. She obtained her master's of public health at the Harvard School of Public Health in 1997. She is active both regionally and nationally in the field of sexually transmitted disease in adolescents. Dr. Shrier is currently supported by a K23 five-year research career development award from the National Institute of Mental Health for her work on the role of mental health in sexual risk behavior and sexually transmitted disease in adolescents. She continues to see patients for both primary and specialty care, including a large practice of patients with eating disorders. In her "spare" time, she enjoys competitive volleyball, scuba diving, and fine dining.

Maryella Desak Sirmon, M.D., is Clinical Associate Professor of Medicine at the Univ. of South Alabama College of Medicine (USA) where she has been awarded Best Clinical Attending. She is now in the private practice of nephrology after 15 years in academics but continues to teach medical ethics and serve on ethics consultation services. She completed her M.D. at USA; internal medicine residency at the Univ. of Alabama, Birmingham where she was Chief Resident; nephrology fellowship at Duke; and medical ethics training at Georgetown. Married to her college sweetheart she is the mother of two teenage sons. She enjoys rafting, sailing, and camping with her guys, but especially loves the challenges and joys of watching boys become men. Having a passion for both reading and writing, she is the author of numerous poems and several short stories.

Marjorie Spurrier Sirridge, M.D., is Professor of Medicine and Director of the Office of Medical Humanities at the University of Missouri-Kansas City School of Medicine. She was also the former Assistant Dean and Dean of the School. An only child, she was born in a small Kansas town in 1921. She attended Kansas State College and medical school at Kansas University, graduating in 1944 with six other women. She married a classmate the day before graduation. Her postgraduate training was intermittent during the next 10 years because of the birth of three children followed by a fourth just before she started private practice of hematology in 1955. Dr. Sirridge has been vitally involved in women's issues, particularly those of women physicians. Recent publications have been about autobiographies of women physicians.

Nancy L. Snyderman, M.D., combines an active practice of head and neck surgery at the California-Pacific Medical Center with her role as a medical correspondent for ABC News. She is a frequent contributor to *20/20* and *Good Morning America*. She attended medical school at the University of Nebraska and completed residencies in pediatrics and ear, nose, and throat surgery at the University of Pittsburgh. Dr. Snyderman has authored two books, *Dr. Nancy Snyderman's Guide to Good Health for Women Over Forty* (1996) and *Necessary Journeys: Letting Ourselves Learn From Life* (2000). Her third book, *Girl in the Mirror: Raising Adolescent Daughters,* will be published in spring, 2002. She resides in San Francisco with her husband Doug and their children Kate, Rachel, and Charlie. Her passions include her five horses, skiing, and hiking.

Gertrude Russack Sobel, M.D., received her M.D. from Columbia University, College of Physicians & Surgeons in New York City in 1940. She had a private practice in allergy in New York City in the 1940s, later continuing in Rockville Center, New York, until 1985. Her medical research and publications focused on the different modalities of densitization. Now retired, she was an Associate Professor of Clinical Medicine at the State University of New York at Stony Brook and former director of the Adult Allergy Clinic at the Nassau County Medical Center, New York. She has been a member of numerous honor and professional societies and received mention in *Who's Who of American Women* in 1970. She has three children and six grandchildren.

Barbara R. Sommer, M.D., is Assistant Professor of Psychiatry and the Director of Geriatric Psychiatry at Stanford University School of Medicine where she is developing her academic interest in factors that affect cognitive reserve across the life span. After her fellowship, she and her husband moved across the country several times to optimize career goals, and after 22 years, her present job of five years is her longest held job. She has two sons, ages 15 and 12.

Roberta E. Sonnino, M.D., is Professor of Surgery and Pediatrics and Chief, Section of Pediatric Surgery at the University of Kansas School of Medicine. She is also Assistant Dean for Student Affairs, Executive Director of the Women in Medicine Program, Chair of the Dean's Advisory Group on Professionalism, and Director of one of the school's academic societies. She currently serves on the Women in Medicine Coordinating Committee of the AAMC. Dr. Sonnino received her B.S. from the University of Michigan and her M.D. from the University of Padova, Italy. Her interests include congenital anomalies and surgical problems of the intestinal tract. Her non-medical passions include photography, scuba diving and underwater photography, alpine ski racing (in the old-ladies age group), opera, and her two cats.

Renda Soylemez, M.D., is currently a resident in the internal medicine program at New York-Presbyterian Hospital. She was born in Boston and grew up in Atlanta. She attended Harvard College and then went on to medical school at Columbia University College of Physicians & Surgeons. Dr. Soylemez wrote the poem included in this anthology about an experience she had shadowing a gynecologist during her first year of medical school. In what little time she has outside of the hospital, Dr. Soylemez enjoys squash, tennis, reading novels, and, of course, creative writing.

Martha Stitelman, M.D., a rural family practitioner, feels luckier than many women because medicine has allowed her to work part-time and still support her family. A graduate of Columbia University, College of Physicians & Surgeons, she has found medicine to be an interesting, useful, and reliable career that has never been dull. She is now looking forward to semiretirement.

Joan Stroud, M.D., works for Community Healthcare Network, providing family planning and prenatal care to young women in Brooklyn. She completed her medical school training at Temple University School of Medicine, Philadelphia, in 1993 and attended the Residency Program for Social Medicine at Montefiore Hospital, finishing a family practice residency program in 1996. She feels that her greatest accomplishment has been to be a Soka Gakkai, a Buddhist organization member, for the last 16 years and now a district leader in Brooklyn.

Lori E. Summers, M.D., is a resident in neurological surgery at Tulane University in New Orleans. She completed an internship in general surgery at Northwestern University in Chicago. She was born and raised in Kansas City, Missouri, and attended the combined BA/MD six-year program at the University of Missouri–Kansas City. Her main interests outside of medicine include training and showing horses. She owns one rehabilitated racehorse, Ocean of Emotion.

Christina M. Surawicz, M.D., is Professor of Medicine at the University of Washington and Section Chief in Gastroenterology at Harborview Medical Center. She was born in Munich, Germany, in 1948 to European physician parents who emigrated to the United States in 1951. She grew up in Vermont and Kentucky and attended Barnard College. Following medical school at the University of Kentucky, she completed internal medicine residency and a gastroenterology fellowship at the University of Washington in Seattle, following which she joined the faculty at the University of Washington as the first woman in the Gastroenterology Division. In addition to patient care, clinical research, teaching, and administration, she served as the first woman president of the American College of Gastroenterology.

Juliana Swiney, M.D., was brought up in a home attached to her father's small hospital, Swiney Sanitorium. Her premedical degree was obtained from Trinity College in Washington, D.C. in 1931 and her medical degree from Columbia University, College of Physicians & Surgeons in 1935. She had a general practice for 56 years. For the first 25 years, she assisted her father and brother in running the family's hospital. She retired in 1986.

Alexandra Symonds, M.D. (1918-1992), graduated from New York Medical College in 1948 and completed her training in psychiatry (Bellevue Hospital) and psychoanalysis (American Institute of Psychoanalysis, Karen Horney Center). She was Associate Clinical Professor of Psychiatry at New York University School of Medicine and a leader in addressing the issues faced by women in the aftermath of women's liberation. Her landmark papers explore the conflicts of women within the contexts of relationships, family, career, and medicine. She was founding President of the Association of Women Psychiatrists and editor of its newsletter, *News for Women in Psychiatry*. Widely known as an educator and activist, she was a friend and mentor to many women in her field. She was the recipient of numerous honors and the namesake for many more.

Patricia Collins Temple, M.D., M.P.H., is Professor of Pediatrics at Vanderbilt University Medical Center. She was born in Oregon in 1942 and raised on the family cattle ranch in central Oregon. She graduated from Mills College (Oakland, California) and from Oregon Health Sciences University in 1969 where she earned a master's of science degree and an M.D. After completing her pediatric residency at Boston City Hospital, she received her M.P.H. from Harvard, in 1974. She and her husband, Dr. Steven G. Gabbe, have four children and one grandson.

Rebecca Tennant, M.D., became a wife, a mother, and a doctor in the span of four years and continues to enjoy and be challenged by the different roles. She went to Columbia University, College of Physicians & Surgeons for medical school and the University of California, San Francisco, for residency in family practice. Currently, she is not practicing clinical medicine but is a stay-at-home mom and freelance writer. She lives in Berkeley with her husband and two sons, Joseph and James.

ABOUT THE CONTRIBUTORS

Emily R. Transue, M.D., works as a general internist at the Polyclinic, a multispecialty group in downtown Seattle; she also has an adjunct clinical faculty appointment at the University of Washington. She graduated from Yale College in 1992 and from Dartmouth Medical School in 1996. She completed her residency and chief residency in internal medicine at the University of Washington in Seattle. Dr. Transue began writing stories about her clinical experiences as a medical student and has continued writing through residency and into practice. She has published pieces in *JAMA*, the *Dartmouth Medicine* magazine, and elsewhere.

Amy A. Tyson, M.D., has a private practice of adult and child psychiatry and adult psychoanalysis in San Francisco and is on the clinical faculty of the University of California, San Francisco and teaching faculty at SF Psychoanalytic Institute. She graduated from Yale University School of Medicine in 1989 and completed a residency in adult psychiatry and a fellowship in child/adolescent psychiatry at Langley Porter Psychiatric Institute, UCSF in 1994. She is a graduate of San Francisco Psychoanalytic Institute (2001).

Katherine Uraneck, M.D., has taken a sabbatical from the chaos of emergency medicine and is pursuing a master's degree in journalism at Columbia University in New York City. She graduated from Washington University School of Medicine, St. Louis, in 1984 after which she attended the Medical College of Pennsylvania, Philadelphia, for her residency in emergency medicine. Since completing her residency she has led a varied career. She has practiced clinical and academic medicine in Philadelphia; Albany, New York; and finally Bennington, Vermont, where she worked for most of the last 10 years. She has published articles in *Salon*, *Praxis Post*, and *The Scientist* and is continuing as a freelance medical journalist.

Bertha Van Hoosen, M.D. (1863-1952), received her M.D. from the Uni- versity of Michigan in 1888. She was Professor of Gynecology at the North- western University Woman's Medical School, Professor of Clinical Gynecol- ogy at the University of Illinois College of Medicine, and Professor and Head of Obstetrics at the Loyola University Medical School. She was the founding President of the Medical Women's National Association in 1915 (now the American Medical Women's Association). Dr. Van Hoosen pioneered the "buttonhole surgery" appendectomy and the use of Scopolamine Morphine "twilight sleep" in childbirth. Her life story is recorded in her autobiography, *Petticoat Surgeon* (1947). The Rochester Hills Museum at Van Hoosen Farm in Michigan, is the home where she was born and raised.

Sondra Vazirani, M.D., M.P.H., works as a hospitalist at the University of California, Los Angeles attending on the general medicine wards and performing internal medicine consultation. She is also an Assistant Medical Director for the UCLA Medical Group and is currently working on a NIH-funded grant. She has lived in Los Angeles since the age of 12 and wanted to be a doctor since the age of 4. She went to Brown University for undergraduate studies where she met her husband, Steven. Dr. Vazirani attended medical school at the University of California, San Francisco, and went on to internal medicine internship and residency at UCLA. She completed an MPH also at UCLA and joined the faculty there. She resides in Brentwood and enjoys traveling, fine dining, and boogie boarding in the summer.

Lila A. Wallis, M.D., is Clinical Professor of Medicine, Cornell University Weill Medical College; past President, Amer. Medical Women's Assoc.; founding President, National Council on Women's Health; Master, Amer. College of Physicians; and an international expert on hormone replacement therapy and osteoporosis. Director of the Advanced Curriculum on Women's Health, she founded the teaching associates program whereby non-MD subjects teach competent, painless genital exams. She is author of *The Whole Woman: Take Charge of Your Health in Every Phase of Your Life*, Editor-in-Chief of the *Textbook of Women's Health*, and recipient of numerous awards. The Dr. Lila Wallis Distinguished Visiting Professorship in Women's Health and the Dr. Lila Wallis Women's Health Research Fund, both at Cornell, and AMWA's Dr. Lila Wallis Women's Health Award have been established in her honor.

Livia Shang-yu Wan, M.D., is Professor of Obstetrics & Gynecology at the New York University (NYU) School of Medicine. Born in Nanking, China, she graduated from the National Taiwan University in 1958. She completed a rotating internship at Kings County Hospital in Brooklyn, an obstetrics and gynecology residency at Philadelphia General Hospital, and a fellowship in gynecologic fertility research at Pennsylvania Hospital. Since 1969, Dr. Wan has been Director of the Family Planning Division at NYU and later Director of the Division of Endoscopic Pelvic Surgery. She was the first surgeon to perform laparoscopic surgery at NYU in 1970. She is still active in gynecologic practice and surgery, teaching and research and has published over 50 papers in peer-reviewed journals. Dr. Wan is married to Francis C. Lui and has two children.

Rebekah Wang-Cheng, M.D., is Professor of Medicine at the Medical College of Wisconsin where she enjoys taking care of patients and teaching medical students and residents. Listed in the 2000 *Guide to the Best Doctors in America*, she also writes a question-and-answer column, "Dear Dr. Becky," in the *Milwaukee Journal-Sentinel* newspaper, which has been one of their most widely read columns over the past six years. A 1974 graduate of Andrews University in Michigan, she received her M.D. from Loma Linda University School of Medicine in California where she also completed a residency in internal medicine. Mother of three boys, Christopher, Andrew and Ryan, she strives to live a balanced life by enjoying time with them, tennis, biking, piano, reading, and being active in her church.

Michelle Palmieri Warren, M.D., is Medical Director of the Center for Menopause, Hormonal Disorders, and Women's Health; Professor of Medicine and Obstetrics and Gynecology; and the Wyeth Ayerst Professor of Women's Health at Columbia University College of Physicians & Surgeons. She was first to identify the skeletal problems that result from menstrual irregularities and eating disorders in young women and athletes and has published over 150 articles and several books on these subjects. She is a graduate of Mount Holyoke College and Cornell University Medical College. Before her current position, she was head of reproductive endocrinology both at George Washington University Hospital and St. Luke's-Roosevelt Hospital. A recipient of numerous awards, she has been named one of *New York Magazine's* "Best Doctors in New York City."

Melanie M. Watkins is a third year medical student at Stanford University School of Medicine. She completed her undergraduate degree in health sciences at the University of Nevada, Reno. She enjoys spending time with her seven-year-old son, Jonathan, and even though she will be known as "doctor" in the year 2003, she really enjoys simply being known as "Jonathan's mommy" by the neighborhood kids. Her previous work and life story have appeared in *USA Today, Woman's World* magazine, and *Chicken Soup for the Single's Soul.* Ms. Watkins would like to pursue a career in obstetrics and gynecology, combining a career in academia with her community and international concerns. She also plans to continue her interests in writing short stories and motivational speaking.

Dorothy V. Whipple, M.D., is a pediatrician in private practice in Washington, D.C.

Alfreda Withington, M.D., (1860-1951) graduated from the Women's Medical College of the New York Infirmary in 1887. After completing her internship, she spent several years abroad in Europe studying medicine. She led an active, varied career, working for some time in the Deep Sea Mission in Labrador, the American Red Cross efforts in France during and after the war, where she became the Medical Field Director overseeing a number of tuberculosis dispensaries, and finally as a rural practitioner in the Kentucky mountains where she lived in a cabin and made house calls by horse.

Marianne Wolff, M.D., now works part-time at a large commercial laboratory. She graduated summa cum laude from Hunter College in 1948 and A.O.A. from Columbia University College of Physicians & Surgeons in 1952. After medical internship and pathology training, she worked first at Roosevelt Hospital and then at Presbyterian Hospital in the Department of Surgical Pathology, rising in rank to Professor of Clinical Surgical Pathology. She later moved to a Columbia-affiliated hospital in New Jersey. She was awarded the gold medal in 1995 for "meritorious service to the College of Physicians & Surgeons" and a medal in 1997 for "conspicuous Columbia Alumni Service." Her husband, Herbert Schainholz, now deceased, was a mechanical engineer / inventor. She has two sons, both Columbia University graduates, one in law and one in medicine.

Note

1. Adapted from the book jacket for *Doctor Nellie: The autobiography of Helen MacKnight Doyle,* by Helen MacKnight Doyle (Mammoth Lakes, CA: Genny Smith Books, 1983).

If you have stories, poems, or essays to share
about your experiences, please send them to

Eliza Lo Chin, MD
P.O. Box 10906
Oakland, CA 94610-0906
ThisSideofDoctoring@yahoo.com